THIS BOOK
BELONGS TO:

Reprinted 2018

PUBLISHED BY Little Green Frog Publishing

Art direction and publication design:
Stephanie Antill

Photography:
Sabine Bannard

Shot at:
The Farm, Byron Bay

ISBN: 978-0-473-41971-4

Printed in China

For the farmers who tend to the soil with such care, and grow our food.

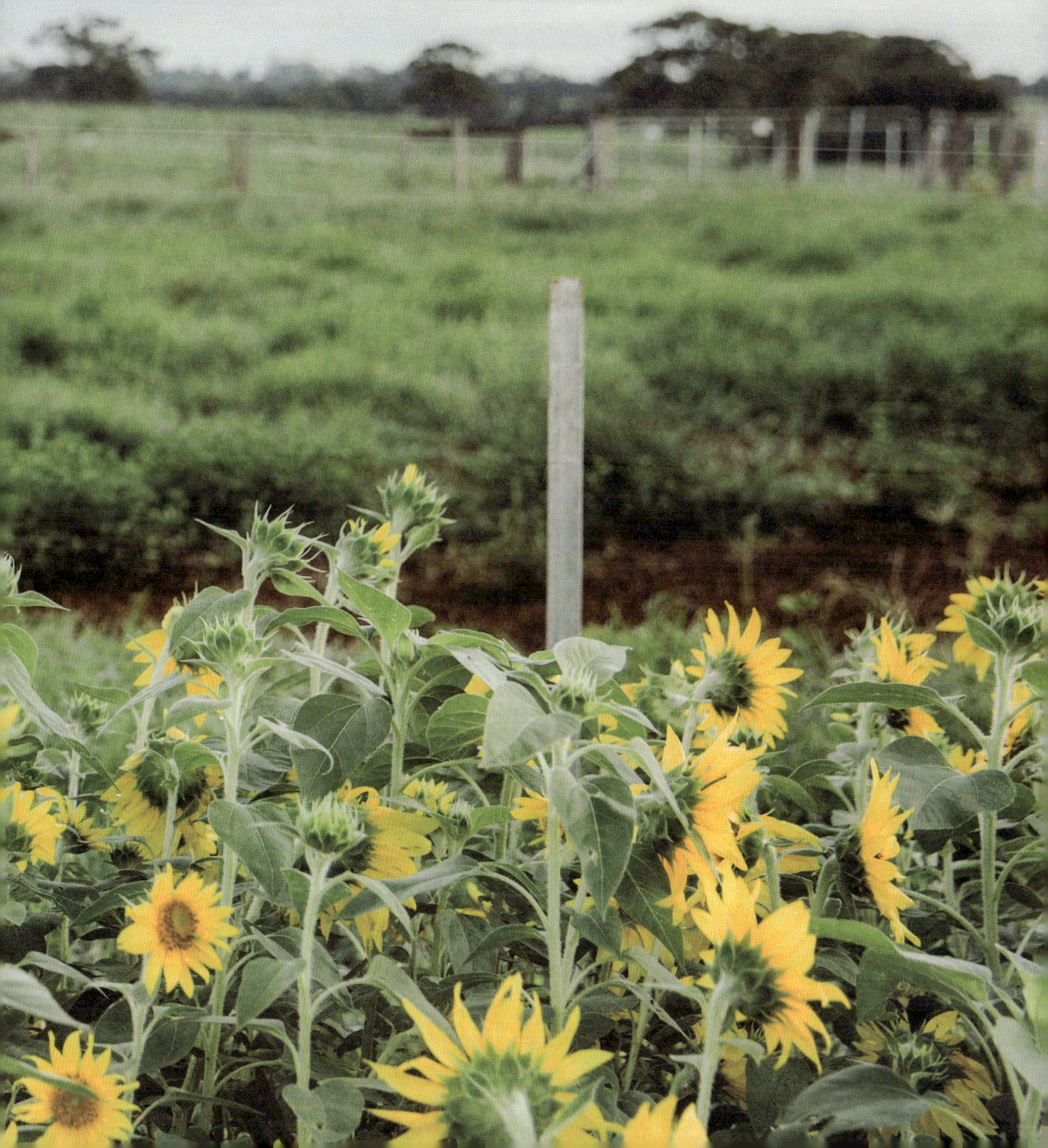

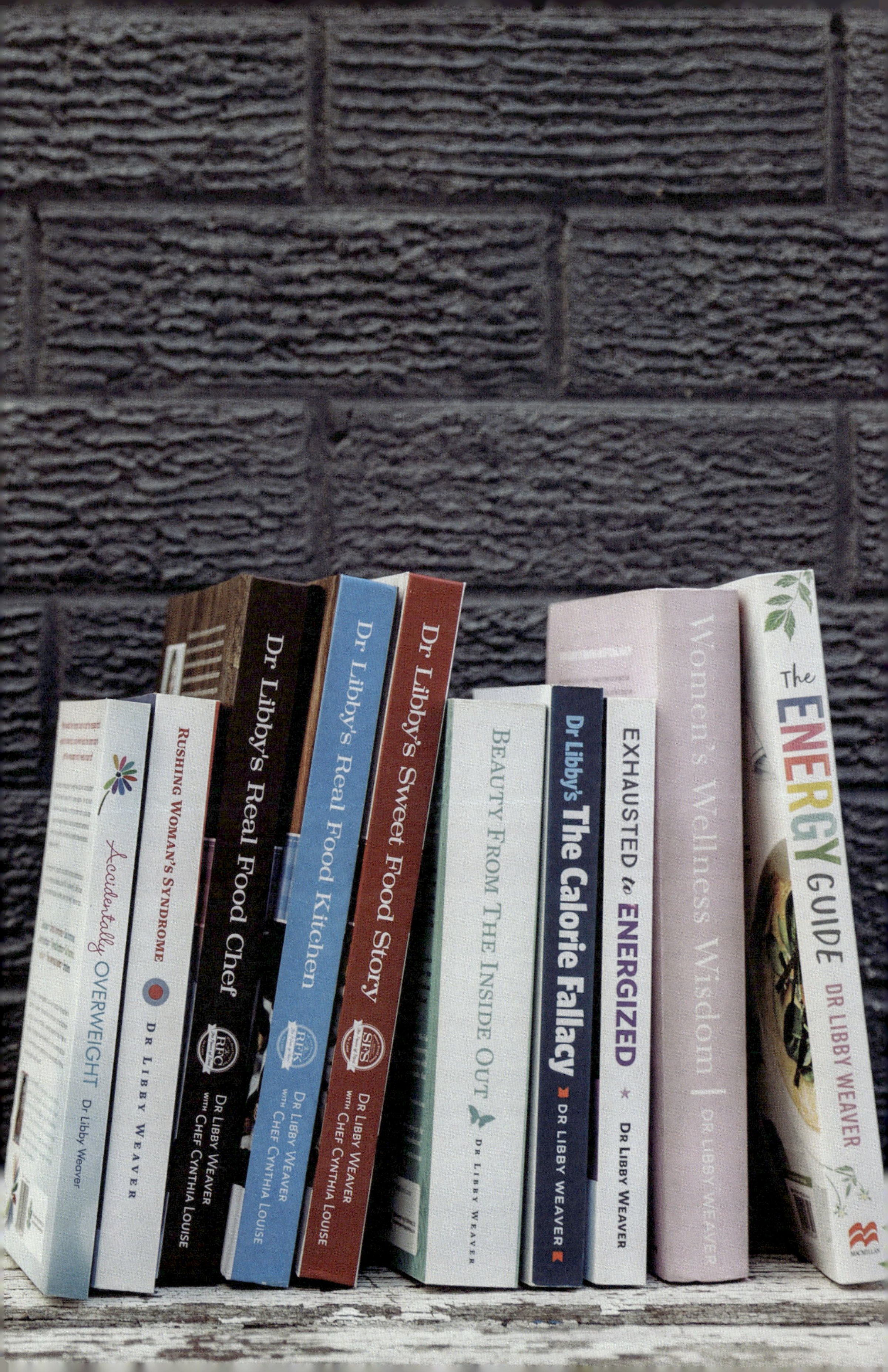
Accidentally OVERWEIGHT
Dr Libby Weaver
RUSHING WOMAN'S SYNDROME
DR LIBBY WEAVER
Dr Libby's Real Food Chef
DR LIBBY WEAVER WITH CHEF CYNTHIA LOUISE
Dr Libby's Real Food Kitchen
DR LIBBY WEAVER WITH CHEF CYNTHIA LOUISE
Dr Libby's Sweet Food Story
DR LIBBY WEAVER WITH CHEF CYNTHIA LOUISE
BEAUTY FROM THE INSIDE OUT
DR LIBBY WEAVER
Dr Libby's The Calorie Fallacy
DR LIBBY WEAVER
EXHAUSTED to ENERGIZED
DR LIBBY WEAVER
Women's Wellness Wisdom
DR LIBBY WEAVER
The ENERGY GUIDE
DR LIBBY WEAVER
MACMILLAN

Also by
DR LIBBY WEAVER

Accidentally Overweight (2011)

Rushing Woman's Syndrome (2011)

Dr Libby's Real Food Chef, with Chef Cynthia Louise (2012)

Beauty from the Inside Out — 3rd Edition (2017)

Dr Libby's Real Food Kitchen, with Chef Cynthia Louise (2013)

The Calorie Fallacy (2014)

Sweet Food Story, with Chef Cynthia Louise (2014)

Exhausted to Energized (2015)

Women's Wellness Wisdom (2016)

The Energy Guide (2017)

Contents

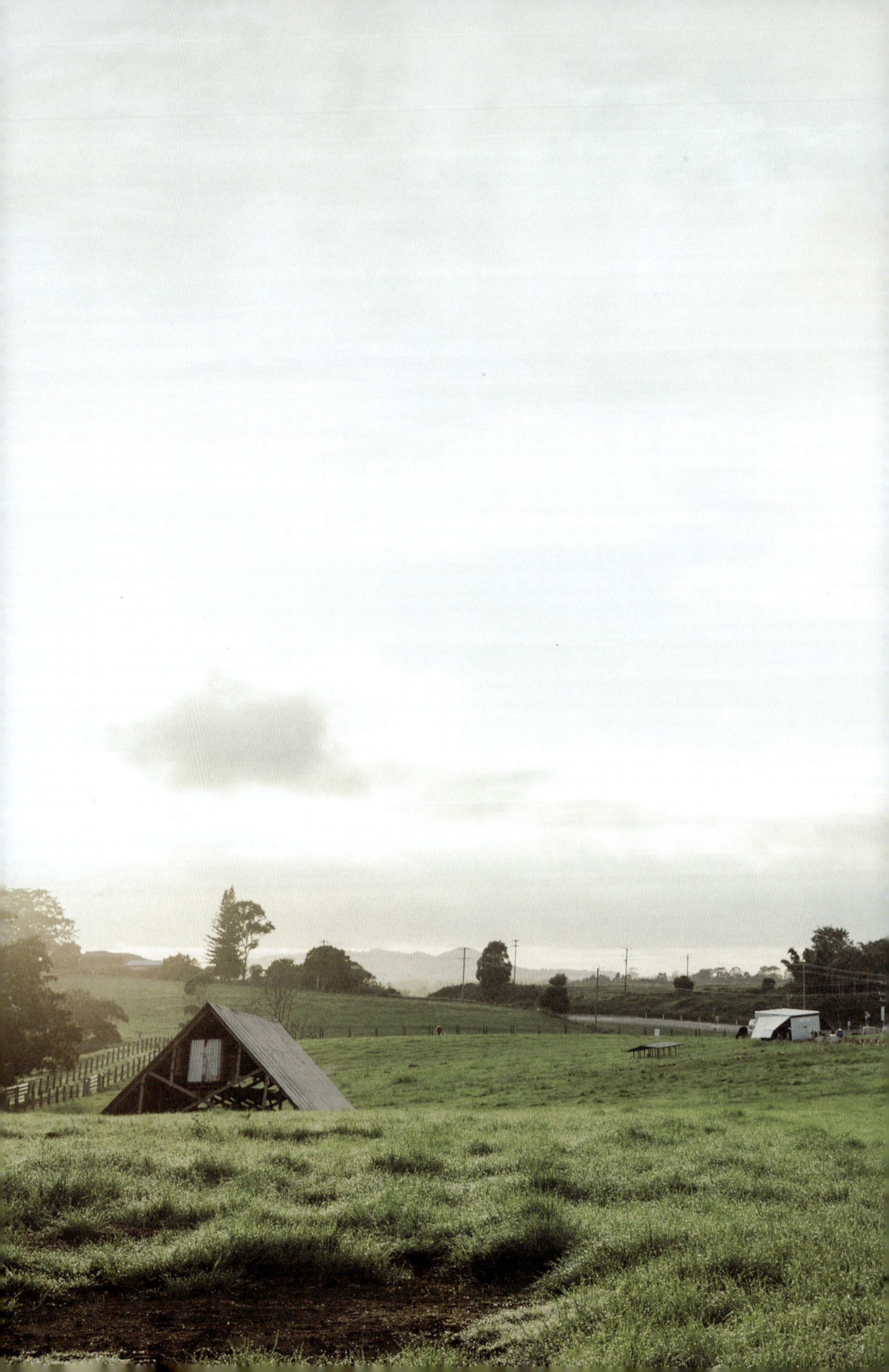

My mission is to educate and inspire, enhancing people's health and happiness, igniting a ripple effect that transforms the world.

DR LIBBY WEAVER

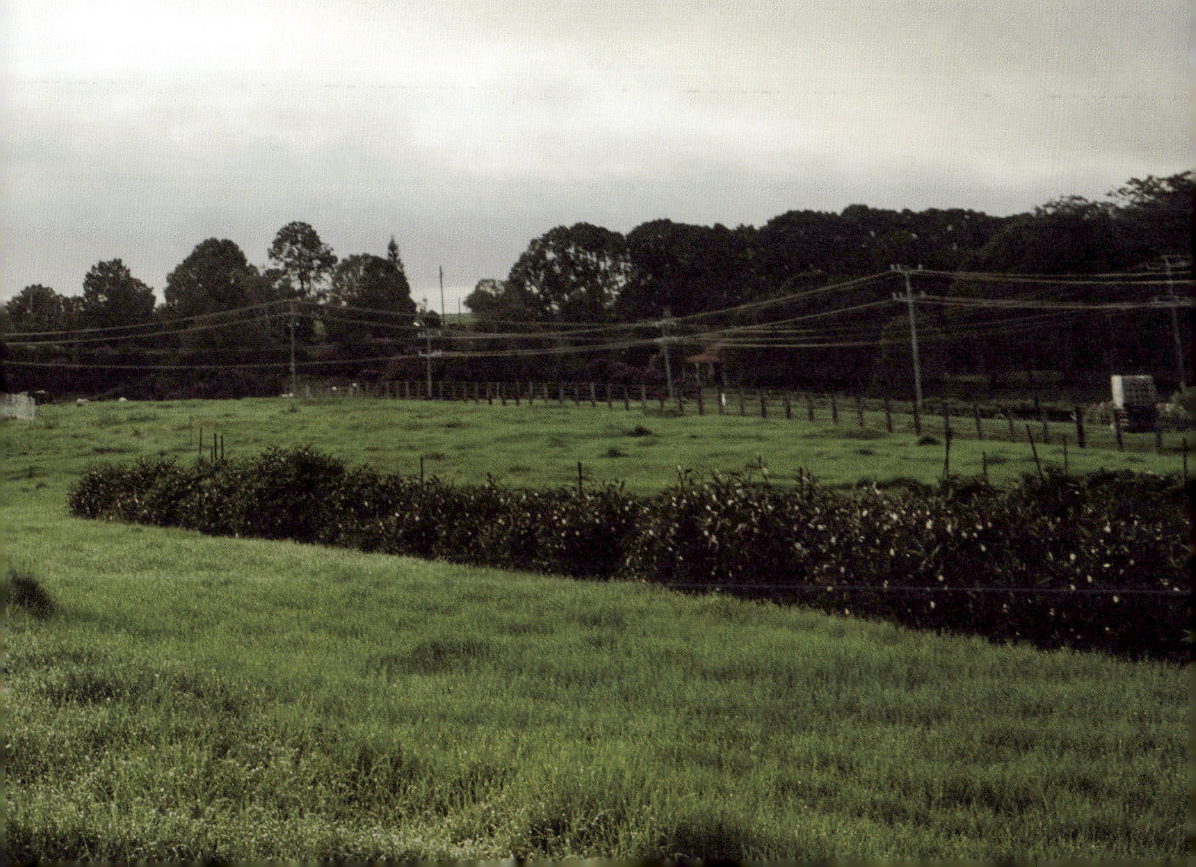

Introduction

SHIFTING YOUR FOOD CONFUSION

There is no one way for every human on the planet to eat, despite that holy grail having been searched for, for aeons.

This book is not about metabolism and body systems. It is about food and eating and appetite, and all of the things that influence what we choose. Its aim is to help you find what is right for you.

It's about how so many of you no longer trust your own instincts and desires, and that you feel like your taste buds and your body betray you.

My goal with this book is to help you get back in touch with how to best meet your own nutritional needs, rather than insist you follow a prescribed dogma without consideration for your bio-individuality.

I'm not denying for a second that guidance and nutritional advice is not useful — of course it can be. Even more so when there is a health condition involved. Allergies and many illnesses require specific, precise and accurate advice, and guidance from a nutrition professional might literally change your life.

For example, if someone has irritable bowel syndrome (IBS), an experienced practitioner can work out from their symptoms whether they need to eat in a way that is gluten-free or dairy-free or low FODMAPs or no raw food or no processed food… And they might be stunned at the positive changes in their energy or their sleep quality or how their clothes fit after switching to a way of eating that better suits their body. But there are now people sharing what they do, with the best of intentions, in the belief that if this worked for them, it will work for everyone, which is not the case.

My approach has three pillars to it: the biochemical, the nutritional and the emotional. That third pillar is there because, let's face it, for many people today it is not a lack of education that leads them to polish off a tub of ice cream after dinner. No one does that thinking they are going to feel fantastic afterwards.

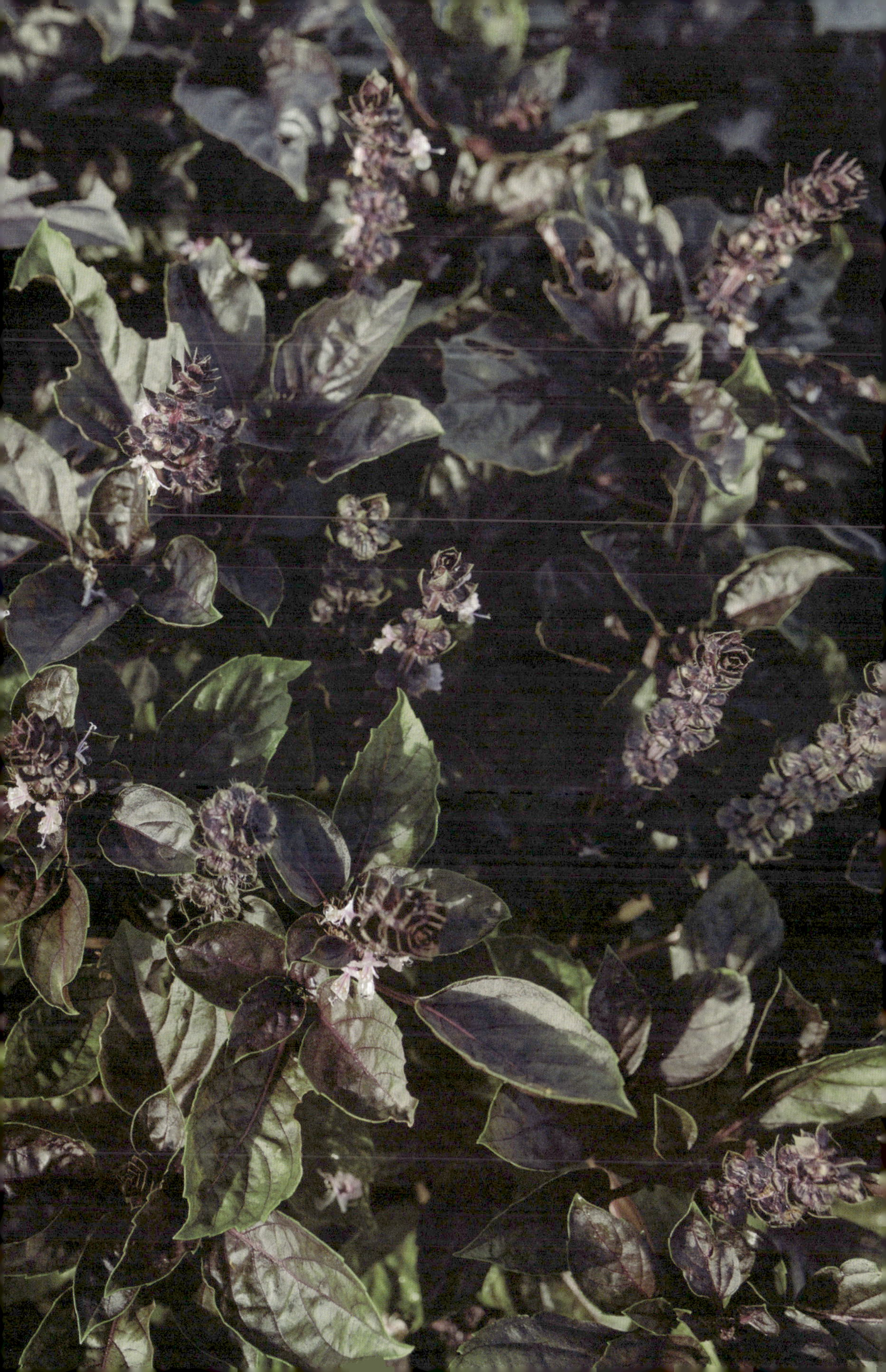

You often aren't aware of why you do it though. While my other books examine the biochemistry of body systems, this book will look at the biochemistry of food. Of course, we will explore in depth the nutritional pillar and then we'll examine as many of the reasons that drive people to eat as I have determined over 14 years of study and twenty years of practice — reasons other than hunger.

The way you are supposed to eat is influenced by many factors including:

- your heritage
- your medical history
- current disease/illness
- your emotional state
- symptoms you are currently presenting with (e.g. regular headaches are not an illness, but a symptom)
- your metabolic rate (impacted by many factors, including thyroid function, brown fat mass and autonomic nervous system function, to name a few).

We will explore some of these in more detail throughout the book to help begin to guide your food choices and return you to living from a place of trusting your own instincts and desires.

It is very difficult to be in touch with what your body needs — as opposed to your taste buds — when you eat processed food. Eating concentrated, refined sugars on a regular basis makes you hungry and you have little chance of innate appetite regulation when you include these processed foods in how you eat.

When you eat whole, real food, you don't even have to think about how much you eat. You just eat. The right amount for you at that time. And then you stop. You're not bursting or still hungry. You simply know it's time to stop and that you've had elegant sufficiency. The finishing of your eating does not stem from a conscious thought along the lines of "Oh, I had better stop now." It arises from a feeling and you simply stop.

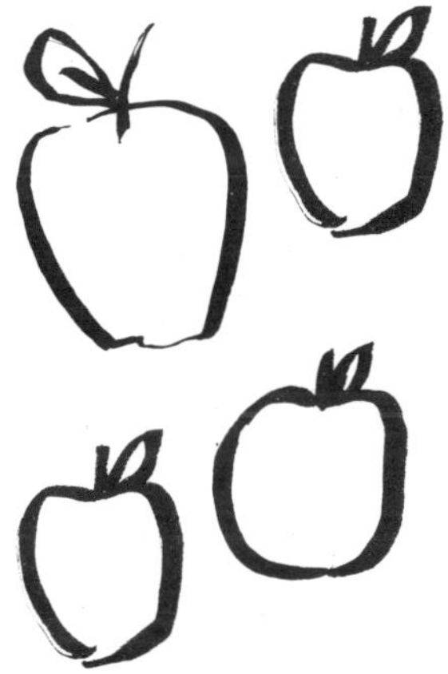

Some sections throughout the book are for you to form your own opinion; however, at the end of the book I will also summarise what I cover in the chapters to provide guidance for you with your food choices. I want you to finish this book feeling empowered to make informed decisions. There may also be times when you wonder why I'm guiding you with something, when the goal of the book is to get you back in touch with your body and its needs. As I've already mentioned, it's hard to hear what your body needs when its messages are masked by the taste bud conflict that processed food and emotional challenges generate. So, for these latter scenarios, I aim to gently guide you by offering information and thoughts to prompt your own insights.

Throughout these pages, we will also contest the assumption that you have to lose weight to be healthy, instead replacing it with a paradigm-shifting statement that, in fact, you have to be healthy to lose weight. This will transform how you view your body and enhance your understanding of what your body needs to function at its best.

This book is not about weight loss. But for all of you who have been making an enormous effort and commitment to weight loss with little or no sustainable outcome, and for those who simply want to understand how to live happier, healthier lives, allowing your body to efficiently use body fat as a fuel — this book will arm you with the wisdom to stop dieting and depriving yourself (if that's what you currently do), and instead to start thriving.

Stop dieting and start nourishing yourself, and watch the transformation occur.

The word "diet" used throughout this book does not refer to a restricted diet, based on deprivation. Instead, it is used to refer to the way a person habitually eats.

It is my hope that the information shared within this book will help to put you back in touch with your own inner knowing, able to know what serves you in this moment, not because some diet or set of guidelines told you that is how you are supposed to eat.

We regularly hand over responsibility for how to eat to others, taking on their knowledge or beliefs. Sometimes this helps us — or helps us start to eat in a more nourishing way — while it can be a sticking point for others.

There is no one way for all humans to eat. My desire with this book is not to prescribe anything to you, but simply to teach you principles, to encourage you to go within, and start to observe how you feel when you eat the way you do.

I have lost count of the number of times I have had people say to me, "I don't know who to listen to" when it comes to their food choices. Sure, you might need some initial guidance if gaining accurate nutrition knowledge (not information based on fads) has not been a focus for you, but then it is up to you to pay attention to how you feel eating that way. If I've had to ask someone to stop eating apples because I am suspicious that apples are the source of their stabbing gut pain, many reply along the lines of "But I thought apples were healthy." Not for you they aren't, if they give you chronic gut pain. Or someone would see me for help to determine whether food was playing a role in their child's behaviour challenges. Among many other questions, I would ask: "When is his behaviour most challenging?" "Well, he runs laps of the backyard and can no longer hear my requests to come inside, after he gets home and has afternoon tea, but he doesn't eat any sugar or anything processed for afternoon tea." "So what does he eat for afternoon tea?" "One to two punnets of cherry tomatoes — a really healthy food." "Possibly not for him, though, if some of the compounds in tomatoes are actually behind his intense running and/or inability to listen."

In other words, what is nutritious to one person may not be to another.

Another story, from someone I'll refer to as Helen, who works as a health coach.

> **Me:** When did the gut pain first happen?
>
> **Helen:** When I was at a health retreat.
>
> **Me:** What were you eating there?
>
> **Helen:** Only raw food. The pain subsided after I left, but then when I got home I was hospitalised for severe gut pain.
>
> **Me:** What did you eat when you got home?
>
> **Helen:** Well, I was motivated by what I learnt at the retreat, so kept the 100 per cent raw food thing going.
>
> **Me:** *(with kindness)* Have you ever considered that perhaps you do better with mostly cooked food?
>
> **Helen:** No, because I was just taught that raw food is best.
>
> **Me:** Not for you at the moment by the looks of things.

Your body is your best evidence for what works for you and what doesn't. While your body (which I lovingly refer to as an 'Earth suit') doesn't have a voice, it will let you know with symptoms whether or not your choices support its best function. And if your Earth suit gives you grief, I cannot encourage you enough to go within and explore whether it is asking you to eat, drink, move, think, breathe, believe or perceive in a new way. And you will know. You might not love the answer, but the answer is there.

Now you need to act on it. The thing is, *you have to care enough about yourself to act on it,* and for some of you that is your biggest hurdle to eating more intuitively. I hope this book also supports you with that.

When you listen to external sources and take that to be gospel, you stop listening to the voice within that knows what is best for you at all times. I want you to start to listen to, and act on, that.

I hope this book helps guide your way home.

A gentle approach

A NEW DESTINATION

Imagine your destiny is like a set of parallel lines. Envisage railway tracks if you like, although they are going to be railway tracks that can cross the ocean! These railway tracks are leaving the top of South America and are on a direct path heading south to Chile. If you continue to make the choices you make today, you will end up at that destination.

Let the left railway track represent your life with no changes and your right track represent your life with some subtle, sustained changes that you make to your choices after reading this book.

The compounding effect of making small incremental changes sees your new destiny initially shifting by one degree, yet continue that new track out into the future and the left and right tracks will be metres apart. By changing your relationship with food, by addressing how you eat, drink, move, think, breathe, believe and/or perceive, your right track (your new destiny) ends up in a completely new destination than where your left (old-paradigm) track would end up.

Small, sustained incremental change can make an enormous difference to your quality of life and long term sustainable, excellent health.

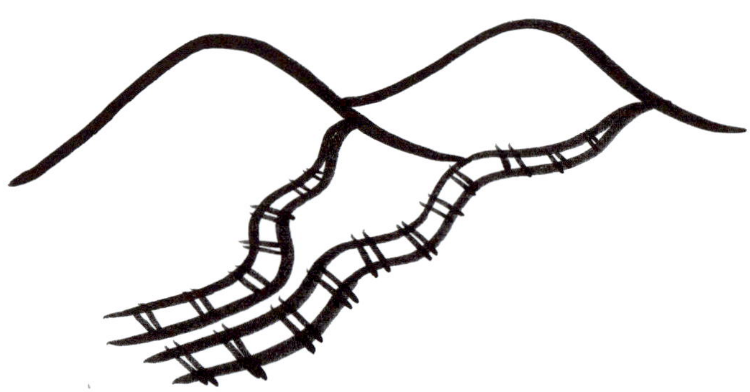

EXAMPLE

To make this even clearer, stand up and hold your hands out as if they are parallel lines in front of you. Now move your right arm a centimetre to the right. Now imagine that line continuing out into the future. You can now see how your right arm is directionally different to your left.

You can now imagine if you are standing at the top of South America with your left arm pointing directly at Chile, the small changes that you may make after reading this book means that, over time, your right arm is now pointing at New Zealand, a completely new destination.

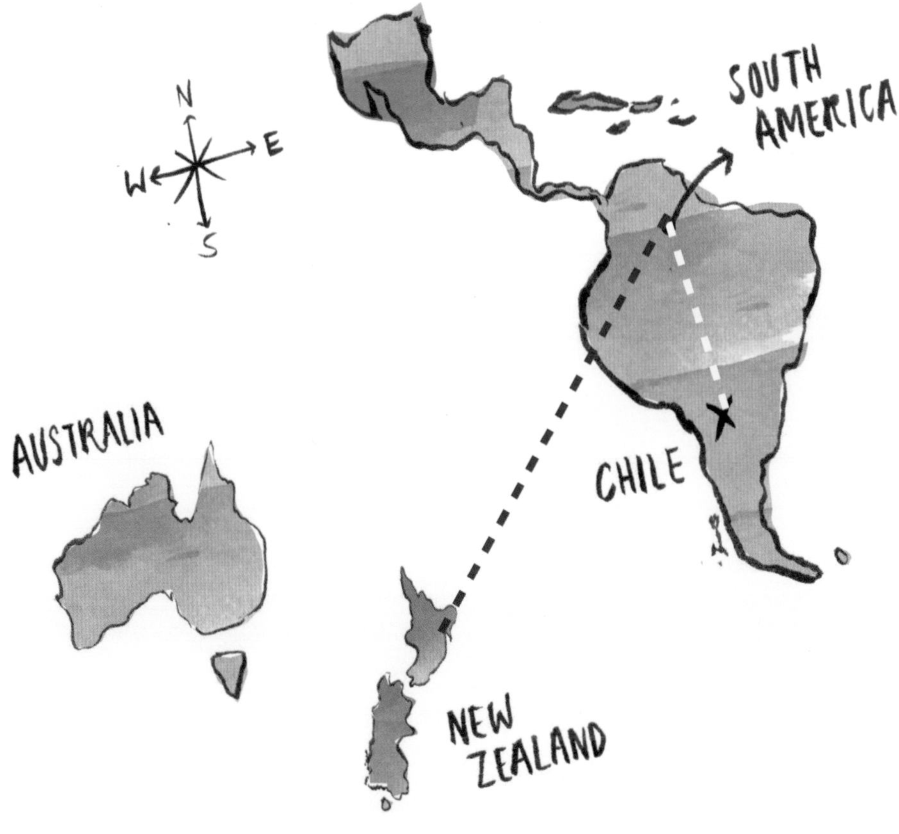

Where are your roots?

YOUR HERITAGE TELLS A STORY

When I was at university, we were taught that all people needed to follow the dietary pyramid. In the middle of that pyramid it says that everyone needs to consume three serves of dairy products per day. Yet it is well documented in scientific journals that 98 per cent of people of Asian heritage are lactose-intolerant, so why would I suggest that they include these foods?

Another example. There is a genetic typing that has been strongly linked to autoimmune diseases, of which coeliac disease is one. That genotype occurs more in people of Irish heritage. Think about this: up until 1845, the major source of starch for Irish people was potatoes. However, once the potato famine hit, they then started to eat gluten-containing grains in much greater quantities than ever before, to provide starch for energy for their labour.

Now Ireland has one of the highest incidences of coeliac disease in the Western world. Given the combination of gluten consumption in any large quantities being relatively new to their way of eating — 1845 is only about six or seven generations of people ago and we don't evolve that quickly — with a gene profile that is common among people of Irish descent, you have a scenario where gluten is likely not to support health; in fact it can be harmful.

In my clinical practice, if someone has an autoimmune disease or was of Irish heritage and having health problems, particularly challenges with their gut, the first place I would start in guiding them with food was to do a four-week strict gluten-free dietary trial. In many instances, the results never ceased to amaze me. For many, this was all they needed to change to get their outcome.

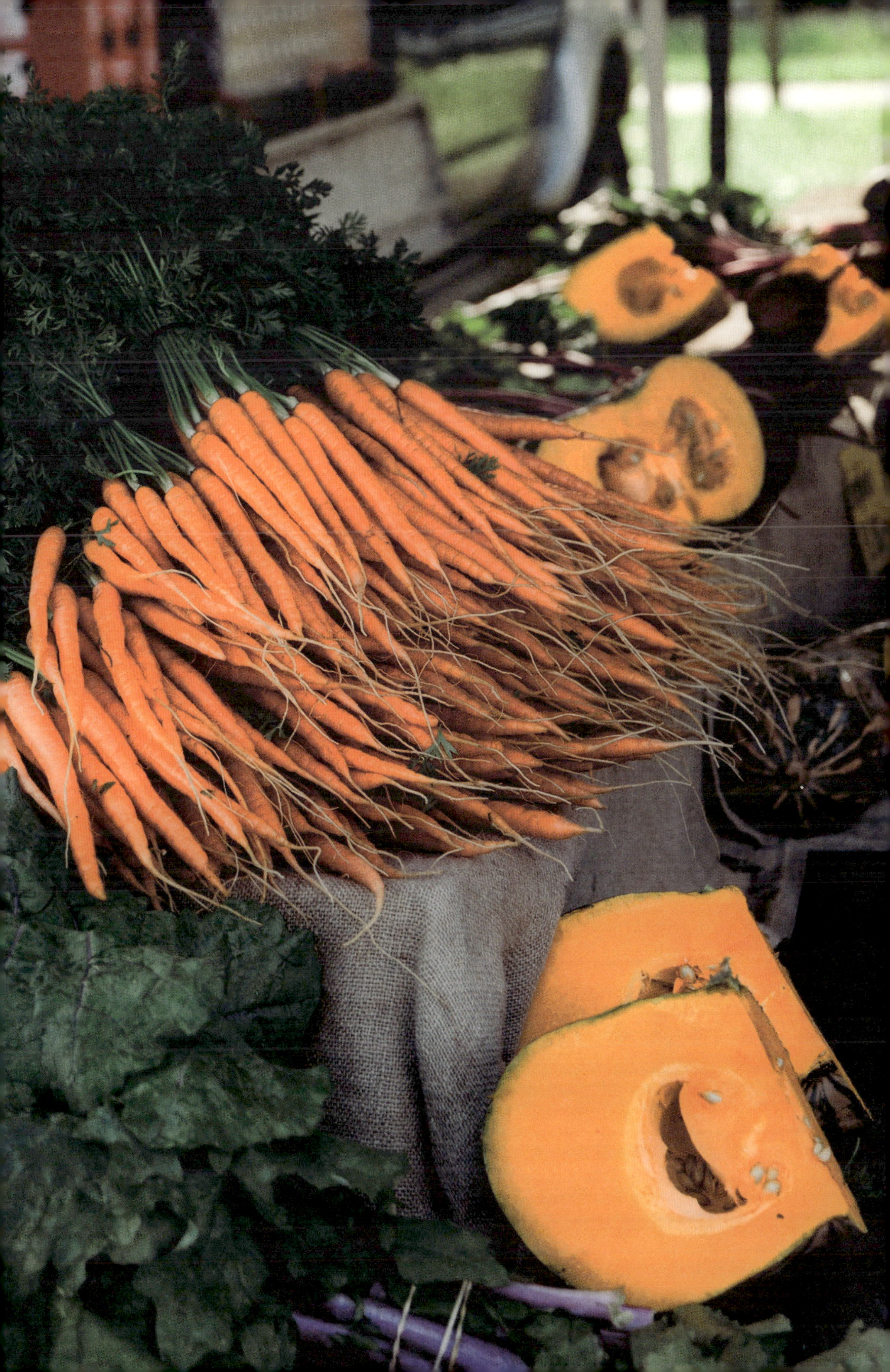

If you have grown up in one of the Pacific Islands, generally speaking, your meals traditionally consisted of predominantly vegetables, fruit, starchy root vegetables and fish, which is why from a digestive capacity perspective people with this heritage do the best health-wise eating this way now, regardless of where they live.

So what does your heritage suggest to you? How does it influence what will best serve you? What has your digestive system been used to handling when you consider your family's history?

Symptoms

If you experience reflux after eating, do you think your body is rejoicing and letting you know it is thrilled with the choice you just made? No. It is regurgitating what you swallowed so that it doesn't go any further into your body. Plus, it burns you on the way back up, to make sure you are really paying attention! Yet so often our brain (or taste buds!) kick in and, despite knowing that that food does not agree with us, we cry, "Oh, but I love it!", denying that any changes need to be made. It doesn't mean you necessarily have to avoid this food forever. It means right now (or maybe for a week or a month) it is not your friend, and continuing to consume it potentially puts you at risk in the long term for greater, more serious problems.

> *What if the parts of your body that frustrate or sadden you are simply messengers trying to get you to wake up? To make some different choices in how you eat, drink, move, think, breathe, believe and/or perceive?*

See your body as the gift that it is. It enables you to live this life, and its function impacts dramatically on your quality of life.

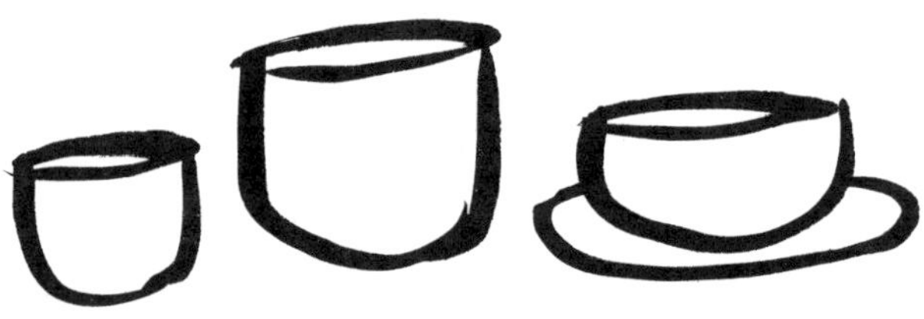

Fundamentals

There are, of course, some dietary fundamentals that apply to all people — eating plenty of plants is one of them. In other words, we all need to eat more vegetables. Some studies in New Zealand and Australia suggest that less than 10 per cent of the adult population eats the recommended five serves of vegetables per day. This is the minimum amount required for average health. Not amazing health, but basically to prevent diseases. And pockets of too many countries are not getting close to this minimum recommendation. Vegetables contain a plethora of substances that are highly protective against many lifestyle diseases. Always keep in mind how important it is to amp up your vegetable consumption for better nourishment and better health.

> “Studies in New Zealand and Australia suggest that less than 10 per cent of the adult population eats the recommended five serves of vegetables per day.”

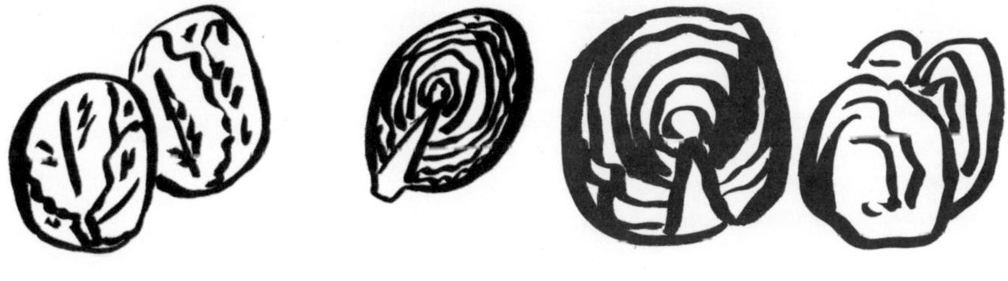

Focus on nourishment, not calories

HOW YOU PERCEIVE FOOD, MATTERS

Your perception of food impacts the information you are prepared to consider about the way that is best for you to eat. One of the blocks to eating in a highly nourishing way is counting calories, as the mindset of this is about restriction, deprivation and what you *can't* have. There is no health with such a fear of food, and it's unlikely you'll be getting the nutrients required for great physical wellbeing.

So if you have been someone who has, at times, counted calories, based on a belief that this is the best road for you to work out how you are supposed to eat, it's time to let that go.

Here's why:

The idea that body shape and size is 100 per cent due to how many calories you eat versus how many you burn is inaccurate. The concept does not consider all of the many facets that determine our body size and weight. What's more, you miss out on life when food, a fear of food and body fat, rule your thinking.

The calorie counting concept prevents you from knowing — from being able to listen to — your own inner knowing, of what is right for you to eat. Counting calories is also not a sustainable way to live, and many people mistakenly believe that they constantly fail at this food thing, because they can't stick to how they think they need to eat, and they never feel like they do enough exercise to justify their food intake. So they live with feelings of guilt and hopelessness most days of their lives.

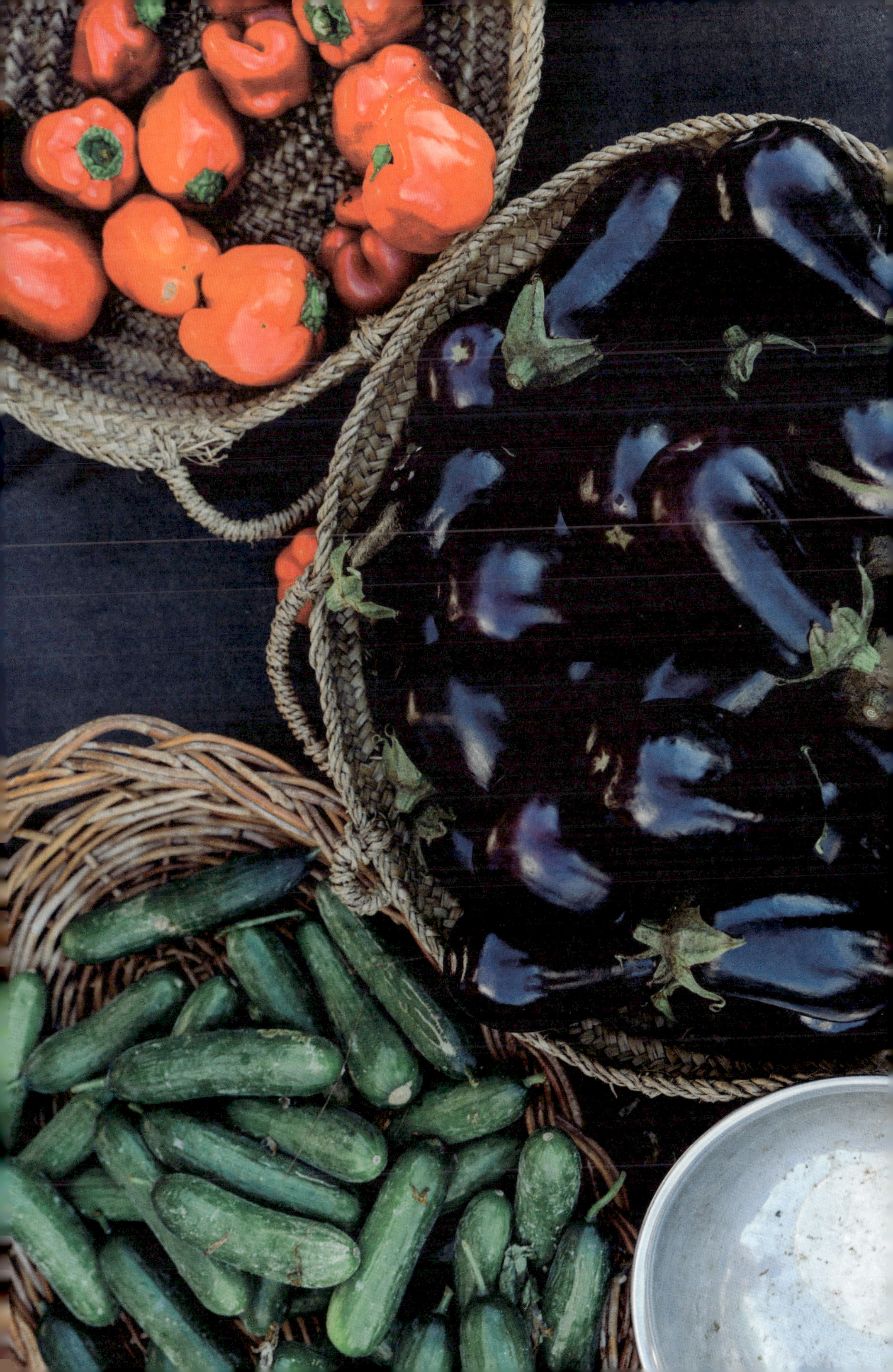

The calorie equation, which was first published in 1918, and on which today's diet mentality is still based, fails to factor in crucial elements of the modern world.

For example, it does not consider the metabolic consequences of modern day food. It continues under the false belief that all that matters to body shape and size is your fat, protein and carbohydrate (and alcohol) intake: the macronutrients from where you obtain your calories. But food for too many people today is no longer real. With each mouthful they get a host of different synthetic chemicals added to enhance shelf life or taste, which is one of the factors potentially messing with our ability to live with optimal health, and even lose weight (if that is desired).

I want you to experience a freedom with food from these pages. I want your relationship with food and your body to be based around the deepest self-care imaginable, and the belief that nourishing food choices stem from wanting to take care of yourself — to have amazing health — not because of a number on a scale that only weighs your self-esteem.

DR LIBBY

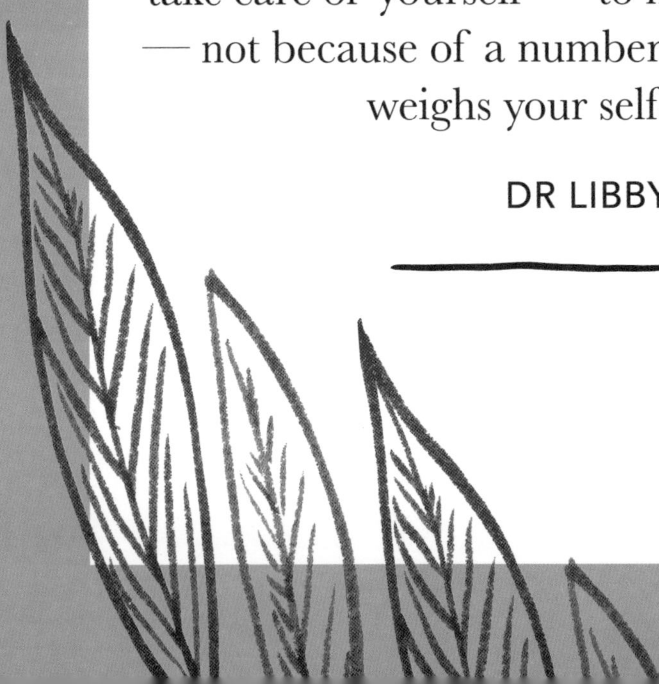

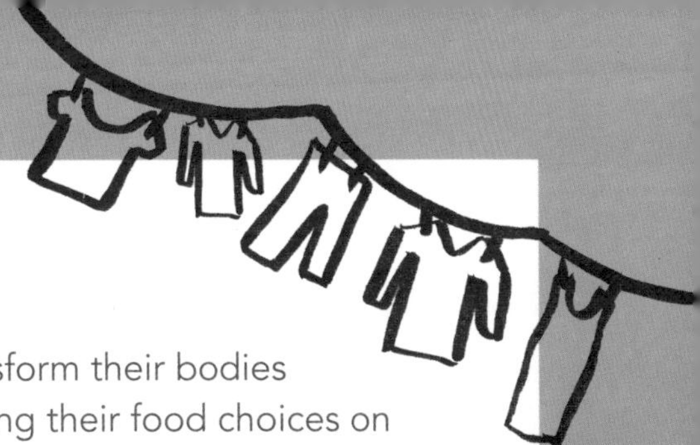

A new paradigm for you

I have witnessed countless people transform their bodies by relaxing and moving away from basing their food choices on the calorie equation. These are people who were eating a diet low in fat and high in complex carbohydrates, based on the food pyramid, and working hard doing five to seven cardiovascular gym workouts each week. They were in caloric deficit, and yet still constantly battling with their weight, experiencing fluctuations that they didn't understand, and that the calorie equation could not explain.

By shifting to a whole, real food way of eating, much higher in fat, doing resistance training, gentle forms of yoga, stretching, qi gong, gardening and/or walking, plus eating from 1200 to 2200 more calories per day than before, I have seen these people lose weight, then stabilise their weight, and the results of any resistance training become noticeable after one to two sessions, not after months of hard slog. They no longer focus on this, and instead simply focus on eating nourishing, nutrient dense real, whole foods. They never weigh themselves. Their clothes always fit. They have great energy and excellent health. Day after day. Year after year. It is truly transformational when you shift your focus from weight and calories to health and nourishment. It is, after all, nutrients that keep us alive.

WORKSHEET

Whole, real foods provide high levels of nourishment, in contrast to foods that might be low in calories, yet contain relatively little goodness or problematic substances that can interfere with the body's inner processes working optimally.

WHAT FOODS (IF ANY) DO YOU CHOOSE SIMPLY BECAUSE YOU KNOW THEY ARE LOW IN CALORIES?

DO THEY NOURISH YOU?

IF THEY COME OUT OF A PACKET, DO THEY HAVE NUMBERS ON THE INGREDIENTS LIST, OR WORDS THAT DON'T LOOK LIKE THEY ARE FOOD?

WHAT FOODS COULD YOU REPLACE THESE WITH THAT MIGHT OFFER YOU THE SATISFACTION YOU'RE AFTER BUT BE A MORE NOURISHING OPTION?

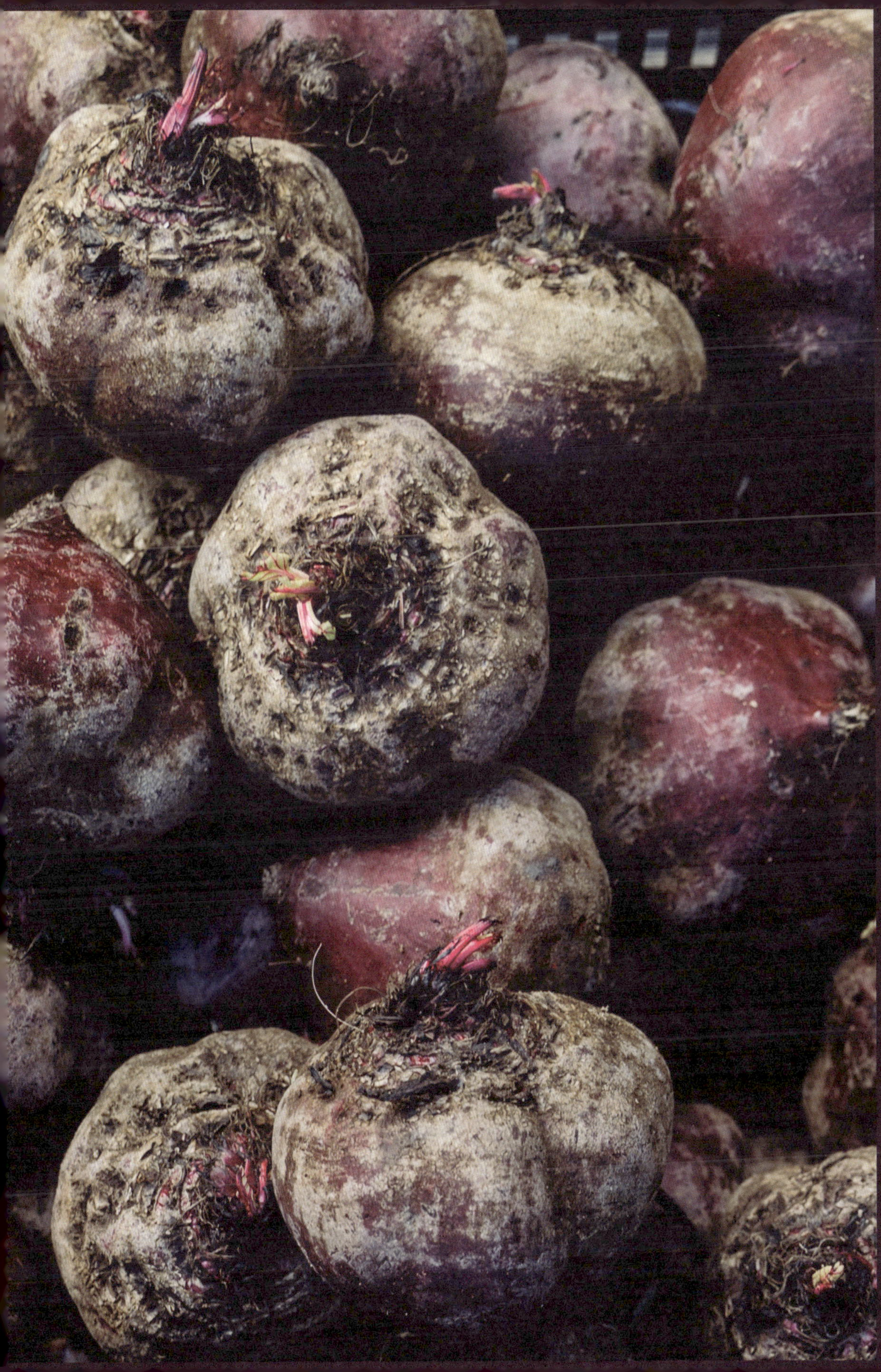

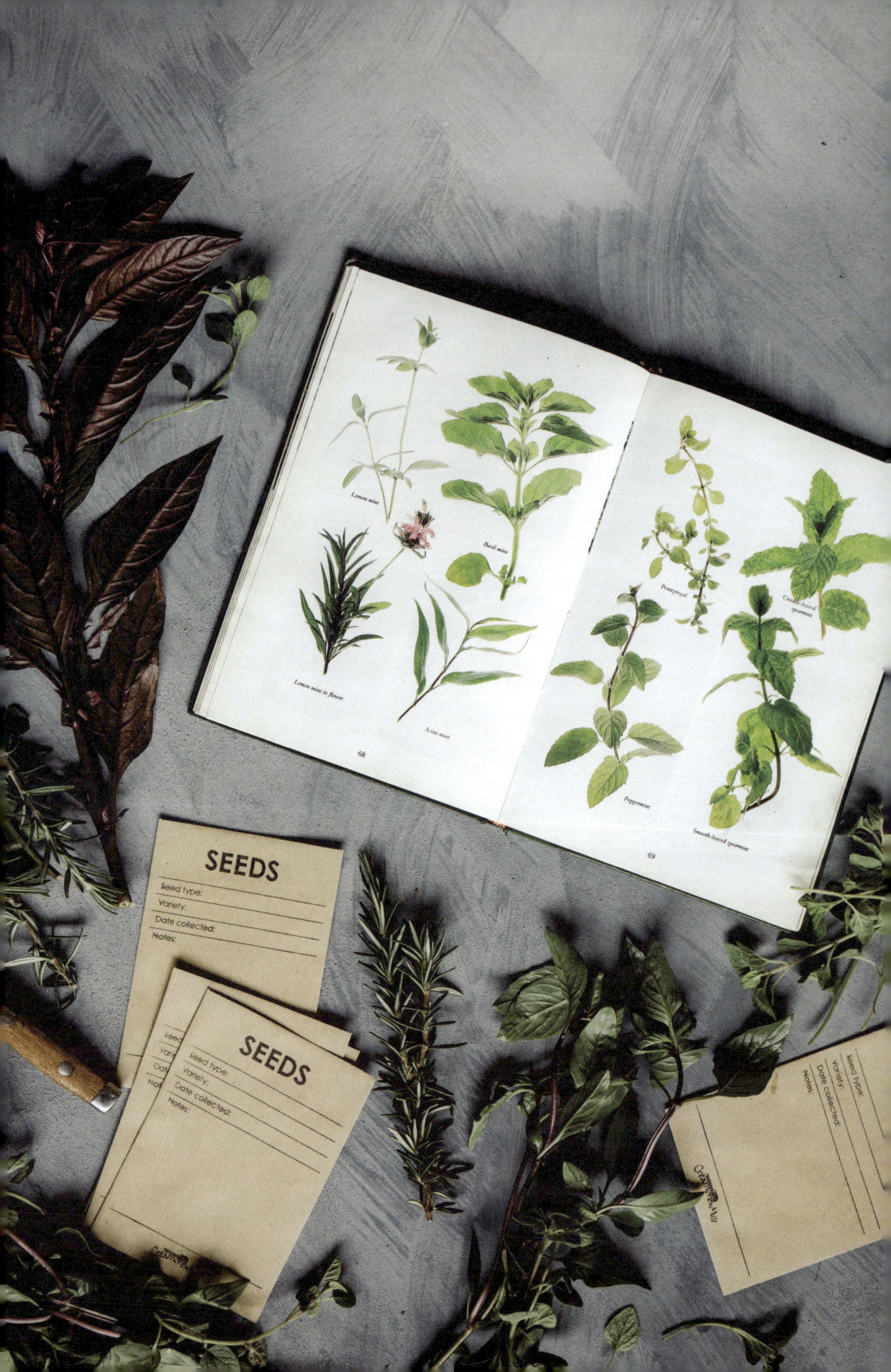

Lemon mint
Basil mint
Lemon mint in flower
Asian mint
68
Pennyroyal
Peppermint
Smooth-leaved spearmint
69
SEEDS
Seed type:
Variety:
Date collected:
Notes:
SEEDS
Seed type:
Variety:
Date collected:
Notes:
Seed type:
Variety:
Date collected:
Notes:

A need for nutrients

OUR FUEL FOR LIFE

When you consider how to eat, do you think about why you need to eat well? There are many reasons, with one of them being that nutrients are essential — yes essential — to drive many of the biochemical reactions that occur inside you that determine so much about your level of wellness.

It's nutrients that keep us alive, yet I feel that most people don't appreciate the immensity of this. The adult body is made up of about 50 trillion cells. That is a number that can easily go over our head with its enormity, so let's use currency to establish the enormity of one trillion, which is only one fiftieth of 50 trillion. If you were to save one dollar a second, it would take you 12 days to save one million dollars. In 32 years you would save one billion dollars but to save one trillion dollars, it would take you 32,000 years! And we are made up of about 50 trillion cells. Hopefully now you can grasp what an enormous number this is.

Imagine these cells as 50 trillion tiny little circles. They don't work alone, they work together by communicating information between them — and they can only do that when there are nutrients present. So when a person is not getting adequate nutrients, some of the most basic processes are compromised, and those that help us to experience optimal health are hindered even further.

The cells of the body don't live forever. They are always in a cycle of replication, repair and death. Some cells go through this cycle quicker than others. For example, eye cells replicate quickly, whereas the bones do so slowly. Our whole outer layer of skin is replaced every 28 days. The health of the next generation of cells is dependent on the information they pick up on in their environment. That environment will either be flush with nutrients or lacking them. It might be one nutrient that's deficient or it might be many.

There are also hormones at work — stress hormones, sex hormones, thyroid hormones — which have an impact too. The health and quality of each new cell is powerfully influenced by this information.

Every second, there are billions of biochemical reactions taking place within you. These reactions involve the conversion of one substance to another, and micronutrients (vitamins and minerals) are often required for these conversions to occur. Nutrients are also needed for the construction of other substances in the body and are sometimes even incorporated into these new structures.

As an example of this, I'll use vitamin C — a vitamin that's utilised in the body for many different important functions; the list is nearly endless! Our adrenal glands love vitamin C and it's used in the biochemical reactions that build our stress hormones. Vitamin C is also needed for the reaction that creates carnitine, a substance that allows us to burn fat as fuel, and for the creation of serotonin, our happy, calm, content hormone. It also keeps our immune system responding appropriately to stimuli and acts as a powerful antihistamine.

But what happens if we aren't consuming enough vitamin C? Without its presence, or in the quantity required to maintain optimal functioning, these reactions can't occur efficiently. You might get a build-up of one substance and not enough of another. You can imagine how undesirable it would be if the substance you were building up was histamine, and the substance you weren't getting enough of was serotonin! When we eat a food that's filled with vitamin C, our body prioritises where it gets used first. So think of it this way, what if we're feeling completely overwhelmed or we're anxious about something and so our body is signalling the need to create stress hormones, but the pollens have come out and they're stimulating our sinuses towards hay fever — what takes priority in the use of vitamin C? How is our optimum health going to be affected by a lack of vitamin C? This is just one example of how a lack of one nutrient can impact on our overall health.

> The way you feed yourself is the most basic, most fundamental way you demonstrate care for yourself.

Due to the incredible advances of Western medicine we are going to continue to live longer and longer. We are so fortunate to live in a time where we have access to such extraordinary emergency medicine. Yet, please consider this: are we living too short and dying too long? It is an important question to ponder, for what I care about so sincerely is the quality of that life. Imagine what life would be like if you had to rely on someone else to tie your shoelaces? How would this reliance feel?

You don't want this to happen because your food choices have led to your tummy growing too large for you to be able to reach your feet, and so you sit back and wish you had made changes sooner. You don't want to not be able to reach your feet because your spine is relatively inflexible from a sedentary lifestyle and so you can't bend to put your socks on. You want to maintain your independence. And the ways you eat, drink, move, think, breathe, believe and perceive don't just impact on how you feel, function and look today — they are going to influence how you feel, function and look in the future. And the power to change all of that is in your hands, and in your hands only.

Let that empower you.

The way you feed yourself is the most basic, most fundamental way you demonstrate care for yourself.

If you've had a dieting mentality, I encourage you to shift your focus from dieting to nourishing. It is time to stop counting calories; if you need to count anything, count nutrients and amp them up, and count synthetic substances and omit them. You will see why, and how, throughout the pages of this book.

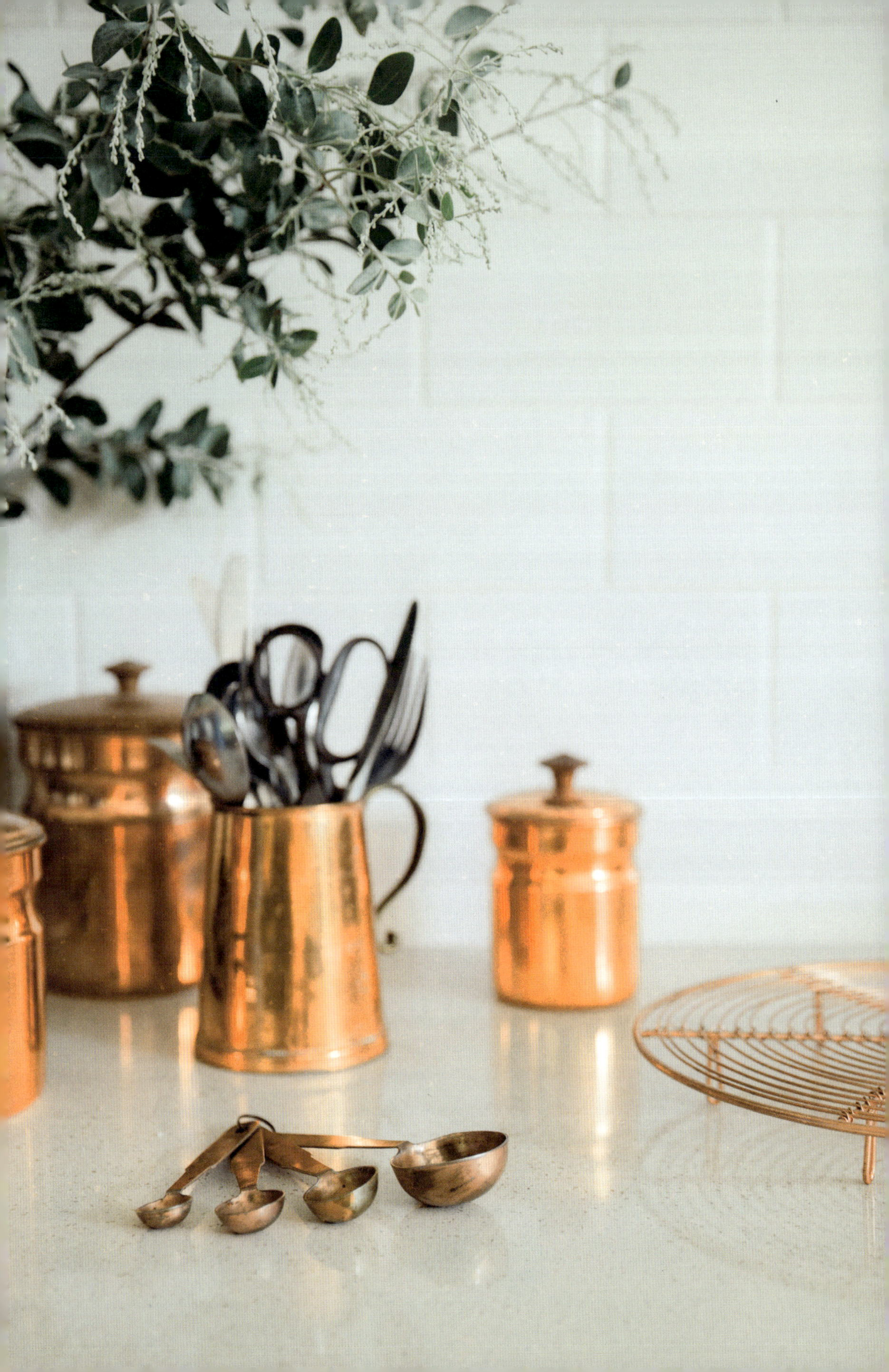

Is it really a slow metabolism?

WHY THE CALORIE EQUATION IS OUTDATED

The discovery that there was a basic level of energy (measured as calories or kilojoules) required for the body to survive, and the subsequent creation of a mathematical equation that could calculate this, was groundbreaking in its day. In 1918, it literally saved lives. If you think about what was happening around that time, World War I was only just coming to an end and for many people, food was scarce. I too have been fortunate to see it in action in modern times, when I worked as a dietician in the emergency department of a hospital and, at times, with athletes.

However, many inaccuracies and problems arise when we apply this calorie equation in more modern times. For starters, an equation that was founded on a minimum level requirement for survival is now used conversely to help people keep their energy consumption down. If people believe that this equation holds the answers to their weight loss or energy needs, we need to address them.

Where the problems lie are:

- In the extrapolation of the data that the calorie equation offers to the general public.
- The restrictive, deprivation mindset that the calorie equation drives in those who adopt it (the majority of female clients I have worked with over the past two decades), and that this deprivation is not sustainable.
- It leads too many people to believe that they constantly have to be on a diet — living from deprivation and feeling guilt or shame if they deviate from that way of eating, whenever they aren't following it strictly or feel as though they have eaten too much or exercised too little.

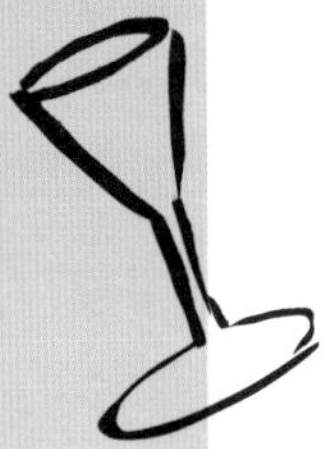

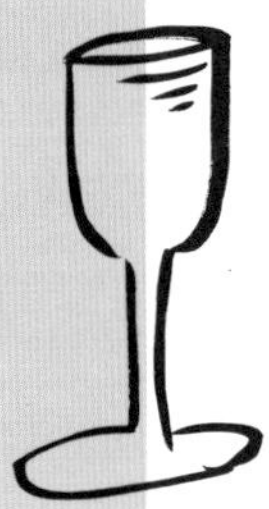

- It can lead body or weight conscious people to restrict calories too much, to the point that their metabolic rate slows (the point at which this happens will be different for everyone).
- It does not consider how significantly the food supply has changed since 1918 when the equation was first published (and the 1984 revised version does not consider the change in food supply either).
- It does not consider the stress hormone production of modern life via caffeine consumption (this mechanism is explained in my other books) and the perceptions of pressure and urgency.
- It does not consider the impact of concentrated (refined) carbohydrates — both sugars and starches — on metabolism via insulin, and also its subsequent blocking of leptin, an appetite regulating hormone.
- It does not factor in fat accumulation in the liver from alcohol consumption and a diet high in processed foods and drinks, and the impact of this on metabolism.
- It does not consider the impact of the increase in estrogen-like compounds in the food chain and environment, and their impact on metabolism.
- It does not consider the impact of adrenalin or cortisol and their differing impacts on metabolism and given the acute and chronic stress experienced by too many people today, this is a major oversight.
- It does not consider that science has now clearly demonstrated that the bacteria inhabiting the large intestine can influence what calories are worth.
- It does not consider the impact of sub-optimal (or diseased) thyroid function, a major oversight given the significant rise in autoimmune thyroid conditions.
- It does not consider the impact of constant upper-thoracic breathing, instead of diaphragmatic breathing and the impact

of how an individual's natural way of breathing on a daily basis influences the body's fuel utilisation via the autonomic nervous system (ANS).

- It does not get to the heart of the matter if someone emotionally overeats.
- It does nothing to address why, if you see and feel your clothes getting tighter and you don't like it or you feel uncomfortable, you do nothing about it — why doesn't your self-care kick in?

In other words, the calorie equation fails to consider the bigger picture, physically, environmentally and emotionally, based on the world in which we now live. It is time for an update, as the foundation of nutritional philosophy — that the calorie equation is the sole determinant of body size — is completely outdated.

> "Eat real food. Eat fat from whole food sources."

Therefore, I propose that it is time to be done with the calorie concept as a way of educating the public about what they are supposed to eat. It is time to stop dieting and start nourishing. It is time to stop counting calories.

Eat real food. Eat fat from whole food sources. Eat carbs from real food sources. It is easy to eat protein from real food sources, and, if it is animal protein, make sure that animal has been raised eating the food it is supposed to eat — not what humans have decided makes them grow faster — as well as being raised outside, partaking in its natural behaviours, and being cared for.

You can now demand this through how and from whom you purchase.

Change your mentality, change the way you approach how you feed yourself to a focus on your health and energy, not your weight. Positive not negative. A focus on what you can eat, not what you are not 'permitted' to eat. Do not let it take a health crisis to remind you of what you already know: that without your health, you have nothing. Listen to your body.

When you stop eating processed foods that interfere with your body's natural rhythms and signals, you will get back in touch with what your body, not your taste buds, wants. You will learn to trust yourself again. You have your own inner compass. Allow yourself to tune in.

“You have your own inner compass. Allow yourself to tune in.”

Make your health a priority, and watch your health and body transform, and, just as wonderfully, free yourself from a life lived in the fear of weight gain, calorie counting, deprivation and never feeling good enough.

A curious experiment

Up until the time I wrote *The Calorie Fallacy*, I hadn't analysed my caloric intake since 1999. So I used software to calculate my caloric intake and energy equation needs from Australian and New Zealand food tables. Based on the equation, I need 1812 calories for weight maintenance, and to lose weight it suggested I eat 1582 calories per day. I eat on average 2500 calories per day and my body size rarely changes. Of that, 50 per cent of my calories are coming from fat, 25 per cent from carbohydrates, and 25 per cent from protein. I am not suggesting you eat this way, as everyone is different, and I certainly haven't always eaten this way. It is what nourishes me now. I feed my body what it wants, and I have witnessed this change over time.

It is just that I trust my body. I don't doubt it; I don't believe it has ulterior motives. It knows better than me.

I simply share this with you to show you an example of a discrepancy in a number that an equation generates (that many people take as gospel) to how someone with a stable body size eats. I hypothesise, however, that if I ate 2500 calories of poor quality, processed, highly-refined foods, my body size would most likely increase. And that would have more to do with how the non-food ingredients would interfere with my detoxification processes, and what I'm missing out on by not eating whole real food (nutrients), and less to do with calories.

Starting the transition away from counting calories

When I am asked for my number one health tip, my answer often surprises people, as it has nothing to do with food. It is to diaphragmatically breathe.

Consider this. The way we are created, we live for the shortest time without oxygen. Next comes water, and thirdly comes food. How you breathe plays a significant role in the information your body picks up on about what must be occurring in your environment. This is explained in detail in my other books, but the detail right now doesn't matter; I simply want to point this out to you here.

You'll see it is at the top of the list over the page, which is designed to help you focus on giving your body what it needs for vibrant health. Some of the reasons why I am suggesting that these rituals be embraced are listed too.

11 tips for vibrant health

1 **Breathe diaphragmatically.** Long and slow, in and out through your nostrils, moving your lower tummy only as you breathe (not your upper chest). This communicates to the body that you are safe via a part of your nervous system (the autonomic nervous system — ANS), and you use body fat as a fuel effectively when the body knows it is safe.

2 **Drink water.** Rarely anything else. Hydration is critical to life, but also to the effective detoxification, filtration and elimination work done by the body.

3 **Eat whole, real food.** Your body has the enzymes to break this down, providing your cells with the nutrients they need for optimal health and function.

4 **Build muscle.** This increases metabolic rate, improves insulin sensitivity, and improves blood glucose management.

5 **Stretch/deep tissue massage.** Fascia is the specialised connective tissue layer surrounding muscles, bones and joints, giving structure to the body. It aids muscle movement, but also provides a passageway for nerves and blood vessels, and hence the exchange of nutrients, waste and energy. Therefore, flexibility is a conduit to good energy, hormonal function and detoxification. If the cells aren't receiving the nutrients they need, or aren't able to mobilise waste away from themselves efficiently, this too can cause toxin storage, stress and inflammation within the body — all of which interfere with vibrant health and body fat utilisation.

6

Adopt restorative practices. Practices such as Stillness Through Movement (STM), restorative yoga and qi gong are excellent for activating the part of the nervous system (the parasympathetic nervous system — PNS) that communicates safety to the rest of the body, allowing efficient body fat utilisation.

7

Sleep. Get eight hours sleep per night, and do your best to get two of those before midnight for hormonal balance and appetite regulation.

8

Reduce alcohol consumption. Only drink alcohol on super special occasions, thereby supporting efficient detoxification processes and hormonal balance, and avoiding fat accumulation in the liver.

9

Swap coffee for green tea or herbal tea. Unless you are naturally very calm and/or don't have many demands on your time, caffeine reduction will support an appropriate stress response rather than amping you up to feel anxious and utilise predominantly glucose.

10

Avoid refined flours and sugars, artificial sweeteners, colourings, flavours and preservatives. Doing so will help avoid the development of a fatty liver. These aren't whole, real foods.

11

Focus on health, not weight. This shift in focus will help give you great energy, vitality, happiness and freedom, as well as optimal health.

If the tips on the previous page overwhelm you, begin by choosing one of those factors to focus on and incorporate additional new habits as you feel ready. You may choose to focus only on eating more real food, for example. You will certainly see why this is of such importance throughout the pages of this book.

This is not a book about rules or perfection though, for they alone are not healthy. It is about holding a high standard for yourself and what you allow into your amazing body; for if you knew who you really are, you would be in awe of yourself and you would treat yourself accordingly.

I believe that the way we feed ourselves is our most basic form of self-care. It is what you do every day that impacts on your health, not what you do occasionally.

It is how you consistently live that matters: how you eat, drink, move, think, breathe, believe and perceive all impact on your wellbeing. It is time for the dawning of a new era in how people approach their self-care, ending the vast array of confusion that surrounds food and how to best nourish ourselves.

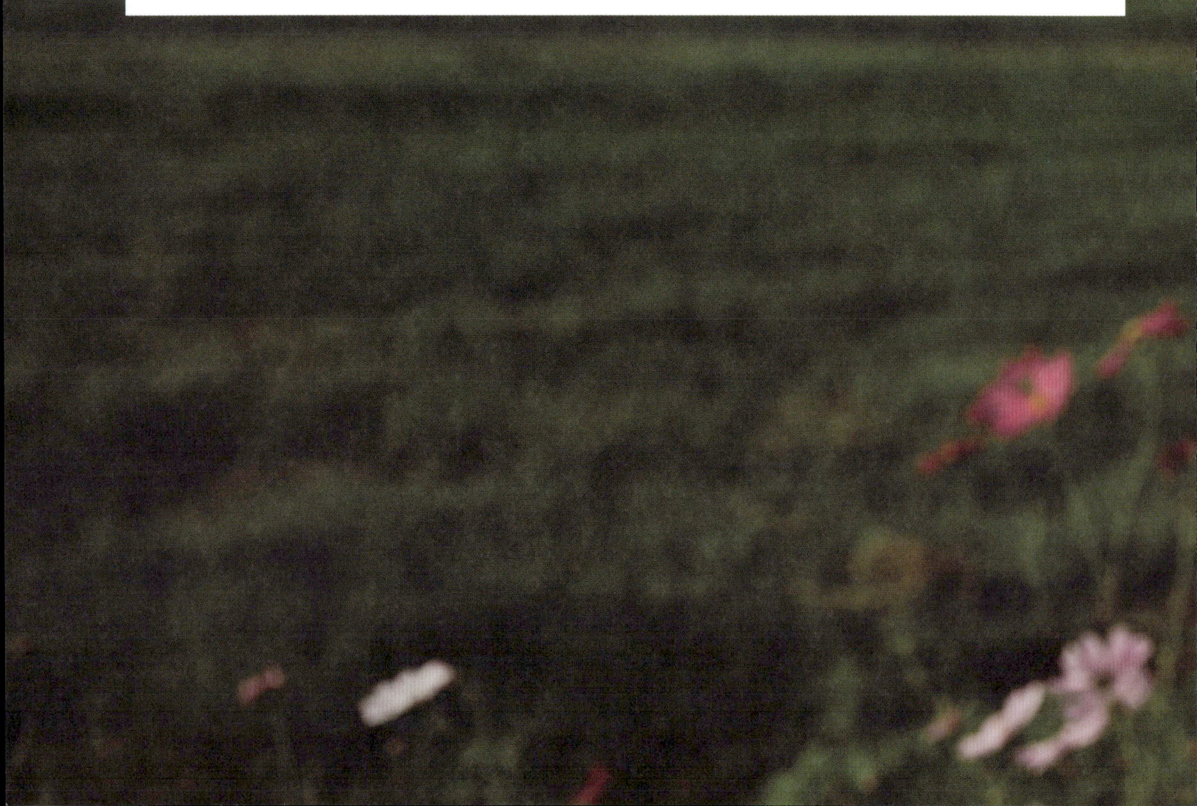

Your tomorrow depends entirely on what you do today.

MAHATMA GANDHI

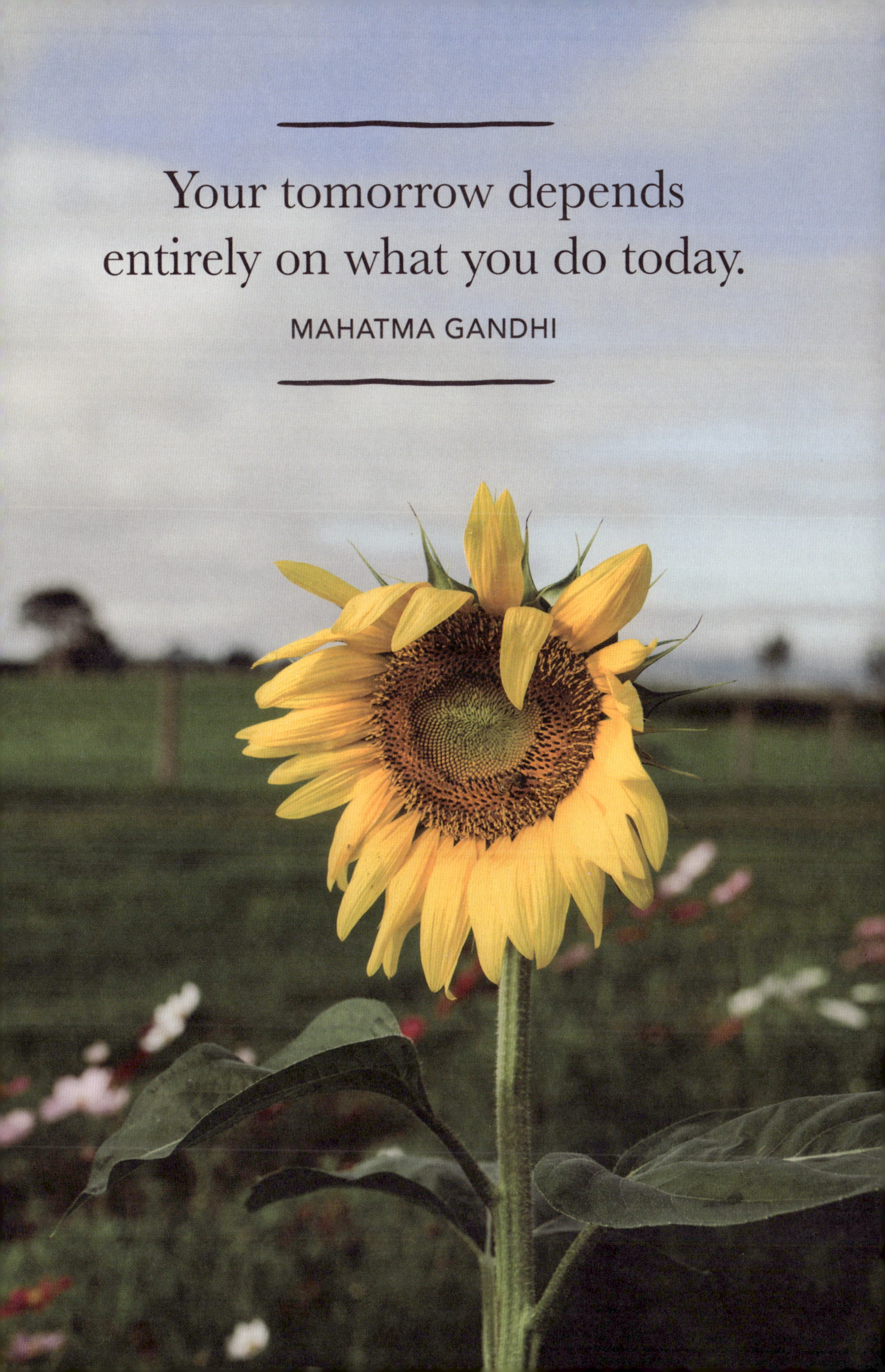

WORKSHEET

Of the previous tips, which ones did you resist the most? Reflect on why this might be the case. Then circle three below you are going to incorporate into your life, over time.

Remembering that often what we resist is what needs addressing.

Adopt a restorative practice

Drink more water

Build muscle

Stretch/deep tissue massage

Breathe diaphragmatically

Sleep

Swap coffee for green tea or herbal tea

Avoid refined foods, artificial sweeteners and preservatives

Eat whole, real food

Focus on health, not weight

Reduce alcohol consumption

Now you've identified your top three, how are you going to start incorporating these into your daily or weekly routine?

1

(e.g. drink more water)

I am going to incorporate this into my life by

2

I am going to incorporate this into my life by

3

I am going to incorporate this into my life by

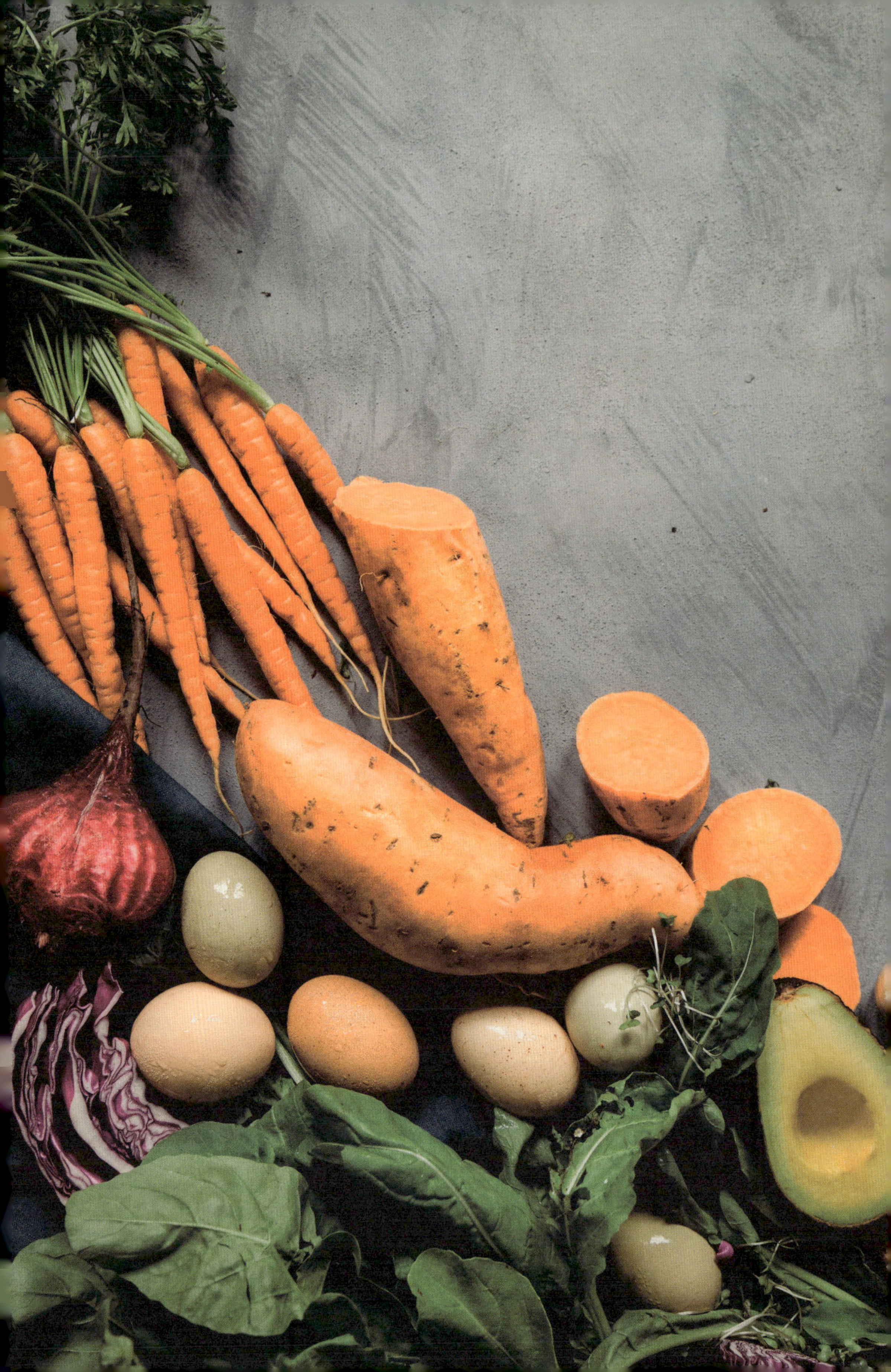

Fats, proteins and carbohydrates

YOUR ENERGY SOURCE

Macronutrients are where you obtain your energy from.

They are:

- carbohydrates
- proteins
- fats
- alcohol.

Yes, it seems weird including alcohol in a section with the word "nutrient" in the title, but by definition it is. Ideally it is not a large contributor to your daily intake of macronutrients since it is not needed for survival, nor does it provide nutritional benefits. Macronutrients provide energy, and this form of energy is measured as calories or kilojoules: calories being the imperial and kilojoules being the metric way to measure energy.

Macronutrients are substances needed for growth and metabolism and for many other body functions, and they allow us to experience energy in our daily lives — provided a host of other processes function optimally.

Since "macro" means large, macronutrients are substances required in large amounts, while the micronutrients — vitamins and minerals — are needed in smaller amounts and don't contain energy themselves.

There are only two fuels for the human body: glucose and fat. The body typically uses a combination of both, and the nervous system plays a major role in the best ratio for you to use in any given moment to which the way you eat, drink, move, think, breathe, believe and perceive all contribute.

CARBOHYDRATES

Carbohydrates supply the body with glucose, the fuel you use first when you start to exercise, and the fuel that your brain, kidneys and red blood cells prefer. One gram of carbohydrate supplies the body with four calories of energy. It is, however, important to note that when the number of calories a food contains is measured, it does not reflect what I refer to as the "metabolic consequences" of that food. For example, when you consume foods that contain carbohydrates, your pancreas secretes insulin to deal with the increase in blood glucose, and insulin signals to the body to store fat. Dietary fat, on the other hand, does not drive an insulin response, so the calories you obtain from foods rich in fats do not hormonally signal the body to store fat.

Science has attempted to distinguish carbohydrates from one another, as explained below. I simply want you to understand that the source of the carbohydrates matters, and I encourage you to obtain your carbohydrates from whole foods, as they come with a range of different nutrients, some of which enhance their digestion and hence their ability to supply you with what you need for vibrant health.

Carbohydrates can be sweet or starch-based. Simple and complex are two of the categories science has divided carbohydrates into, although this happens less often these days. Simple carbohydrates are sugars, lollies, soft drinks, fruit juice and other sweet products. Simple carbohydrates are usually quick energy; they enter your bloodstream quickly and are either used up or stored as fat, and typically offer little or no nutritional value. In fact, they may actually detract from your health.

Complex carbohydrates, on the other hand, are typically sources of more extended energy: sweet potato and brown rice are examples of this category. The energy from complex carbohydrates usually (although not always) takes longer to enter the bloodstream and provides a more sustained form of energy.

WHAT IS SUGAR?

Before answering the question, "What is sugar?" it is vital to clarify the precise definition of the word 'sugar', as it is used loosely in the modern vernacular and given a variety of meanings.

As you now know, sugars and starches are carbohydrates, with one of the main differences between them being the size of their structures and how quickly they enter the bloodstream. The term 'sugar' refers to simple sugars, monosaccharides, such as glucose and fructose, as well as disaccharides, such as sucrose, lactose and maltose, which are two monosaccharides linked together. These sugars are widely spread throughout whole, real foods but in relatively small amounts when compared to the added and/or concentrated sugars found in processed foods. Starches are polysaccharides made up of long chains of monosaccharides. Real food sources of starch include sweet potato, rice (all types) and potatoes, while processed foods that contain starch include bread, pasta and biscuits. Starches are broken down into sugars during digestion.

The simplest way to understand the language used to describe carbohydrates is to think of the 'saccharide' part of the words above to mean 'sugar'. 'Mono' means 'one', 'di' means 'two' and 'poly' means 'many'.

What you need to know about all the different categories of carbohydrates is that the human body has been consuming them for all of history. What has changed dramatically is the amount being consumed. When the only food sources of carbohydrates are root vegetables, legumes, fruit and honey, you eat very little. When the sugars and starches are refined and put into processed food, you can easily eat far too much. Australian statistics estimate that as recently as 100 years ago, people ate about a kilogram of sugar per person each year. Now it is about 35 kilograms per person per year. Do you think that is due to people consuming 35 times the amount of fruit and vegetables they used to eat? Of course not.

The human body has been consuming carbohydrates for all of history, but what has changed dramatically is the amount being consumed.

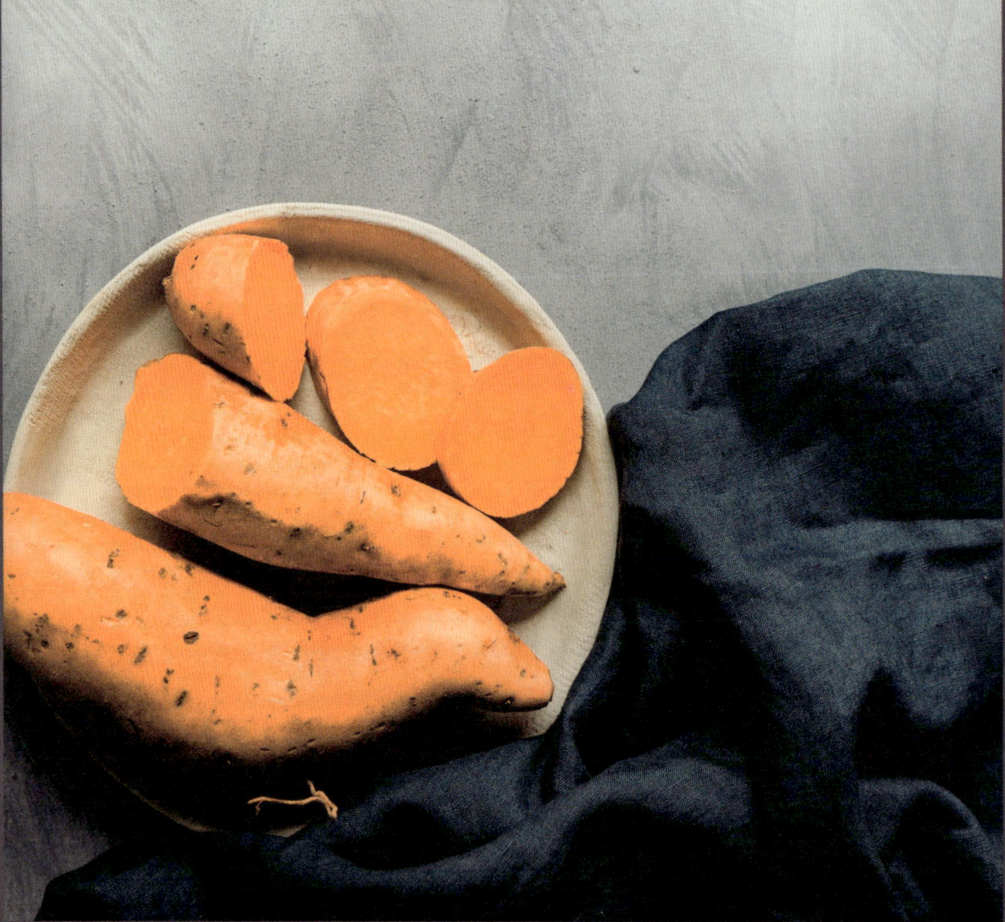

The source of this is processed foods. They are the problem. Not just because of the concentrated carbohydrates they supply, but because they are virtually devoid of nutrients.

What happens when we overconsume carbohydrates?

- The lining of your blood vessels can be damaged and/or inflamed.
- Your clothes can become tight.
- You experience energy slumps regularly.
- You can become insulin resistant, which is a risk factor for type 2 diabetes.
- Blood fats (triglycerides) can become elevated, which is detrimental for your heart health.
- It may contribute to fat infiltration of the liver.

What happens if we don't eat enough carbohydrates?

- It is firstly important you are reminded that many foods contain carbohydrates — even green leafy vegetables (in very small amounts), as the sugars in the vegetables provide the fuel for the plants to survive.
- The body can convert amino acids (from proteins) into glucose when it needs to, but if we don't get this from our food the body may begin to break down muscle. The brain, kidneys and red blood cells, in particular, require glucose to function.
- You may be at risk of nutrient deficiencies, as some carbohydrate-rich real, whole foods also contain other important nutrients, such as B-group vitamins.
- Some people experience an adrenalin surge in the middle of the night, waking them up and making them feel anxious.

What's the best way to consume carbohydrates?

- As they come in Nature. For example, fruit is a better choice than lollies as with fruit you also receive vitamins, minerals, antioxidants and fibre, rather than just sugar with no nutrients. But of course you can eat too much fruit — two pieces a day is ideal. Also note that if you don't digest fructose, or other components of the fruit well, you might feel better without it. I am simply saying that fruit is a more nourishing choice than lollies and guiding you to distinguish between nourishing carbohydrate choices and poor quality ones.

The scientific assessment of carbohydrates

Scientists try to define carbohydrates by what happens to them when they enter our body. A scale you might be familiar with is the glycaemic index (GI). This index is a scale based on how quickly the glucose from the food will hit the bloodstream. Essentially, the faster it gets to the bloodstream, the higher it appears on the index and the more insulin (a fat storage hormone) is required. However, the GI does not take into account the amount of carbohydrate in a food in comparison to the other macronutrients, micronutrients or how much you consume in one sitting.

Another categorisation you might be familiar with is glycaemic load (GL). It is a better indicator of how a carbohydrate food will affect blood glucose levels. GL considers the actual amount of carbohydrate you eat in a sitting. For example, pumpkin is considered a high GI carbohydrate, but it is high in fibre, water, vitamins, minerals and protective phytonutrients, which alters the way it is digested and promotes excellent health. The GL of a serve of pumpkin is low (a good thing).

Fructose has a low GI too. In fact, the way fructose is digested and utilised by the body is different from glucose. It requires an enzyme from the liver to convert it into glucose. Only liver cells can take up fructose, whereas all cells in the body can utilise glucose, and the impact of excessive fructose consumption on liver health is finally coming to light. In other words, the GI can be highly misleading if that is all you use to guide your carbohydrate choices. Common sense is a better guide, or simply embracing the statement "just eat real food". I highly doubt whether the GI would have become a way of assessing carbohydrates if processed foods didn't exist.

When we apply these scientific measurements to real life, however, we begin to see how they fail to take into account the way that other things we consume alongside carbohydrates might affect the way our body responds to them, as well as the nutritional value that particular foods offer us.

Both GI and GL are affected by the protein, fat and fibre content of a meal, as they all slow down the release of glucose into the blood and hence the requirement for insulin — so when combined with protein, fat and fibre, a high GI food is unlikely to reach our bloodstream in the same way. Then consider a piece of chocolate cake that you might buy from a bakery — many of them are low GI and, if following this as way of choosing 'healthy' foods, they would be a 'good' choice. Yet they contain high levels of refined sugars, poor quality fats, virtually no nutrients and are high GL.

Listen to all of this jargon and detail, though! No wonder people feel confused and overwhelmed at times about dietary information! We stop needing concepts like this when we simply eat whole, real food. The need for complication falls away.

Plus, we don't need science to tell us that a pumpkin is a better food choice than a chocolate cake. Let's bring back common sense!

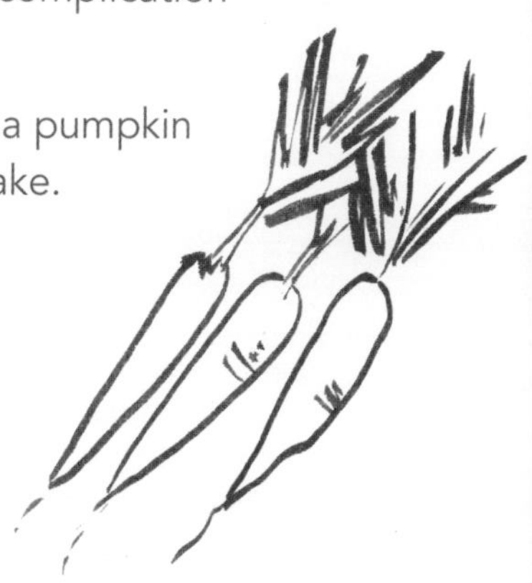

How else is glucose generated inside the body?

Although this is by no means intended to be a complete work on carbohydrate metabolism, it is important to note that there are other mechanisms inside the body that create glucose, such as gluconeogenesis, a pathway via which amino acids (the building blocks of proteins) are converted into glucose.

Starch Digestion

There are some additional steps to the digestion of starch (polysaccharides). If you could see starch, it is made up of glucose units linked together in two different formations. One is called amylose, the other amylopectin.

It takes the body longer to digest starches that contain more amylopectin, as it is a branched molecule and digestive enzymes have to break each bond between the glucose units in the branches before the enzymes can break the links between the glucose units in the backbone. Science suggests that less insulin is therefore required when foods are richer in amylopectin than amylose, and that this leads to less fat storage. However, digestion and metabolism are rarely this straightforward, and very few people can determine from looking at a food whether it contains more amylose or amylopectin!

Around three quarters of the starch in many unprocessed whole foods (such as legumes) is amylopectin, with the remaining quarter being amylose. However, some starch-based food additives — for example, cornstarch — are higher in amylose. But most important to our insulin response is the amount of starch we eat. When we consume naturally occurring starch in real, whole foods as they are found in Nature, the starch is typically packaged up with fibre which can slow down the absorption of glucose into our bloodstream, and therefore requires less insulin to keep our blood glucose levels steady. Fibre also keeps us feeling full, so it may also help to prevent us from over-consuming starch.

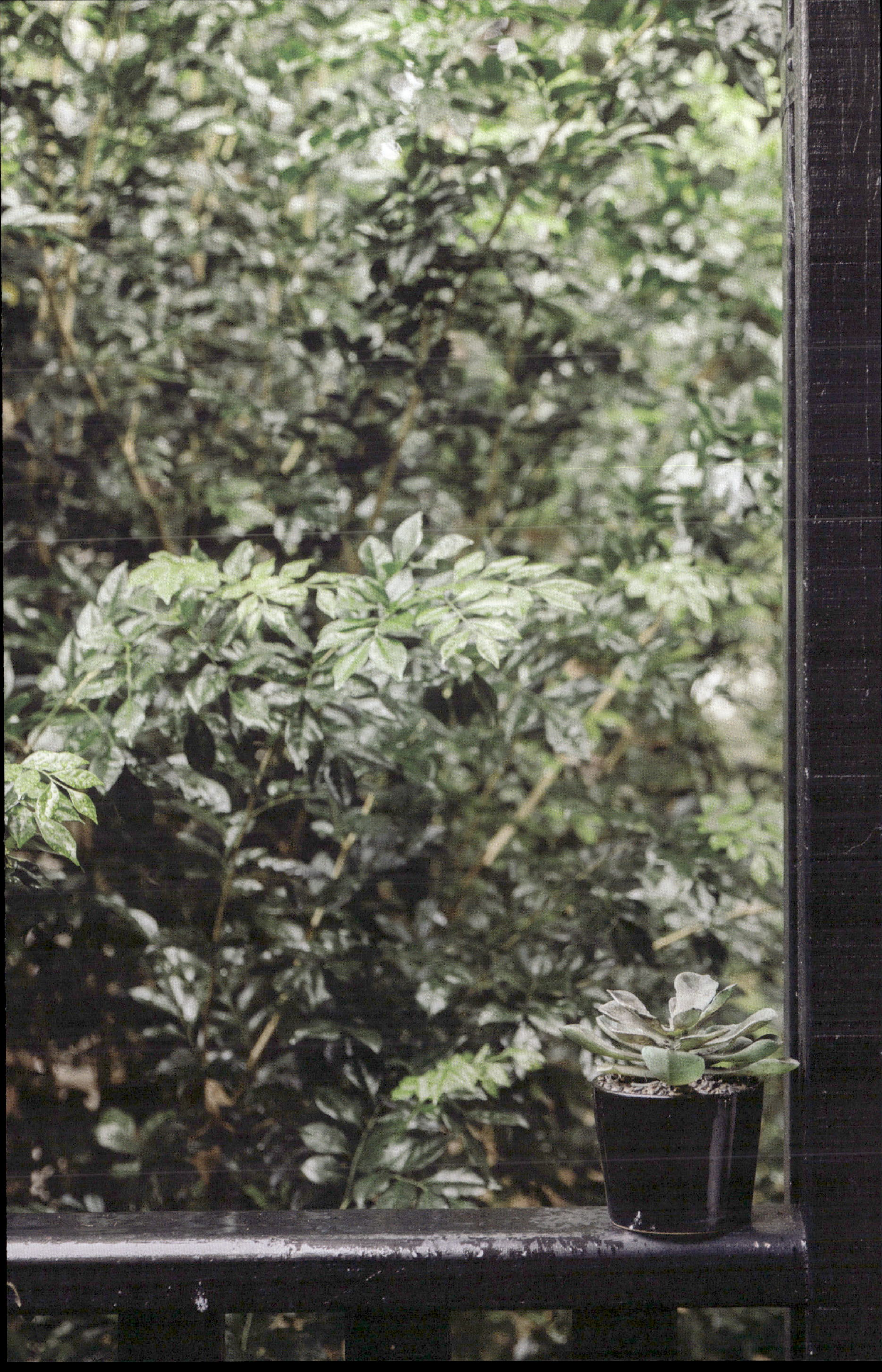

I want the messages offered on the pages of this book to be practical. I share the above with you for those who want to delve deeper into understanding carbohydrate metabolism.

Yet all you really need to know is that glucose is yielded from the digestion of starches and sugars, and that the regular overconsumption of foods that contain refined sugars and flours have the potential to take away from your health. A way of eating that is consistently based on whole, real foods goes a substantial way towards providing your body with the nutrients it needs for optimal health, as well as leaving out the substances that can have a negative effect on your health.

You can see how complicated and confusing carbohydrate messages have been for consumers, so I take this opportunity to remind you again that, when it comes to food, carbohydrates included, Nature gets it right and it is potentially human intervention (HI) — that is, processing — that can get it so wrong. Choose low HI foods. Choose carbohydrates from whole food sources.

FIBRE

Fibre refers to certain types of carbohydrates that our body cannot digest. These carbohydrates pass through the intestinal tract intact and help to move waste out of the body. However, again, I believe the source of the fibre matters.

What happens if we don't get enough fibre?

When we don't consume adequate fibre it can cause problems such as:

- constipation
- haemorrhoids
- may increase the risk of certain types of cancers, such as colon cancer.

One of the most important roles fibre plays is to promote the efficient elimination of waste from the body. If waste products accumulate, we suffer — anything from headaches, liver problems, excessive odorous flatulence, to sex hormone imbalances.

> One of the most important roles fibre plays is to promote the efficient elimination of waste from the body.

How much fibre is best to consume?

Diets that contain more fibre have been shown to decrease the risk of colon cancer. Over the many years I have worked with people, I have seen what works for people and what doesn't. Despite the mainstream advice that encourages high fibre diets for good bowel health, this can work against optimal bowel health for some people with specific bowel problems (such as IBS). There are no hard and fast rules here — nutrition advice in this case is truly best tailored to the individual.

For some people with IBS, they cannot tolerate even moderate amounts of fibre when their gut is exhibiting symptoms. Or for others the source of the fibre matters. Soluble fibre seems to be better tolerated in those with IBS than too much insoluble fibre.

Sources of soluble fibre include:

- legumes, such as lentils
- vegetables, such as carrots, artichoke and broccoli (with the skin of the stalk removed)
- fruits, such as berries and bananas
- oats
- flaxseeds.

Foods that contain insoluble fibre include:

- wholegrains
- nuts and seeds
- the skins of fruits and vegetables.

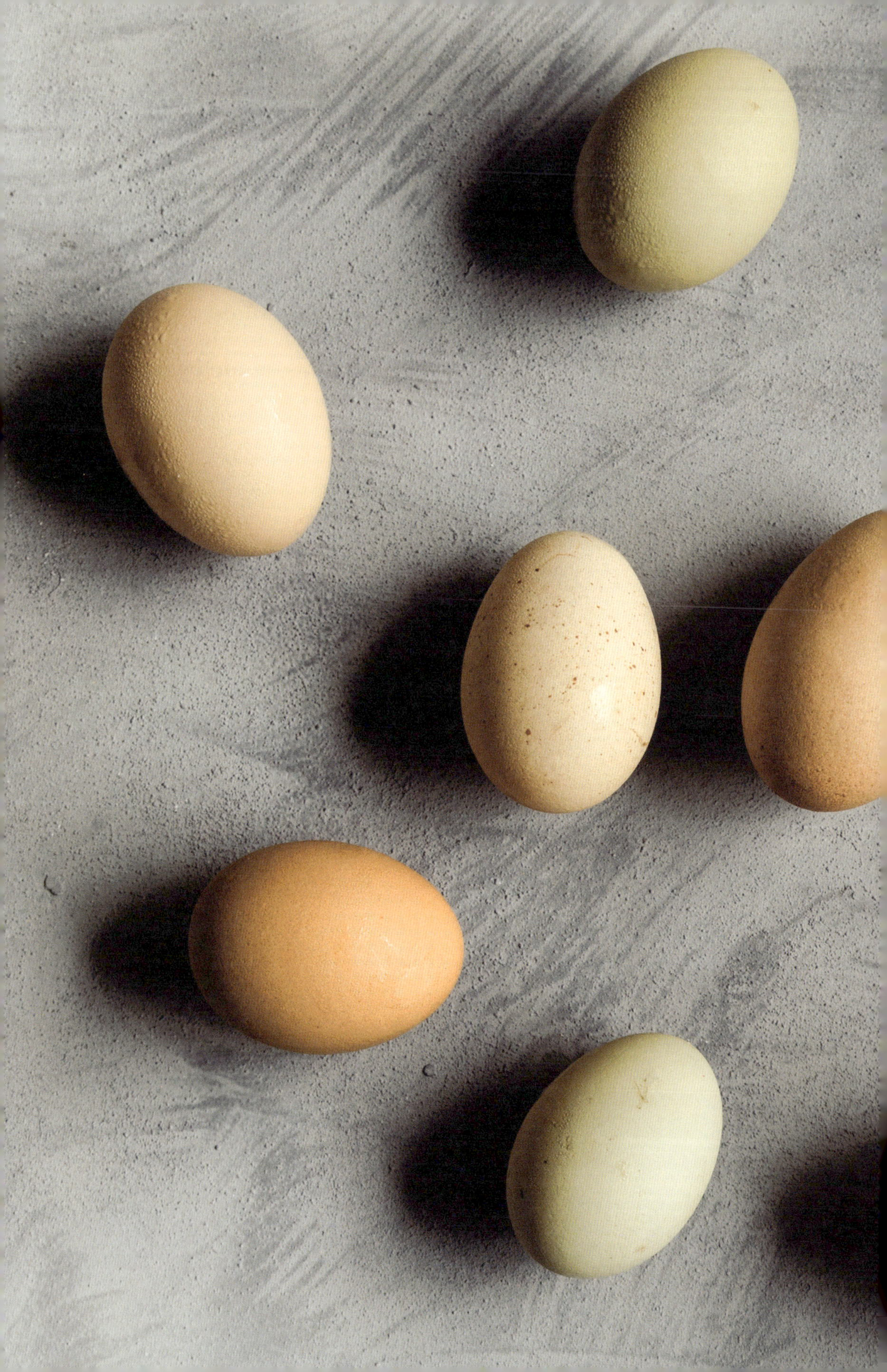

What happens if we get too much fibre?

Too much fibre, particularly without adequate water consumption, can lead to constipation as fibre absorbs water to keep the waste soft and move it. As fibre intake increases, so must water intake. Large amounts of fibre for some people with gut problems assists them, while for others, it can add to their gut symptoms. Notice how the amounts and different types of fibre (soluble and insoluble) affect you to determine your best way forward, as it is highly individualised.

Good whole food sources of fibre that tend not to aggravate the bowel include some starchy carbohydrates such as sweet potato, vegetables and some, but not all, fruits.

PROTEIN

When we talk about protein, people tend to think about the animal-based options. Chicken, beef, lamb and fish are all complete proteins. However, there are many people who choose not to consume meat for numerous reasons and there are those who would benefit from cutting down on the amount of meat they currently consume. There is an array of non-meat foods out there that also contain protein, including eggs, legumes, pulses, nuts, seeds, wholegrains such as brown rice, and even green leafy vegetables contain amino acids.

A gram of protein offers the body four calories of energy, and it supplies the body with amino acids, substances that can become part of us. For example, the amino acids from foods go on to create the cells of your immune system, which helps defend you from colds and flus, as well as forming part of the anti-tumour response. Amino acids also create the neurotransmitters in your body, which influence your mood, and they create the muscles that provide you with the strength to carry your groceries and your children.

Of the 20 amino acids, 10 are considered essential (some research papers suggest nine are essential); in other words your body is unable to create them itself from other substances so you need to consume them in your diet. When a protein food contains all of the essential amino acids it is referred to as "complete". Most vegetable-based protein sources are "incomplete"; however, different vegetable-based protein sources from different botanical families can be combined to be completed, as the essential amino acid lacking in one of the foods will often be high in the one from the other family.

> Keep in mind that no food in Nature is 100 per cent protein, which is why I am usually concerned when people consume drinks containing much higher levels of protein on a regular basis.

An example of this is adding sunflower seeds to a vegetable stir-fry that you serve with lentils: the seeds and the lentils are from different families, and their amino acid profiles complete each other.

Combinations of complementary plant-based protein foods include:

- Lentils + brown rice (for example, lentil dhal served with brown rice).
- Beans such as black beans or kidney beans + brown rice (for example, a Mexican-inspired dish).
- Chickpeas + seeds (for example, a vegetable pattie made with chickpeas and sunflower seeds or sesame seeds).
- Nuts/seeds + buckwheat (for example, a cashew vegetable stir-fry served with buckwheat noodles, or a buckwheat porridge topped with mixed seeds).
- Hummus made from chickpeas and tahini.
- Quinoa (quinoa is one of the few plant-based proteins that contains all of the essential amino acids, so is considered 'complete').

Keep in mind that no food in Nature is 100 per cent protein, which is why I am usually concerned when people consume drinks containing much higher levels of protein on a regular basis. Again, for me this seems like common sense, but if we needed highly concentrated serves of protein, Nature would have created it.

All animal meats are 25 per cent protein, meaning that 100 grams of meat contains 25 grams of protein. Even the World Cancer Research Fund's (WCRF) position statement on the consumption of red meat to reduce the risk of cancer — in particular, colorectal cancer — is to "limit intake of red meat to no more than 500 grams per week" (something I discuss further on page 217).

Yet I meet people who consume more than this every day. I personally don't believe the problem is the red meat itself. It can be part of a bigger health picture for a person, particularly if they don't have efficient bowel evacuation or liver detoxification pathways, or are what is known as 'estrogen-dominant'.

Plus, they may be consuming meat from poorly raised animals, who have been fed poor quality diets.

Add to this the consistent lack of vegetable intake reported across many Western diets, which means that too few cancer-protective substances are being consumed.

What happens if I don't get enough protein?

- Your muscle mass may decrease, which consequently decreases your metabolic rate.
- You may lose strength so carrying your groceries and picking up your children or grandchildren may become more difficult.
- You will likely feel less full and satisfied after your meals.
- Your immune function may be compromised.
- Your body won't have the building blocks it needs to be able to make all the enzymes, hormones and neurotransmitters you need to maintain your health and wellbeing.

- Your body will not prioritise hair, skin and nail health.
- Your mood can be adversely affected.

What is the ideal amount of protein?

This depends on the individual — protein requirements are influenced by age, how much you move, your body composition (how much muscle mass versus body fat you have) and your current state of health (certain conditions can require higher or lower protein intakes). Generally, a healthy adult needs to consume between 0.8 and 1.0 gram of protein per kilogram of body weight per day. For a person who weighs 70 kilograms, this would be around 55-70 grams of protein per day.

What happens if I get too much protein?

- The load on your liver will be increased as the liver must change components of protein metabolism so that they can be excreted.
- You may become dehydrated more easily (water is lost when the excess protein is excreted).
- Calcium excretion will increase.

Protein foods can supply the body with energy, although not directly. Proteins are broken down into amino acids, and those amino acids can stay in that form, join together with other amino acids to form peptides, and go on to form body proteins. Or amino acids can be converted into glucose to be used for energy. The name of the main biochemical pathway responsible for this is gluconeogenesis.

Because biochemically it is more efficient for the body to use glucose supplied as glucose — it is more labour intensive for the body to convert amino acids into glucose — the body prefers to allow the amino acids to be used for their repair work, their neurotransmitter production work, muscle building and new cell building, as no other substances can do this.

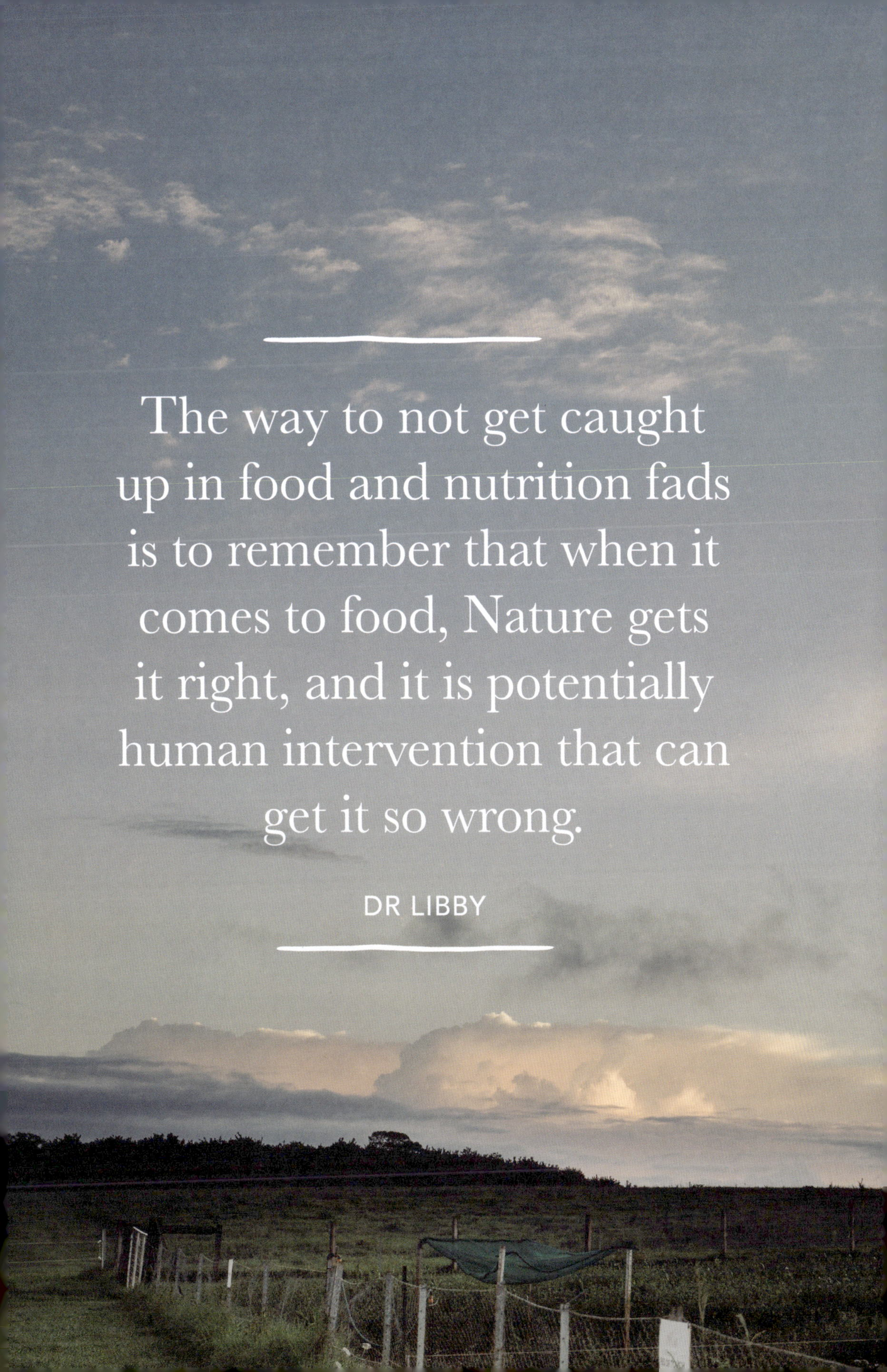

The way to not get caught up in food and nutrition fads is to remember that when it comes to food, Nature gets it right, and it is potentially human intervention that can get it so wrong.

DR LIBBY

FAT

Fats provide us with fatty acids, and they are an important source of energy. They offer us nine calories per gram. Ensuring that your body is efficient at utilising fats as a fuel source is an enormously powerful way to ensure a good and even supply of energy across your day.

Too many people today are unable to efficiently use body fat as a fuel, and rely predominantly on glucose, due to how they eat, drink, breathe, exercise and think. There are immense health and energy benefits from including fats from whole food sources in the diet. However, one of the most commonly asked questions is: "Does eating fat make you fat?"

I have met thousands of clients who are afraid of consuming fat. It is understandable, as for so many years the public was told that eating fat would make you fat. Sadly, for the majority of the population, cutting out or eating less fat didn't make them any healthier or slimmer, for a multitude of reasons.

The first thing to note is that there are different types of fat, so it is important not to generalise and say "avoid fat" or "consume fat" without first identifying and understanding which type of fat is being referenced.

There are three main categories of fats that serve your health — saturated fats, monounsaturated fats and polyunsaturated fats — and all three fats can be obtained from eating whole foods. And the fats that take away from your health? Most concerning are the trans fats and poor quality vegetable oils, which are found mainly in processed foods, particularly deep fried foods, processed cakes, biscuits and muesli bars, and foods with long shelf lives.

Trans fats are created when some types of polyunsaturated fats are damaged due to heat and processing. The ratio of fats consumed can also be a problem. Within the polyunsaturated category, there are two types of fat — omega-3 and omega-6 — with the inflammation promoting omega-6 fats typically too high in many people's diets.

However, one of the most commonly asked questions is: "Does eating fat make you fat?"

DR LIBBY

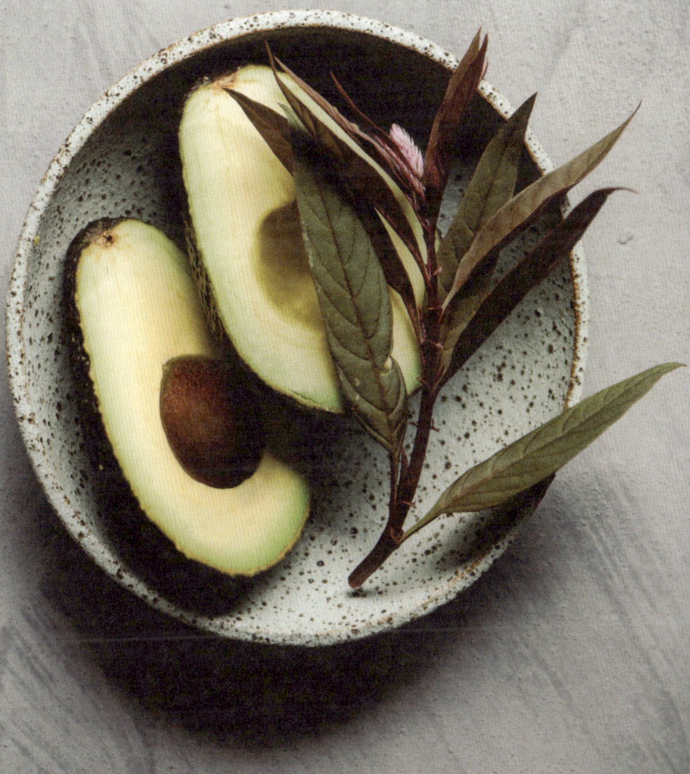

The different types of fats and some of their food sources are:

- Saturated, such as those found in coconut.
- Monounsaturated, such as those found in olives, avocados, and macadamia nuts, as well as the oils from these foods.
- Polyunsaturated, of which there are two types:
    - Omega-6, such as those found predominantly in certain nuts and seeds, and oils from these foods, as well as evening primrose oil, borage oil and whole blackcurrants, seeds included.
    - Omega-3, such as those found in oily fish, linseeds (flaxseeds), walnuts and pecans.

The essential fatty acids: omega-3 and omega-6

The omega-3 fats that must be consumed daily are eicosapentaenoic acid (EPA) and docosahexaenoic acid (DHA), which the body can convert from another essential fatty acid called alpha-linolenic acid (ALA), which also must be consumed. However, the conversion of ALA into the critical EPA and DHA fats is inefficient in some people. Hence, it is wise to include adequate amounts of all of these fats in your diet.

The health benefits of EPA and DHA are well documented: they are powerful anti-inflammatories. They take up residence in the membrane (outside layer) of the cell and are able to exert their anti-inflammatory effects to keep the cells flexible. However, due to their physical structure, they themselves oxidise easily and are best consumed with an antioxidant-rich diet, which is one that is high in coloured plant foods.

The omega-6 essential fatty acid is called linoleic acid (LA), which the body elongates (converts) into the vital gamma linolenic acid (GLA). GLA can also be consumed; a necessary dietary action if people are inefficient at converting LA into GLA. This is usually true for people with eczema as their skin does better having the GLA supplied directly.

The typical Western diet is overabundant in omega-6 fatty acids — found in many processed foods, baked goods, and grains — and usually lacking in omega-3s. DHA and EPA are found in oily fish, such as salmon and mackerel, as well as some algae, while the other omega-3 fat, ALA, is found in flaxseeds, chia seeds and walnuts. A good choice in the omega-6 EFA category is evening primrose oil, which contains GLA and has been shown to help people with eczema take up fat into their skin, allowing it to soften and be moisturised.

Medium-chain triglycerides

Sometimes the language used to describe fats can make the best types to consume seem confusing. To understand this, it is important to remember that all fats and oils are made up of substances called fatty acids and there are two methods of classifying fatty acids. The one most often used describes the level of 'saturation'. As outlined above, there are saturated fatty acids, monounsaturated fatty acids and polyunsaturated fatty acids. The second method of classification is based on the length of the carbon chain (its backbone) in the fatty acid. There are short-chain fatty acids (SCFAs), medium-chain fatty acids (MCFAs) and long-chain fatty acids (LCFAs).

Another word often used in reference to fatty acids is triglyceride. Three fatty acids joined together create a triglyceride creating what are known as short-chain triglycerides (SCTs), medium-chain triglycerides (MCTs) or long-chain triglycerides (LCTs). Almost all of the fats and oils you eat — whether they are saturated or unsaturated, or come from animal or plant-based foods — are composed of long-chain triglycerides.

Studies suggest that at least 98 per cent of all of the fats that most people eat consist of LCT. However, some food, such as coconut, is rather unique as it is composed predominantly of MCT. Organic butter also contains some MCTs, although it contains more LCTs than MCTs.

One of the unique properties of MCTs is that they are broken down almost immediately by enzymes in the saliva and gastric juices, so that pancreatic, fat-digesting enzymes are not essential for their digestion, which can be helpful for people who experience challenges with their digestive system. MCTs are broken down into individual fatty acids (MCFAs) in the digestive system. MCFAs are absorbed directly from the intestines into the portal vein (a vein that goes straight to the liver) and sent immediately to the liver where they are, for the most part, burned as fuel. They can therefore potentially offer the body an energy supply that is highly efficient — provided your body gets the message from your nervous system that it is "safe" for you to use fat as a fuel.

In order for LCTs to be digested, pancreatic enzymes are required. Once these pancreatic enzymes have broken down the fats, they are then absorbed and packaged with a protein molecule to become what's called a lipoprotein. These lipoproteins are transported via the lymphatic system, bypassing the liver, and end up in the bloodstream.

Once in the blood, these lipoproteins move around and deliver their fat components to the various tissues in the body. As they continue to travel in the bloodstream, distributing their fatty components, these lipoproteins eventually become so small there is not much left of them. At this point, they are sent to the liver where they are either broken down to be used for energy or they become part of other lipoproteins and re-enter the bloodstream and the process continues.

Cholesterol, saturated fat, monounsaturated fat and polyunsaturated fat are all packaged together into lipoproteins and carried throughout the body in this form. In contrast, and as mentioned above, medium-chain fatty acids are not packaged into lipoproteins, but go straight to the liver where they are converted into energy, making MCFA an efficient source of fuel for most people.

Types of fats

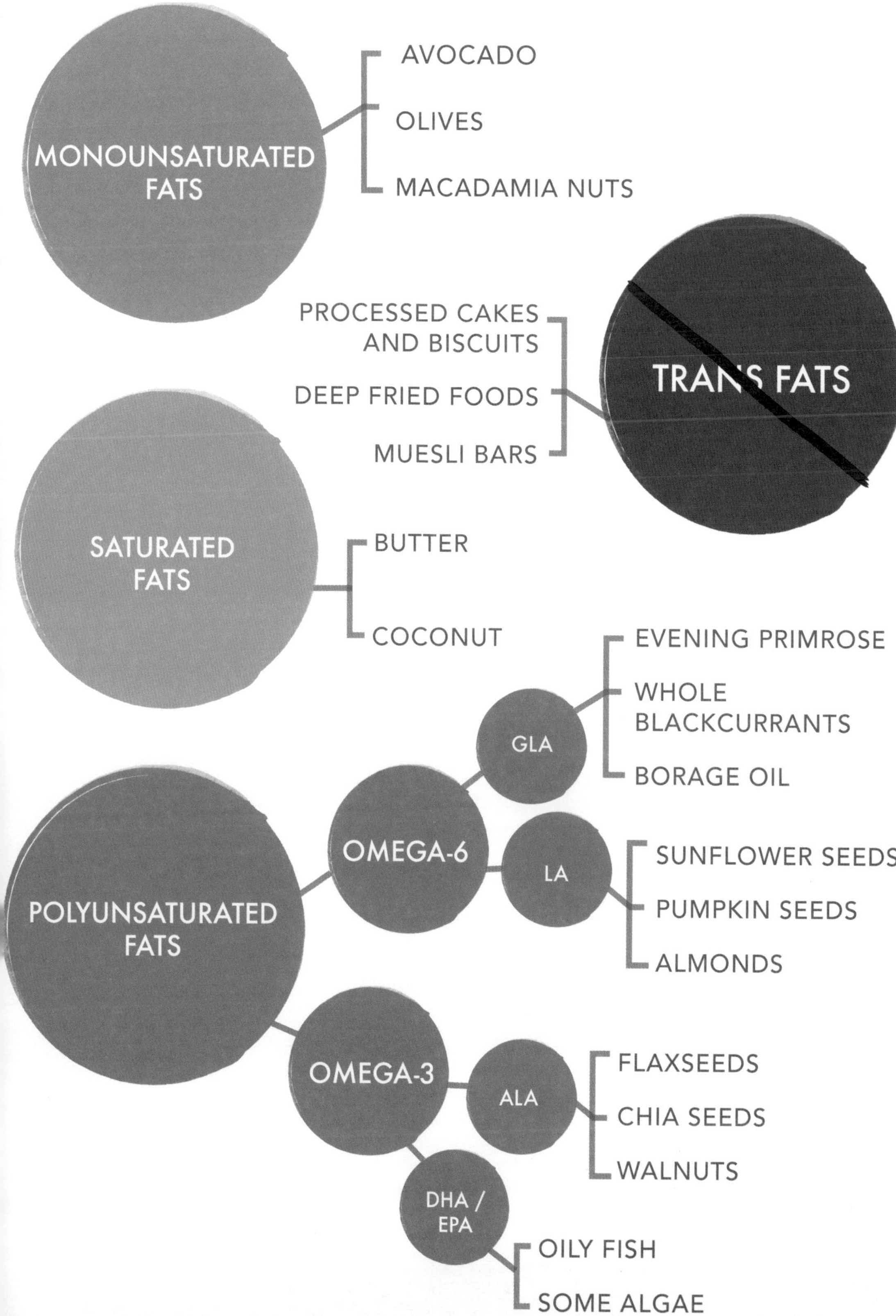

One MCFA that deserves special mention is lauric acid. Both coconut and organic butter contain lauric acid, which is known for its contribution to a healthy gut bacteria profile and immune system benefits. Butter from pasture-fed cows contains yet another special fat known as conjugated linoleic acid (CLA), a relative of LA, which research has shown to have anti-cancer properties as well as anti-inflammatory actions.

What happens if I don't consume enough fats?

An adequate consumption of healthy fats plays a crucial role in maintaining the health of your precious organs and having great energy. Some whole foods are composed of fatty acids that are essential for life, and fatty acids help the body to absorb the fat-soluble vitamins — vitamins A, D, E and K. You also tend to crave more sweet food with inadequate dietary fat intake.

What is a good amount of fat to consume?

Again, this depends on the individual. As a general guide, start with around a handful of real whole foods that are rich in nourishing fats with each meal. For more guidance on this, see the Food Matrix on page 286. You may feel better with less than this, and your body's preferences may change from day to day.

What happens if I consume too much fat?

- You may experience digestive distress or nausea.
- You may feel very full and therefore eat less of other foods that contain important nutrients.
- Even with that tip of the fat-information iceberg, I hope you can begin to see that the 'fat-free' fad took away a much needed food, fuel and nourishment source from too many people.

What is so sad is that 'fat-free' mostly meant that the fat was replaced with refined sugars and, to mask the increase in sweetness in the food supply, a bucket-load of poor quality salt was added! This is discussed further on page 199.

Consuming the right kind of fat will help you feel happy and content and fuller for longer.

Fat chosen from real and whole food sources is imperative for great energy and optimal health.

'Real food fat' is satiating. It can help mediate inflammation in the body, is an integral part of a healthy immune system and is essential for the health of your skin, eyes, nails and hair.

But you see, if you are frightened of fat — likely due to it having the highest number of calories per gram of all of the macronutrients — you won't let yourself eat it, no matter how much you feel like it. Again, this is why I explain all this background to you, so you can remove any bias you may have against a certain food, and get back in touch with what your body needs.

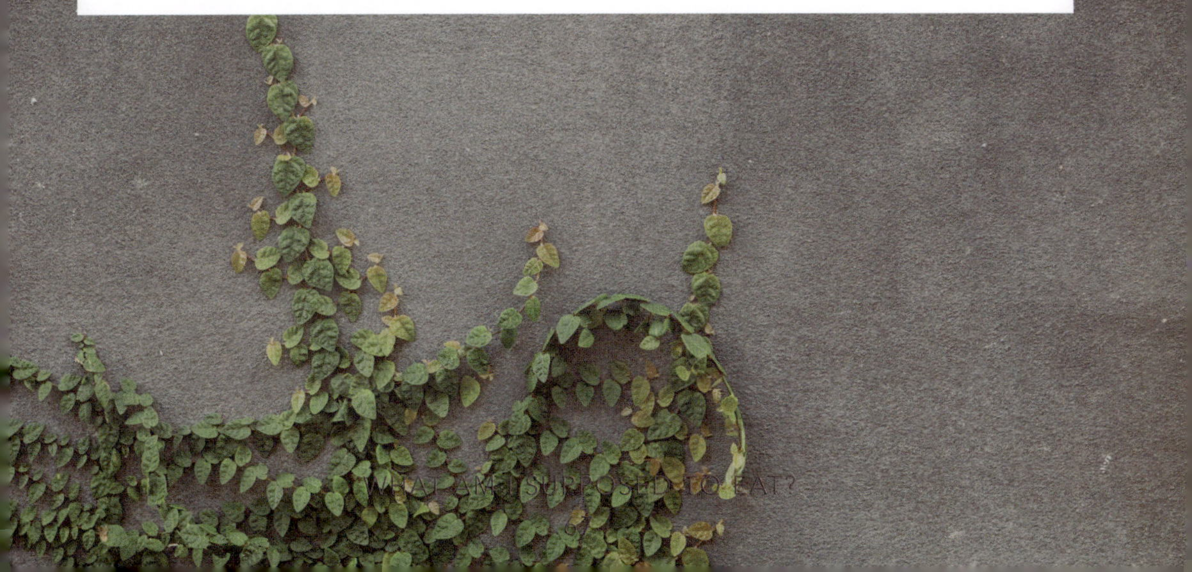

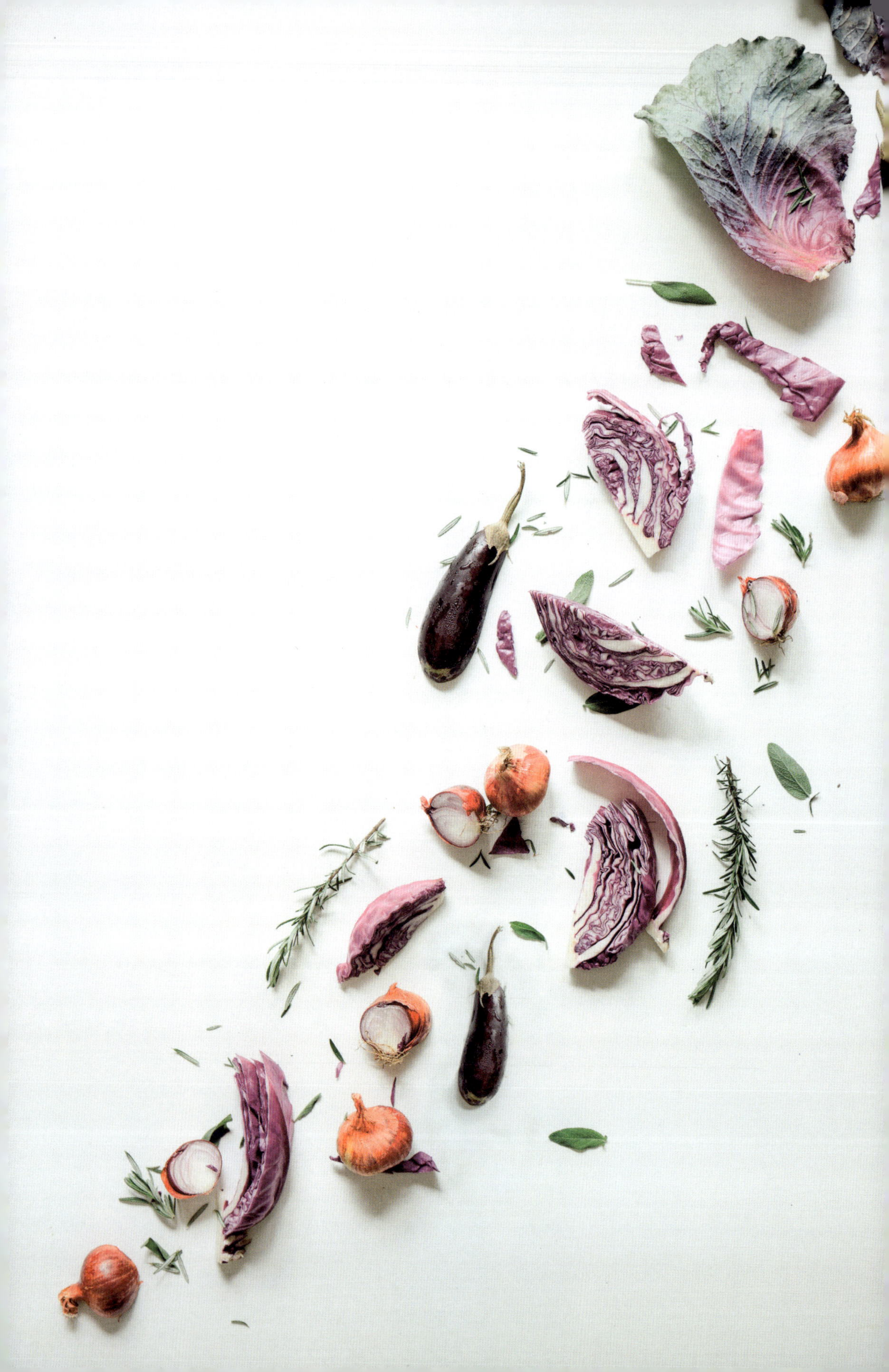

Micro-nourishment

VITAMINS, MINERALS AND TRACE MINERALS

Micronutrients are so named as they are only necessary in small amounts (compared to macronutrients). Nevertheless, micronutrients are essential for both keeping us alive and maintaining our quality of life.

Micronutrients are vitamins, minerals and trace minerals, and they provide the body with nutritive substances which provide the cells with the nourishment they require, and indirectly influence available energy by serving as catalysts to release macronutrients. In other words, the macros give us energy, but the micros allow us to utilise the energy from the macros.

Micronutrients include dietary minerals such as zinc, iodine, selenium, iron and copper. They also include vitamins such as vitamin A, C, D, E and K, as well as the range of B vitamins. They're essential for the healthy functioning of all body systems, from bone growth to brain function. And obtaining them through how we eat needs to be forefront in our minds when making food choices. In other words, if you are stuck and don't know what to choose, ask yourself the question, "Which choice will best nourish me?" and see what you decide. The best choices are always whole and real foods.

Overt nutritional deficiencies don't have to be screaming at you — such as scurvy (vitamin C deficiency) or beriberi (thiamin/vitamin B_1) deficiency — for your body to not be functioning optimally. What is very common these days is what are known as 'sub-clinical' deficiencies, where the cells of the body just aren't getting what they need to function at their best. When you consistently make lifestyle choices that deplete nutrients — think caffeine, alcohol, refined sugar, excess salt from processed foods — or simply make poor nutritional choices through eating processed, packaged foods, you compromise the ability of your cells to not only function well — giving you great energy — but also to defend themselves. When the metabolic function of cells is poor, you get sick, which is why a whole, real food way of eating is so compelling in its capacity to create great energy and less disease.

A D C B E K

Vitamins

Vitamins are essential micronutrients needed for various roles throughout the human body. They are divided into two groups: fat-soluble vitamins (A, D, E and K) and water-soluble (B-complex vitamins and vitamin C). Fat-soluble vitamins are stored in the liver and fatty tissues, and are eliminated much more slowly than water-soluble vitamins which require regular replacement in the body as they are not stored anywhere, except for small amounts of vitamin B_{12} and folate.

FAT-SOLUBLE VITAMINS

Fat-soluble vitamins A, D, E and K are stored in the body, and while diseases caused by a lack of fat-soluble vitamins are rare in the Western world, without adequate amounts of vitamins in the diet, symptoms of mild deficiency can develop; particularly if the diet is low in fat.

A VITAMIN A

Vitamin A, also known as retinol, has many functions in the body. Supporting the ability of the eyes to adjust to changes in light, vitamin A also plays a critical role in gene expression, immune system responses, reproduction processes and bone growth, just to name a few. The skin, eyes and mucous membranes of the mouth, nose, throat and lungs require vitamin A to remain moist.

Real food sources of vitamin A include:

- Meat, fish and liver for retinol, retinal and retinoic acid forms of vitamin A.
- Carrots, pumpkin, dark green leafy vegetables and apricots for the antioxidant beta-carotene (which the body can convert to vitamin A).
- Compared to retinol, we require more carotene-rich foods to meet the body's basic vitamin A requirements. These may also be increased due to hyperthyroidism, infections and exposure to excessive amounts of sunlight.

Signs of deficiency:

Vitamin A deficiency is rare in the Western world. Since vitamin A is fat-soluble and stored in the liver, it may take months for any of the following signs of deficiency to appear.

- eyesight changes or night blindness
- dry, rough, scaly skin
- increased susceptibility to infections
- defective teeth and gums
- slower bone growth
- lack of appetite and vigour
- heavy menstrual bleeding
- cervical problems.

Conversely, there can be too much of a good thing, as vitamin A toxicity (not possible from beta-carotene) can cause severe birth defects and liver damage, although this is rare.

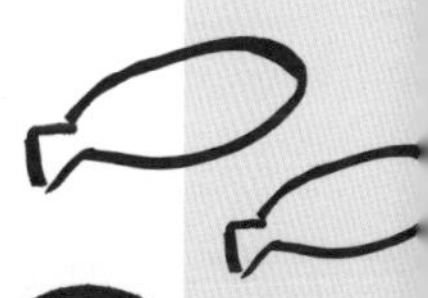

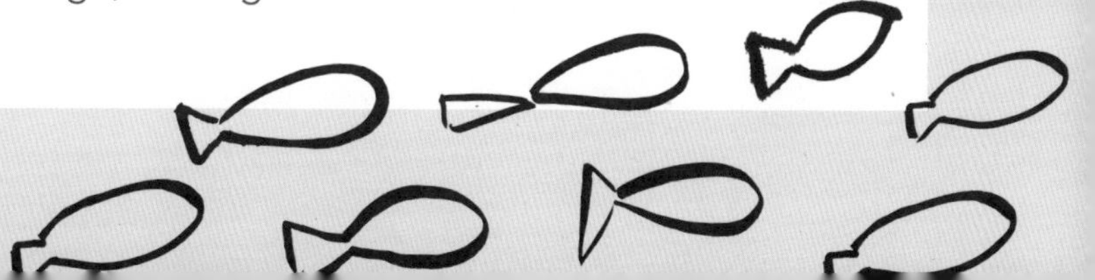

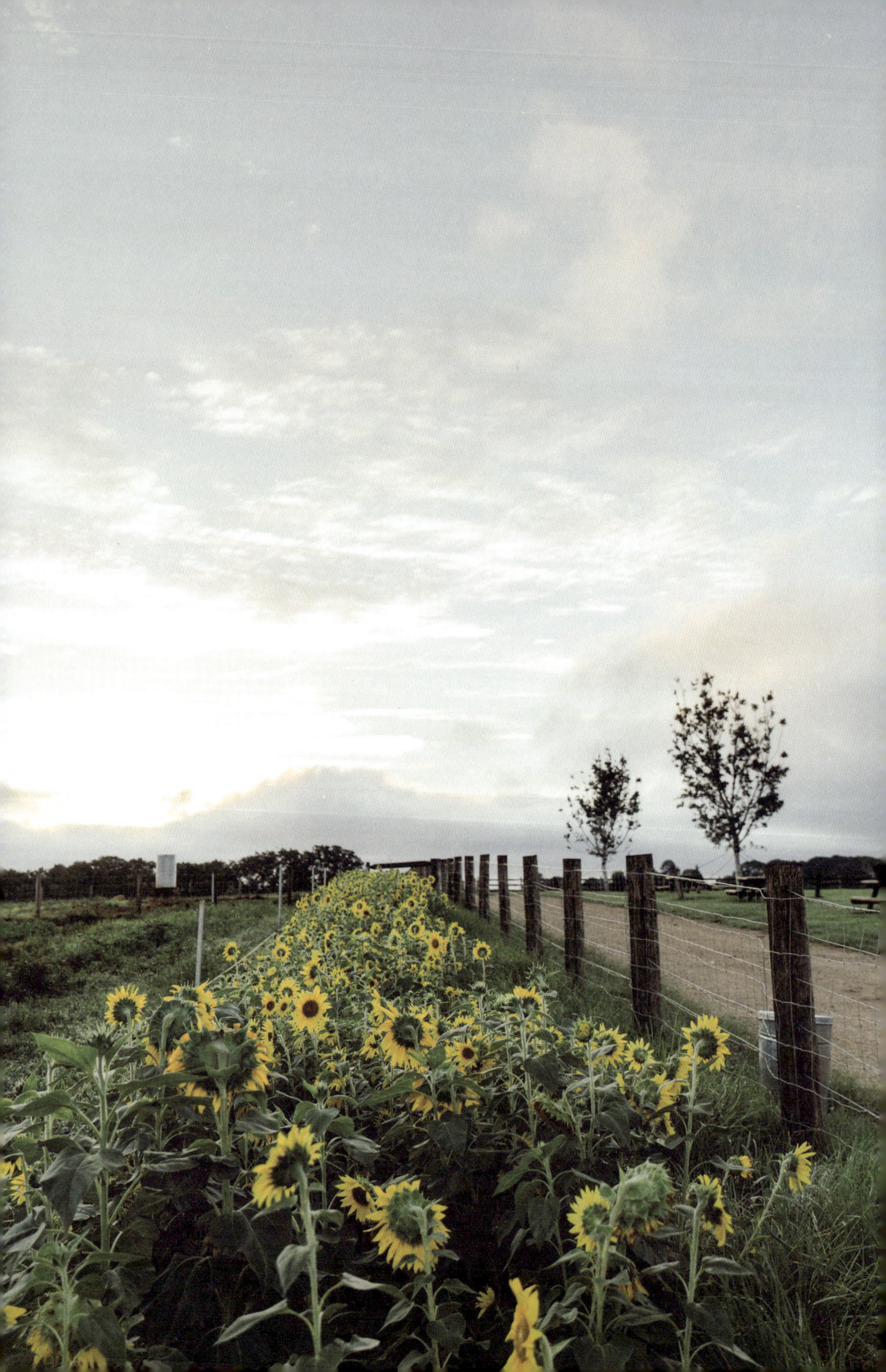

D

VITAMIN D

Vitamin D plays an essential role in the body's regulation and use of calcium and phosphorus. It increases the amount of calcium absorbed from the small intestine, and this helps to form and maintain bones. Vitamin D also supports the immune system. It is a nutrient that is of particular importance for children due to its role in the development of strong bones and healthy teeth.

Real food sources of vitamin D include:

- oily fish, such as herring and sardines
- mushrooms that have been exposed to sunlight
- cod-liver oil
- organic butter.

Most vitamin D is obtained through the skin. Sunlight's action on cholesterol in the skin converts the cholesterol into vitamin D via additional conversions in the liver and kidneys.

Since most foods have very low vitamin D levels, a deficiency may be more likely to develop without adequate exposure to sunlight. Many factors can contribute to vitamin D deficiency, such as overuse of sunscreen, wearing clothes that cover most of the skin, working inside all day, as well as living in climates where little sun is seen in the winter.

Signs of vitamin D deficiency include:

- bone and muscle pain
- deficiency has been associated with increased risk of a variety of cancers, autoimmune diseases, hypertension and infectious disease.
- People with fat malabsorption syndromes, inflammatory bowel disease (IBD) or who are overweight may have a decreased ability to absorb and/or use vitamin D in fat stores.

Conversely, signs of vitamin D toxicity are rare, but include excess calcium in the blood, slowed mental and physical growth, decreased appetite, nausea and vomiting. Due to their small body size, it is especially important that infants and young children do not consume excess amounts of vitamin D regularly. However, this would be difficult for them to do in the absence of supplements or fortified foods.

E

VITAMIN E

Vitamin E is a superstar vitamin that acts as an antioxidant, protecting vitamins A and C, red blood cells, the lining of blood vessels, as well as essential fatty acids from free radical damage. Studies show a link between an antioxidant-rich diet full of fruits and vegetables and a lower risk of heart disease, cancer and several other chronic, degenerative illnesses.

Real food sources of vitamin E include:

- eggs
- wholegrains, such as wild rice
- nuts, such as almonds and hazelnuts
- seeds, particularly sunflower seeds.

Signs of vitamin E deficiency may include:

- anaemia
- muscle degeneration
- fertility challenges
- changes in the menstrual cycle
- hot flushes (flashes)
- increased risk of blood-clot formation
- estrogen excess
- selenium deficiency, as it is needed for the body to be able to utilise vitamin E.

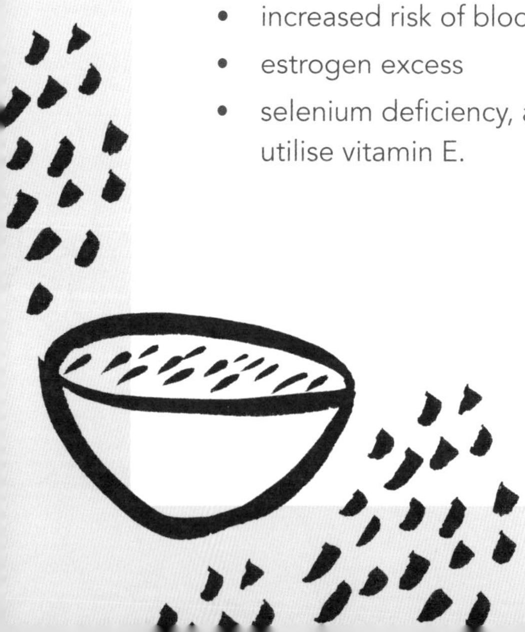

K

VITAMIN K

Food supplies us with vitamin K; however, it is unusual in that the body also makes it internally. Gut bacteria produce vitamin K and regardless of where the vitamin K is obtained, it plays an essential role in blood clotting, bone health as well as helping to produce body proteins. The amount of vitamin K produced by gut bacteria is not enough to meet our requirements, so we must also consume vitamin K rich foods.

Good food sources of vitamin K include:

- green leafy vegetables, such as spinach
- cauliflower
- cabbage
- broccoli
- olive oil.

If vitamin K levels are inadequate haemorrhaging can occur. Deficiency of vitamin K can occur in infants, as initial counts of gut bacteria are small (we are born with an immature gut). People taking antibiotics may lack vitamin K temporarily because intestinal bacteria are killed by antibiotics.

People taking blood-thinning drugs or anticoagulants are advised to moderate their intake of foods with vitamin K, because excess vitamin K can affect blood-clotting ability.

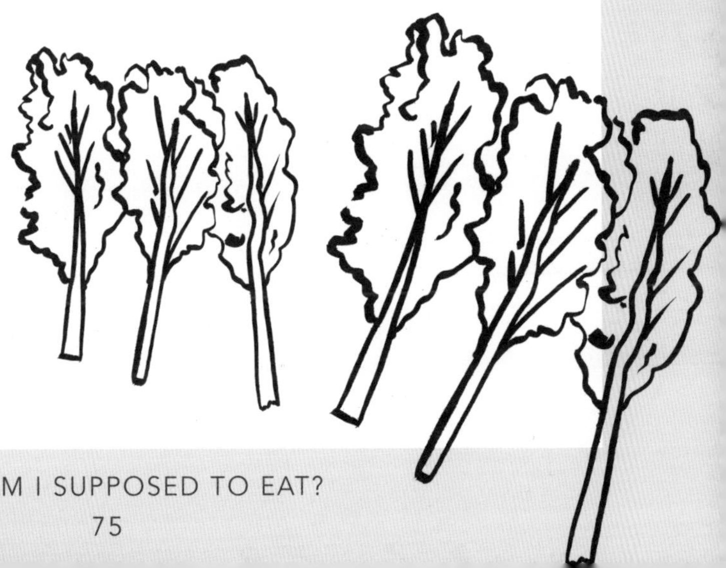

Water-soluble vitamins

B-COMPLEX VITAMINS

Eight of the water-soluble vitamins are known as the vitamin B-complex group: thiamin (vitamin B_1), riboflavin (vitamin B_2), niacin (vitamin B_3), pantothenic acid (vitamin B_5), pyridoxine (vitamin B_6), vitamin B_{12}, folate and biotin. The B vitamins are widely available in foods, and their influence is a critical component of many bodily functions. They function as coenzymes that help the body obtain energy from food, as well as being important for a healthy appetite, energy, good vision, healthy skin, nervous system function and red blood cell formation.

Optimal vitamin B levels allow us to make the most out of the food and nutrients we consume. With low vitamin B levels, our food is unable to energise us effectively. B vitamins are essential to liver detoxification processes, critical for disease prevention as well as great skin. They are also vital to adrenal health, where we make our stress hormones, blood pressure regulating hormones, as well as some sex hormones. Even though the B-group vitamins are found in many foods, they are water-soluble and delicate. They are easily destroyed, particularly by alcohol and cooking. Food processing also reduces the amount of B-group vitamins in foods, making white flours, breads and rice far less nutritious than their wholegrain counterparts.

The body has a limited capacity to store most of the B-group vitamins, except for very small amounts of B_{12} and folate, which are stored for a brief period in the liver. A person who has a poor diet for a few weeks or months may end up with a B-group vitamin deficiency. Some low carbohydrate diets can also lead to a B-group vitamin deficiency, unless care is taken to ensure foods rich in B vitamins are still consumed. Offal meats such as liver are particularly rich sources or you may prefer to supplement the range of B vitamins.

It is important that adequate amounts of these vitamins be eaten regularly for countless biochemical processes inside the body, and so health, energy and vitality can be optimal.

Signs of a general B vitamin deficiency:

Vitamin B deficiency signs are highly varied. Some of the most common and early signs include:

- redness and irritation in the skin, particularly around the nose and mouth
- cracks at the corners of the mouth
- a dermatitis-type rash, particularly when under stress
- for some, a hypo- and hyper-pigmentation may occur with chronic low vitamin B intake. (I have seen this in people eating a very low carbohydrate diet who also don't eat meat or eggs regularly, or take a supplement that contains B vitamins.)

B1

Food sources of thiamin (vitamin B_1) include:

- seeds, particularly sesame seeds
- legumes
- nuts
- savoury yeast
- wholegrains.

It is important to note that many people today feel better without grains in their diet, or with only small amounts.
If your digestion, for example, functions better without grains, try some gluten-free grains, such as brown rice, to see whether they serve you better (than those that contain gluten) and, if not, then go with what your body is guiding you to do. Just know that your dietary intake of vitamin B_1, or most likely all B vitamins, might be low and you may need to supplement.

Signs of deficiency may include:

- fatigue
- weakness
- insomnia
- vague aches and pains
- weight loss
- depressed mood
- irritability
- lack of initiative
- constipation
- oversensitivity to noise
- loss of appetite or sugar cravings
- circulatory problems.

B2

Food sources of riboflavin (vitamin B_2) include:

- mushrooms
- spinach
- liver
- savoury yeast
- eggs.

Signs of deficiency may include:

- gum and mouth infections, often in the corners of the mouth (which can also be due to iron deficiency)
- dizziness
- depressed mood
- eye irritations
- skin problems
- dandruff.

B3

Food sources of niacin (vitamin B_3) include:

- red meat, fish, chicken
- eggs
- wholegrains
- nuts
- mushrooms
- almost all protein-containing foods.

Signs of deficiency may include:

A deficiency can result in a disease called pellagra. The primary symptoms of pellagra include:

- Skin problems, including dermatitis, skin lesions on the face, arms and hands, and inflamed skin.
- Mouth problems, including canker sores, mouth irritation, and ulceration or swelling of the tongue.
- Digestive problems, including diarrhoea, nausea, vomiting, and poor appetite.
- Mental impairment, including disorientation, dementia, depressed mood, irritability, and emotional instability.

These days, pellagra usually occurs due to alcohol abuse, malnutrition (too much takeaway food), and in those who have multiple nutrient deficiencies. Because this vitamin is vital for the production of energy, a deficiency can lead to general fatigue, muscular weakness, and a loss of appetite.

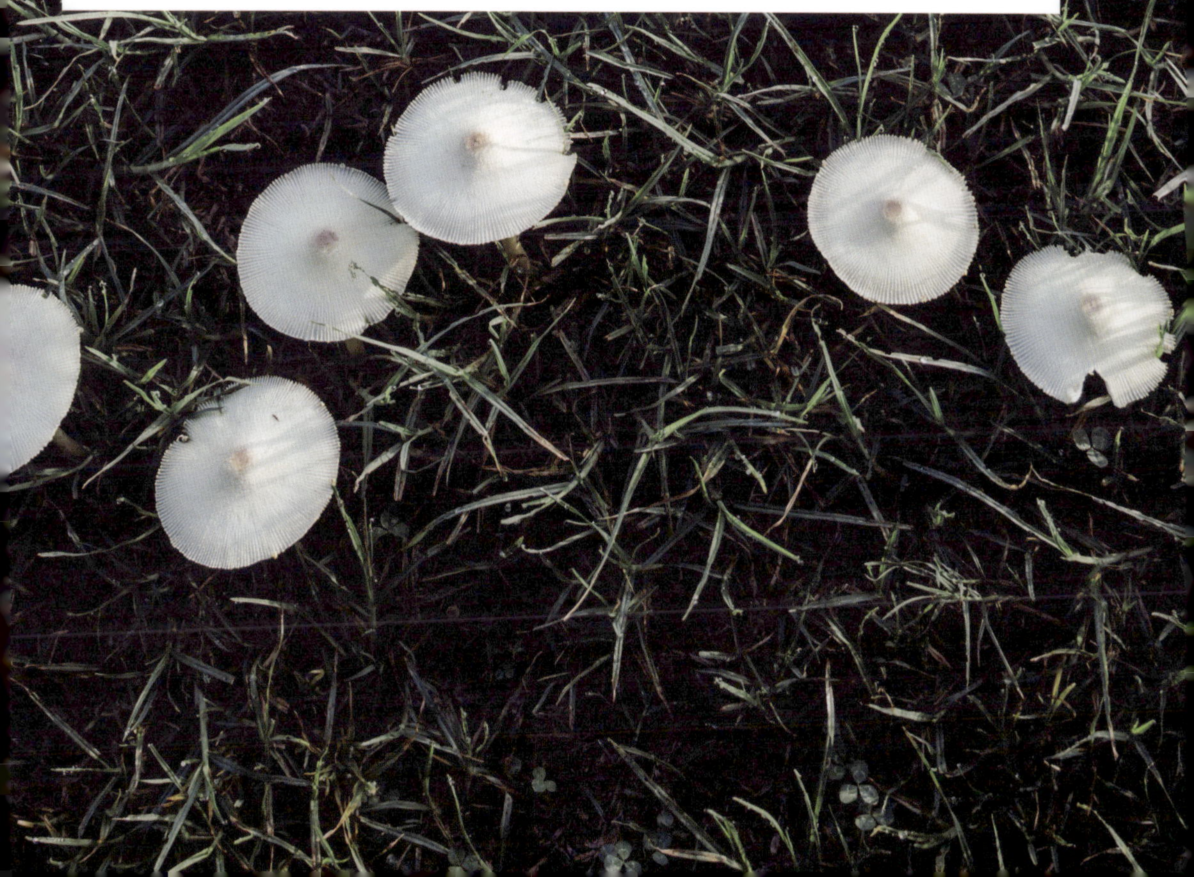

B5

Real food sources of vitamin B_5 include:

Pantothenic acid (vitamin B_5) is found in a wide range of foods, but some good sources include:

- eggs
- liver
- savoury yeast
- almonds.

Signs of deficiency may include:

- burning feet syndrome – numb toes and burning sensation in the feet
- vomiting
- fatigue
- weakness
- irritability.

B6

Food sources of pyridoxine (vitamin B_6) include:

- bananas
- liver
- salmon
- walnuts.

Signs of deficiency may include:

- nausea
- low stress tolerance
- lethargy
- anxiety
- depressed mood
- weakness
- nervousness
- emotional flare-ups
- fatigue
- insomnia
- mild paranoia
- skin eruptions
- loss of muscular control
- eye problems
- swelling/fluid retention (common in the feet and ankles).

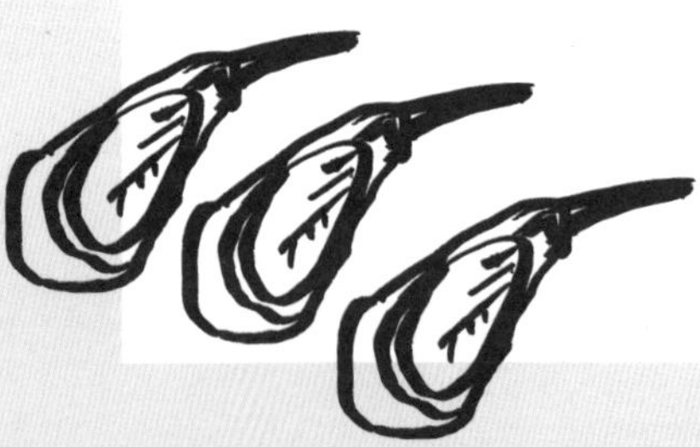

BIOTIN

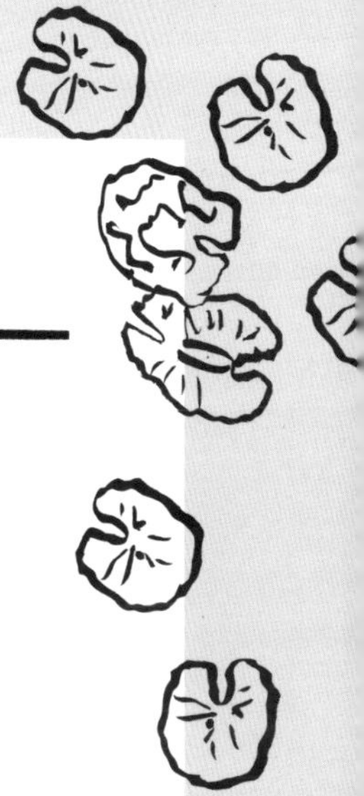

Real food sources of biotin include:

- eggs
- chicken
- savoury yeast
- salmon
- sardines
- avocado
- cauliflower
- raspberries
- nuts such as walnuts, almonds, and pecans
- wholegrains.

Commercial food processing methods destroy biotin, so, like other B vitamins, unprocessed, whole foods are a richer source of this nutrient.

Signs of deficiency may include:

- lethargy
- numbness and tingling in the extremities
- depression
- loss of appetite
- red, scaly dermatitis around the eyes, nose and mouth
- hair loss
- nausea.

FOLATE

Food sources of folate include:

- green leafy vegetables
- beans
- seeds
- eggs
- citrus fruits
- avocado.

If a woman has poor folate status when she conceives, it can result in concerning, or in some cases severe, problems. This is commonly associated with low green vegetable intake and other aspects of a poor quality way of eating. A few years ago I read a book called *The Pill*, which explained that in some women, the oral contraceptive pill (OCP) depletes folate so these concerns can also arise if a

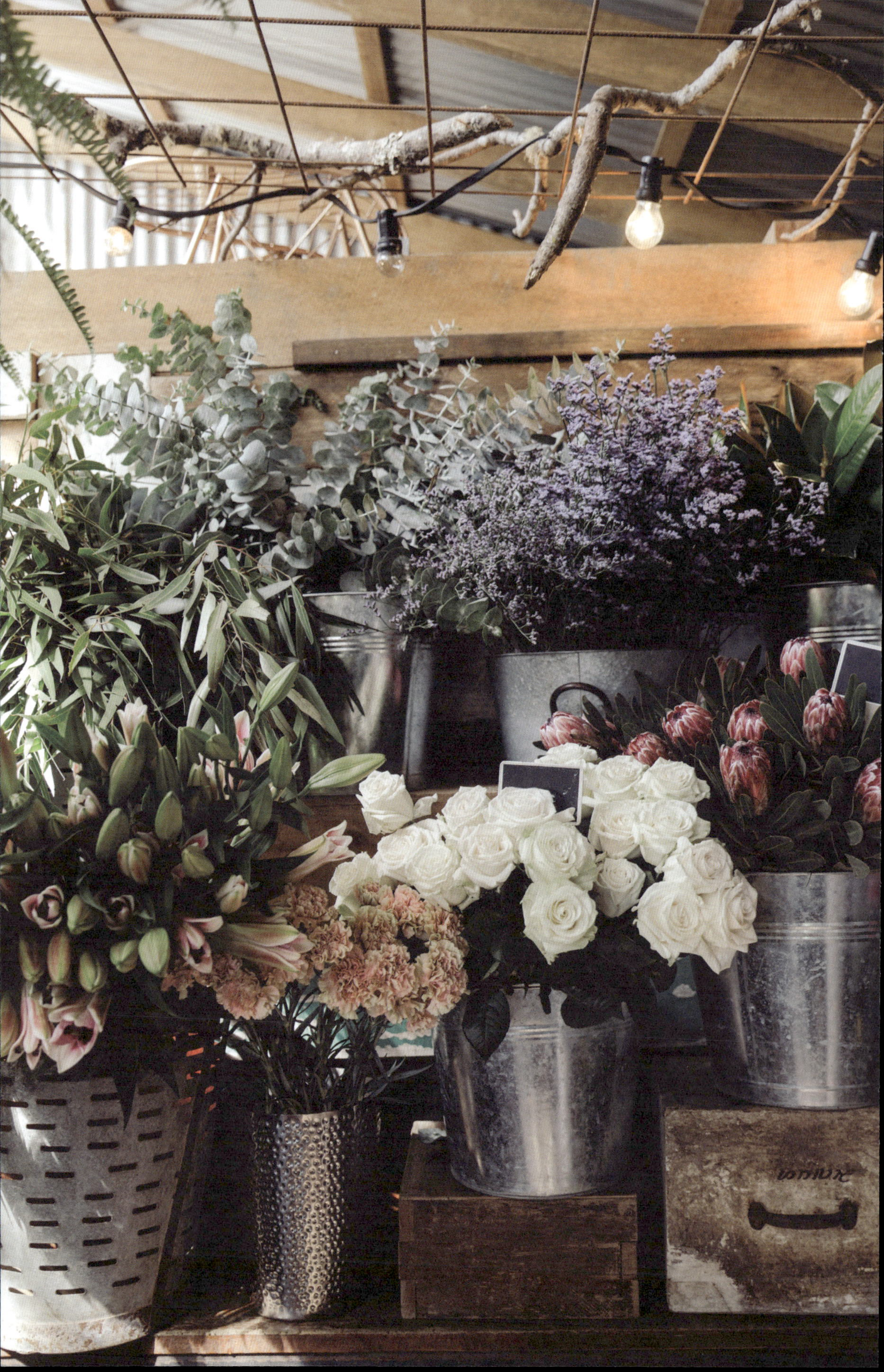

woman conceives in the immediate period following use of the OCP, when the body is still recovering its folate stores.

Signs of deficiency may include:

- damage to the wall of the small intestine
- anaemia
- elevated homocysteine levels.

Elevated homocysteine levels have been associated with heart disease, various gynaecological conditions, and repeated miscarriage. Homocysteine can usually be maintained at healthy levels if folate and vitamins B_6 and B_{12} are in adequate supply.

B12

The only real food sources of vitamin B_{12} are:

- foods from animal origin (except honey).
- Some yeasts are synthetically fortified with B_{12}, giving vegans a B_{12} option.

Vitamin B12 deficiency can be slow to develop, causing symptoms to appear gradually and intensify over time. It can also come on relatively quickly. Given the array of symptoms it can cause, the condition can be overlooked or confused with something else.

Signs of deficiency may include:

- difficulty walking (staggering, balance problems)
- anaemia
- a swollen, inflamed tongue
- yellowed skin (jaundice)
- difficulty thinking and reasoning (cognitive difficulties), or memory loss
- fatigue
- paranoia or hallucinations
- weakness
- weight loss
- depressed mood
- strange sensations, numbness, or tingling in the hands, legs or feet
- elevated homocysteine levels.

B_{12} deficiency occurs in four stages. It begins with declining blood levels of the vitamin (stage I), progressing to low cellular concentrations of the vitamin (stage II), an increased blood level of homocysteine and a decreased rate of DNA synthesis (stage III), and finally, macrocytic anaemia (stage IV). So once you are diagnosed with a B_{12} deficiency, your cells are well and truly suffering.

Causes of B_{12} deficiency:

As with all nutrients, it is essential that you determine why you are deficient. There are multiple causes of B_{12} deficiency, which include:

- poor nutritional intake
- gut dysbiosis
- poor intrinsic factor production (made in the stomach and essential for the absorption of B_{12})
- low stomach acid production (known as "hypochlorhydria")
- undiagnosed coeliac disease
- some medications such as those that suppress stomach acid.

With B_{12} and folate deficiencies, the appearance of fingernails tends to change (dark striations), a reason why I encourage you to allow your body to be the amazing vehicle of communication it is. Instead of getting frustrated with your body, if you don't like your nails or the cracks in the corners of your mouth that won't heal, use these signs as indicators that your body needs you to eat, drink, move, think, breathe, believe or perceive differently. When you listen and take action, not only will the bits that frustrate you tend to clear up, but also many other bodily processes will function more efficiently and be healthier in the process.

VITAMIN C

Vitamin C plays many outstanding roles in the body, and it is hard for it not to be my favourite! Vitamin C aids in wound healing and bone and tooth formation, strengthens blood vessel walls, improves immune function, increases absorption of iron, and acts as an antioxidant, slowing the ageing process. It also holds cells together through collagen synthesis. Many people seem to just think about their face when they think of collagen. It is a connective tissue that holds all muscles, bones and other tissues together. You need vitamin C daily to help your body make this elastic tissue that is found in the skin, ligaments, tendons, cartilage and blood vessels.

Since our bodies cannot produce or store vitamin C, it must be consumed daily to receive enough for optimum health. Vitamin C works with vitamin E as an antioxidant, and plays a crucial role in scavenging free radicals throughout the body. It is also crucial for adrenal gland function and may play a role in reducing the risk of heart disease and cataracts.

The health of your hair depends on vitamin C, as this vitamin supports the blood vessels that feed the hair follicles and is critical for circulation to the scalp and helps slow the formation of split ends. It is also one of the most important nutrients for great skin.

Foods high in vitamin C include:

- berries
- capsicums (peppers)
- citrus fruits
- kale
- kiwifruit
- parsley
- broccoli.

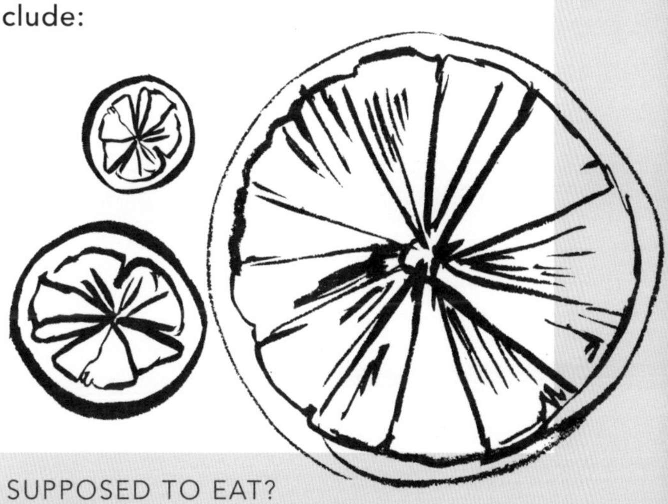

Vitamin C deficiency signs include:

- premature ageing
- dull skin
- hair that breaks easily
- easy bruising
- bleeding gums
- dilated capillaries and spider veins
- heavy menstrual bleeding
- regular colds
- eye problems
- loss of appetite
- muscular weakness
- anaemia
- fatigue
- lowered immune response
- poor sex hormone balance.

Vitamin C is essential for sex hormone production; however, please note that if you are on the OCP and vitamin C is taken in high doses (considered to be more than two grams per day), it can interfere with the effectiveness of the pill. This is because vitamin C increases the potency of the hormones, so when the dosage of vitamin C is reduced, your body can misinterpret this as a reduction in hormone levels, and ovulation may occur.

Vitamin C is a powerful antioxidant that reduces damage and inflammation in the body, helping to protect you from degenerative diseases. I travel regularly for my work, and this is certainly a nutrient I supplement daily.

MINERALS

Minerals themselves fall into two categories based on the requirements of the body. By definition, macro-minerals are those that the body requires 100 milligrams (mg) or more of per day, while trace or micro-minerals are those that the body requires in doses of less than 100mg per day. Although we require smaller amounts of trace minerals, they are just as important to our health as macro-minerals. The macro-minerals outlined below include calcium and magnesium, while the trace minerals include zinc, iron, selenium and iodine.

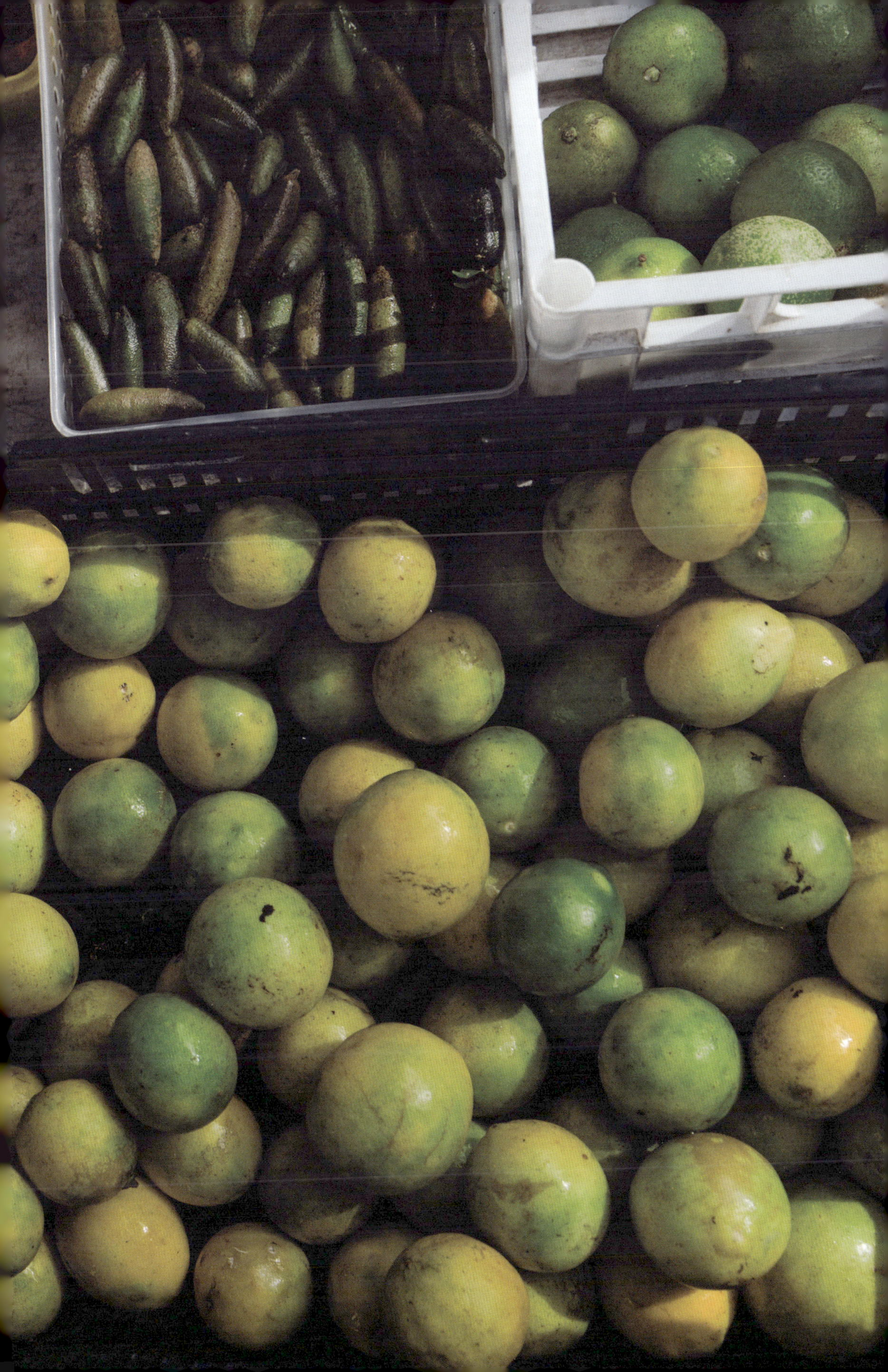

CALCIUM

You are probably familiar with the role calcium plays in bone health, but many people are unaware of the extensive role it plays in countless other processes within the body. Our ability to absorb and distribute calcium throughout the body, for example, impacts on the strength of our hair and nails, and it is actually the liver that makes the decision where nutrients need to be dispersed to, reminding us again of how crucial optimal liver function is.

Pause and consider this: you consume a meal that contains some calcium. The calcium is extracted from the meal and is absorbed from your gut across and into your blood. That nutrient rich blood then travels to the liver, and the liver assesses your body and decides where that calcium will best be used.

The liver will always send the calcium where it is needed most, and the place it is needed most is the task most necessary to keep you alive. For example, if you've been relying too much on processed food and caffeine, and churning out stress hormones, your blood needs the calcium to help maintain the pH. So rather than send the calcium to the areas such as your nails or hair, your liver chooses elsewhere, knowing that your life is not dependent on your nails and hair being in their best shape.

For maximum calcium utilisation, your diet must be nutrient rich, high in plants and not reliant on processed foods. Ideally, you also have stress management strategies in place and your digestive system needs to work well. Caffeine interferes with the absorption of calcium too, so it's best to reduce caffeine consumption.

Food sources of calcium include:

- green leafy vegetables
- nuts
- seeds (particularly sesame seeds)
- tahini
- figs
- sardines.

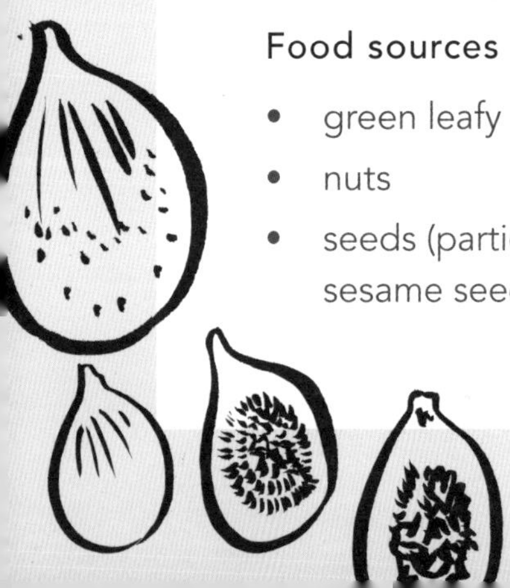

If you take a calcium supplement, it is vital to take one that also contains magnesium, boron and vitamin D, as all of these nutrients are essential for great bone health and nails, as well as countless other processes and functions in the body.

Most calcium in the body is stored in the bones and teeth. You are usually exceptionally deficient by the time the signs of deficiency appear. These may include:

- muscle cramps
- low bone density
- brittle nails
- teeth problems
- premenstrual cramps
- muscle weakness, aches
- fatigue.

Mg

MAGNESIUM

With the European Union authorising a list of the associated health benefits of magnesium, it seems this mineral has finally received the attention it deserves for the positive impact it has on overall health. As the fourth most abundant mineral in the body, around 50 per cent of magnesium is found in the bones. This explains the connection between magnesium and bone density.

What we don't read as much about are the other 300 or more biochemical reactions occurring in the body for which magnesium is an essential cofactor, meaning the reactions inside your body don't happen without it. Unfortunately, due to poor dietary habits, such as too much processed food and caffeine, pharmaceutical drug use and produce grown in nutrient-depleted soils, many people today are deficient in this essential mineral.

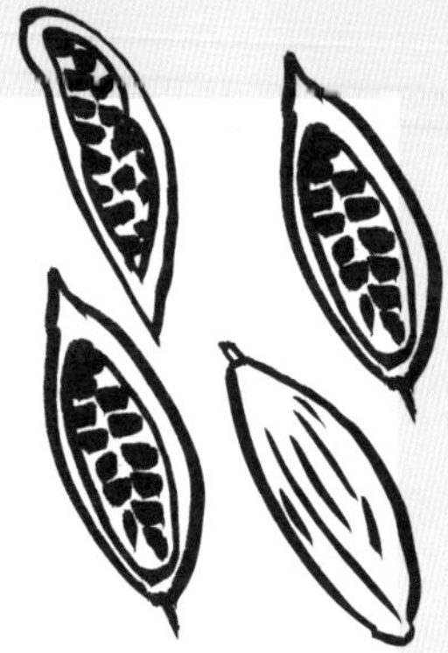

The best food sources include:

- leafy green vegetables
- tahini
- seeds
- nut butter, such as almond butter
- nuts
- seaweed, such as kelp
- raw cacao.

You can also supplement magnesium, and, given magnesium is required for the production of adrenalin, one of your stress hormones, the more stressed you are, the higher your requirements for magnesium.

You are also able to absorb magnesium through your skin. Taking a bath containing magnesium salts such as Epsom salts can be another way to enhance your magnesium levels. Because magnesium is a relaxant, if you have too much, your stools can become loose. If while supplementing, you notice this, see it as a sign that you need less magnesium.

Magnesium deficiency can lead to:

- a variety of premenstrual symptoms
- lumpy breasts
- muscle cramps
- anxiety
- sleeplessness
- chocolate or sugar cravings
- cardiovascular problems.

The health benefits of optimal magnesium intake include better energy, balanced electrolytes (which are essential for hydration and the removal of waste from cells), boosted muscle and nervous system functioning, good protein synthesis, and the maintenance of healthy teeth and strong bones.

Zn

ZINC

What does this mineral not do? Zinc is another superstar among the nutrients, and it contributes to hundreds of processes inside your body, plenty of which are reflected on the outside. Zinc is critical for wound healing. Whether that is a cut on your finger, or the aftermath of a pimple, zinc is necessary for the skin to heal and it helps to prevent scar formation.

Zinc is also required for proper immune system function, as well as for the maintenance of vision, taste and smell. It is essential to the creation of over 300 enzymes necessary for you to have great digestion. Zinc even nourishes the scalp, helping to maintain the integrity and strength of hair, and low zinc levels have been linked with hair loss and a dry, flaky scalp.

If a nutrient is not in the soil, it cannot be in the food. Not even 100 years ago zinc was abundant in many soils; therefore, fruit and vegetables were good sources of it. But because most soils in the world are now zinc deficient, many foods do not contain zinc. This is why I added a food-based source of zinc to my Bio Blends supplement range, because too many people just aren't getting enough of this crucial nutrient.

Foods that contain zinc include:

- sustainably grown oysters from clean waters
- pumpkin and sunflower seeds
- eggs
- red meat.

Many people today are deficient in this vital mineral that is responsible for the taste and texture of food, and it may be contributing to why young children today tend to be fussier with food than in the past.

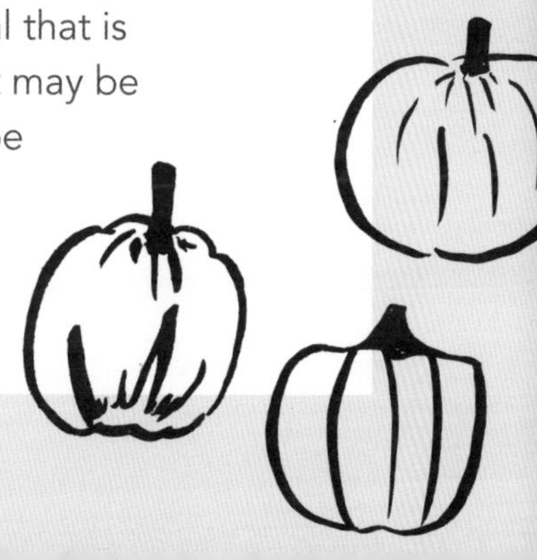

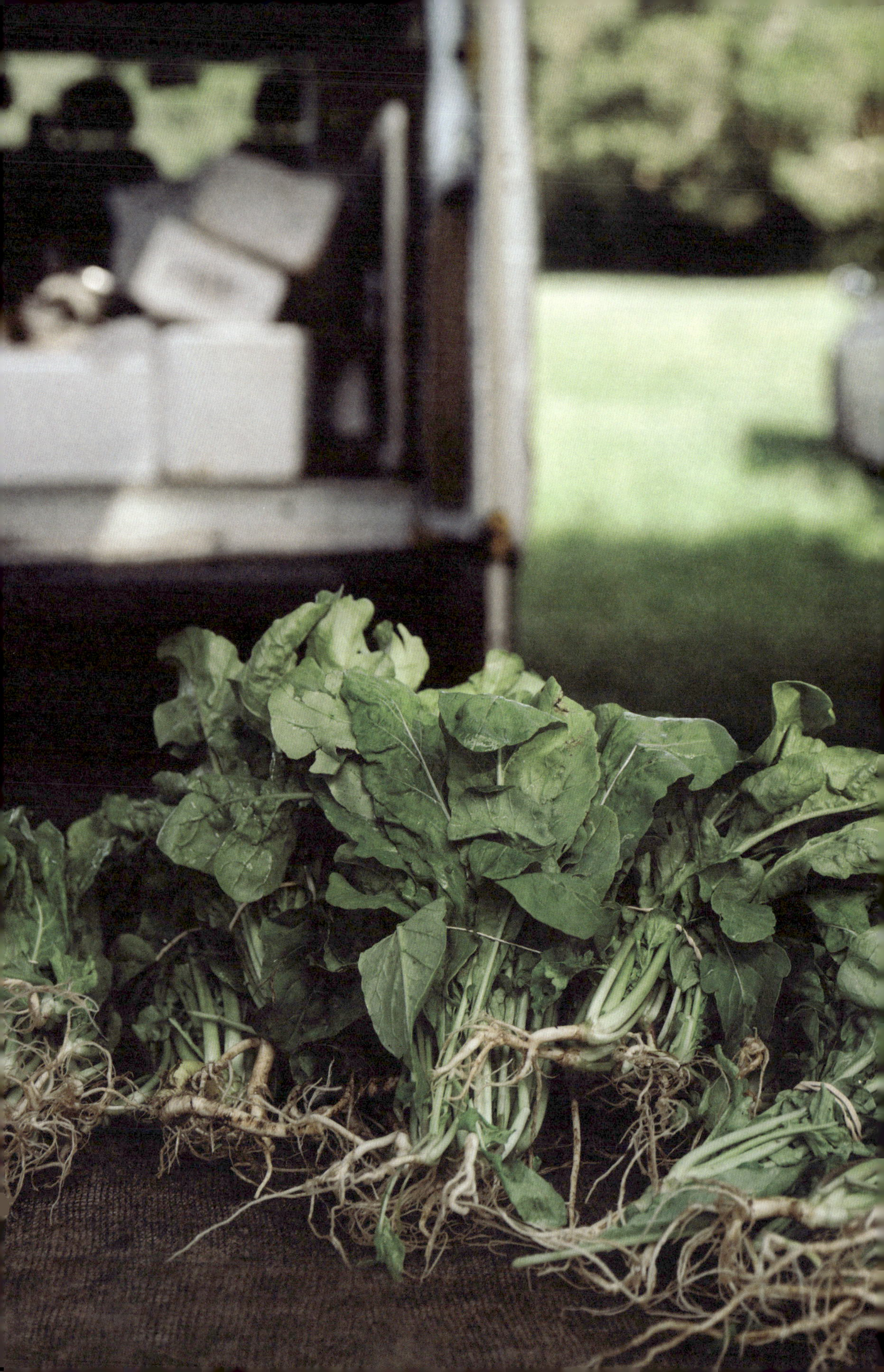

Some signs of zinc deficiency may include:

- poor blood glucose management
- sugar cravings
- loss of appetite
- poor resistance to infection
- skin infections
- easy skin scarring
- lowered fertility
- white spots on finger nails.

Zinc can be supplemented and, if it is, it is best taken before bed to maximise absorption.

Fe

IRON

Iron is another mineral vital to so many aspects of health, particularly your energy and the condition of your hair, yet iron deficiency is reported to be the most common dietary deficiency in the world. It particularly affects children, menstruating women and pregnant women.

In New Zealand, it is estimated that up to 25 per cent of children under the age of three have some degree of iron deficiency — a deeply concerning statistic. According to the World Health Organization (WHO), a staggering two billion people in the world, in both developing and industrialised countries, are iron deficient. It is estimated that between 20 per cent and 30 per cent of women of childbearing age in Australia and New Zealand are iron deficient. Iron deficiency can have a major impact on your quality of life, and that of your children, if you are iron deficient during pregnancy.

Most of the body's iron stores are within the haemoglobin of red blood cells and carry oxygen throughout the body. Extra iron is stored within the liver and is used during times when dietary intake is inadequate.

Your body's iron stores will decline over time if your iron requirements are not met through your diet or via additional supplementation.

Many people are confused about the difference between iron deficiency and another term you may have heard of, 'anaemia'. Immature red blood cells require iron to be converted by the body into a form they can use in order to mature. When fully mature, they will become the oxygen-carriers of the body, distributing oxygen from the lungs to all other cells throughout the body. They have a big and important job to do.

Iron deficiency is the first step towards a decrease in the amount of oxygen-carrying, iron rich haemoglobin within each red blood cell. As red blood cells are deprived of iron, they become contracted and smaller, known in medical terms as becoming 'microcytic'. Anaemia develops when the immature red blood cells, deprived of their quota of iron, fail to survive their infancy. A formal diagnosis of anaemia is made when there is a consequent and significant decrease in the number of mature red blood cells.

Food sources of iron include:

- beef
- lamb
- eggs
- mussels
- sardines
- lentils
- dates
- green leafy vegetables.

The form of iron in animal foods is more bioavailable than vegetables sources. When it comes to sources of iron variety is key, as there is a small amount of iron in many foods. If you do not eat animal foods, do not assume that you are iron deficient. For some vegetarians, the body utilises the iron from vegetable sources very efficiently, whereas for others, it does not. Vegetable sources of iron are better absorbed in the presence of vitamin C.

The main symptoms of iron deficiency include:

- exhaustion
- shortness of breath, especially on an incline
- muscle aches and cramps
- rapid pulse and heart palpitations
- increased anxiety
- brain fog

- poor memory and concentration
- headaches
- depressed mood
- increased frequency of infections
- hair loss
- you sometimes crave crunching on ice.

In children, fussy eating can also be a sign of low iron levels. Children will often have visible blood vessels on their face, which tend to have a blue/purple appearance.

Iron levels gradually decline rather than plummet suddenly (unless there is extreme blood loss).

The stages of iron deficiency include:

- Iron depletion — haemoglobin levels are normal, but the body only has a small amount of stored iron, which will soon run out. Usually no symptoms are noticeable during this stage.
- Iron deficiency — stored and blood-borne iron stores are low and haemoglobin levels have dropped below normal. Some symptoms, such as tiredness, are experienced in this stage.
- Iron deficiency anaemia — haemoglobin levels are so low that the blood is unable to deliver enough oxygen to the cells. Symptoms include looking very pale, breathlessness, dizziness and fatigue. Other symptoms can include reduced immune function as well as impaired growth and cognition.

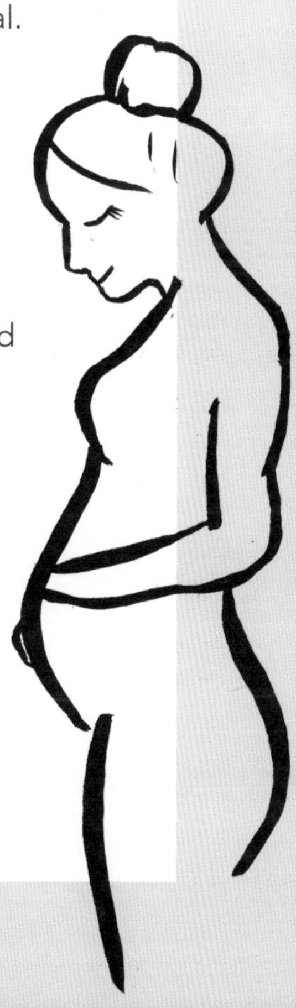

Iron deficiency anaemia is commonly caused by:

- Inadequate dietary intake of iron. There are two types of dietary iron: haem iron (found in animal tissue) and non-haem iron. The body absorbs haem iron much more easily than non-haem iron. Dietary intake of iron could be inadequate. Some examples include chronic fad dieting, a poor quality vegan or vegetarian diet or limited access to a wide range of fresh foods as a result of living in remote areas or low income.

- Poor absorption of iron by the body. Healthy adults absorb about 10–15 per cent of dietary iron, but some people's bodies are unable to absorb or use iron from food efficiently.
- Loss of iron due to bleeding. Common causes include heavy menstrual blood loss, chronic disorders that involve bleeding (such as peptic ulcers, polyps or cancers in the large intestine) and certain medications, particularly aspirin.
- An increased need for iron by the body. For example, the adolescent growth spurt, pregnancy and breastfeeding. In pregnant women, iron stores have to serve the increased blood volume of the mother, as well as the needs of the growing baby. As regular exercise increases the body's need for iron in numerous ways, athletes are also prone to iron deficiency. Iron is lost through sweating, while hard training promotes red blood cell production. If this increased need isn't met, a deficiency can occur.
- The condition can also be caused by untreated coeliac disease. Not everyone presents with the typical bowel symptoms. Sometimes iron, and often vitamin B12, deficiency are the only signs of what is later diagnosed on biopsy as coeliac disease. Once gluten is removed from the diet, iron levels begin to return to normal.
- Fibre interferes with the absorption of dietary iron, so the fibre content of the diet must also be taken into account when determining the basis of the iron deficiency.
- In the gut, calcium and iron compete for absorption, and as calcium is a larger substance, it always wins out. This is great news for your bones, but not always so good for the oxygen-carrying capacity of your blood. A low level of iron is a leading cause of fatigue. Consuming calcium rich foods away from iron rich foods can make a difference to iron absorption.

A simple blood test from your GP will establish whether you are iron deficient or not. It is best to have a test before you supplement. Many ordinary iron supplements are constipating, but this does not tend to happen with food-based or liquid iron supplements. Testing is also important because some people have a tendency to store too much iron in the body and this needs to be avoided or treated if it already exists.

Se

SELENIUM

Selenium's roles are vast and varied. It is an antioxidant mineral responsible for preventing free radical damage to cells. Research suggests that selenium may play an important role in preventing skin cancer, as it appears to protect the skin from damage from excessive ultraviolet light.

Selenium's antioxidant properties regenerate vitamins C and E thereby decreasing the ageing of skin. Other important benefits of selenium are that it boosts the immunological response against bacterial and viral infections, and also against cancer cells, cold sores and shingles. Selenium is also critical for fertility and optimal thyroid gland function.

The need for selenium highlights the critical nature of the quality of the soil. Most of the soil in Australia and New Zealand is deficient, as is the soil in the United Kingdom and China, whereas soils in parts of the United States, Canada and South America still contain some selenium.

The best dietary sources of selenium are:

- Brazil nuts (by far the richest source although the amount of selenium in each nut varies).
- Small amounts of selenium are also found in eggs as well as some seafood and meat.

Research suggests that eating just three to six Brazil nuts per day provides an adequate selenium intake for most people — and what a delicious way to get your selenium.

Selenium deficiency can be hard to recognise; however, some signs include:

- Skin that is prone to dryness and sensitivity, lacking radiance, with possible signs of premature ageing.
- A compromised immune system and/or thyroid function.
- Challenges with fertility.

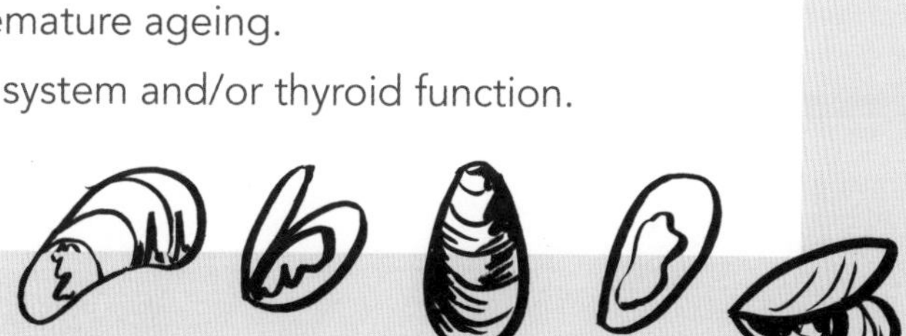

IODINE

Iodine's importance to overall health and wellbeing cannot be overstated. Iodine performs many actions in the body, and I believe we will uncover more as research continues. A shortage of iodine can cause changes to the thyroid gland that directly lead to poor immunity and metabolism. Iodine deficiency puts the gland itself at risk since it promotes free radical damage in the thyroid gland. Iodine blocks various compounds from binding to and accumulating in the thyroid gland, including goitrogens. Research demonstrates that the ingestion of competing substances, such as bromine, fluorine, chlorine and perchlorate, has significantly increased in food, water, medicines and the environment over the past 30 years and that environmental pollution significantly aggravates a lack of iodine and displaces it within the body.

Iodine is also concentrated in the ovaries and breast tissue, acting as a buffer to the growth-stimulating effects of estrogen and as a promoter of proper estrogen metabolism. Iodine assists the functioning of hormone receptors throughout the body, helping hormones communicate more effectively. It is essential for proper brain development and cognitive ability and many studies show the importance of iodine during gestation, when cognitive potential is formed. This is because the rapid rate of growth of the brain during the last trimester of pregnancy and the early postnatal stage makes it vulnerable to an inadequate diet. A deficiency of iodine during this critical period in brain development is associated with reduced cognitive performance. Iodine deficiency is a leading global cause of preventable mental impairment.

Food sources of iodine include:

- Salt (although not all salt contains iodine. Himalayan pink salt and Celtic sea salt contain 84 different minerals, and in most brands one of these is iodine. Always check the label of your salt to be sure).
- Seaweeds, such as kelp and nori (you can add seaweeds such as kombu to soups, stews and casseroles to impart a lovely salty flavour, as well as some iodine — simply remove the stick of seaweed before serving).

Iodine can also be supplemented in the diet. Only a small amount is required, but we must consume it daily.

Iodine deficiency can lead to:

- dull and brittle hair
- balding
- lack of skin tone and/or very dry skin
- low energy levels
- poor concentration
- constipation
- depressed mood
- puffy eyes
- extreme fatigue
- difficulty dealing with environmental temperature change — so much so that you feel "cold in your bones" and find it difficult to warm up.

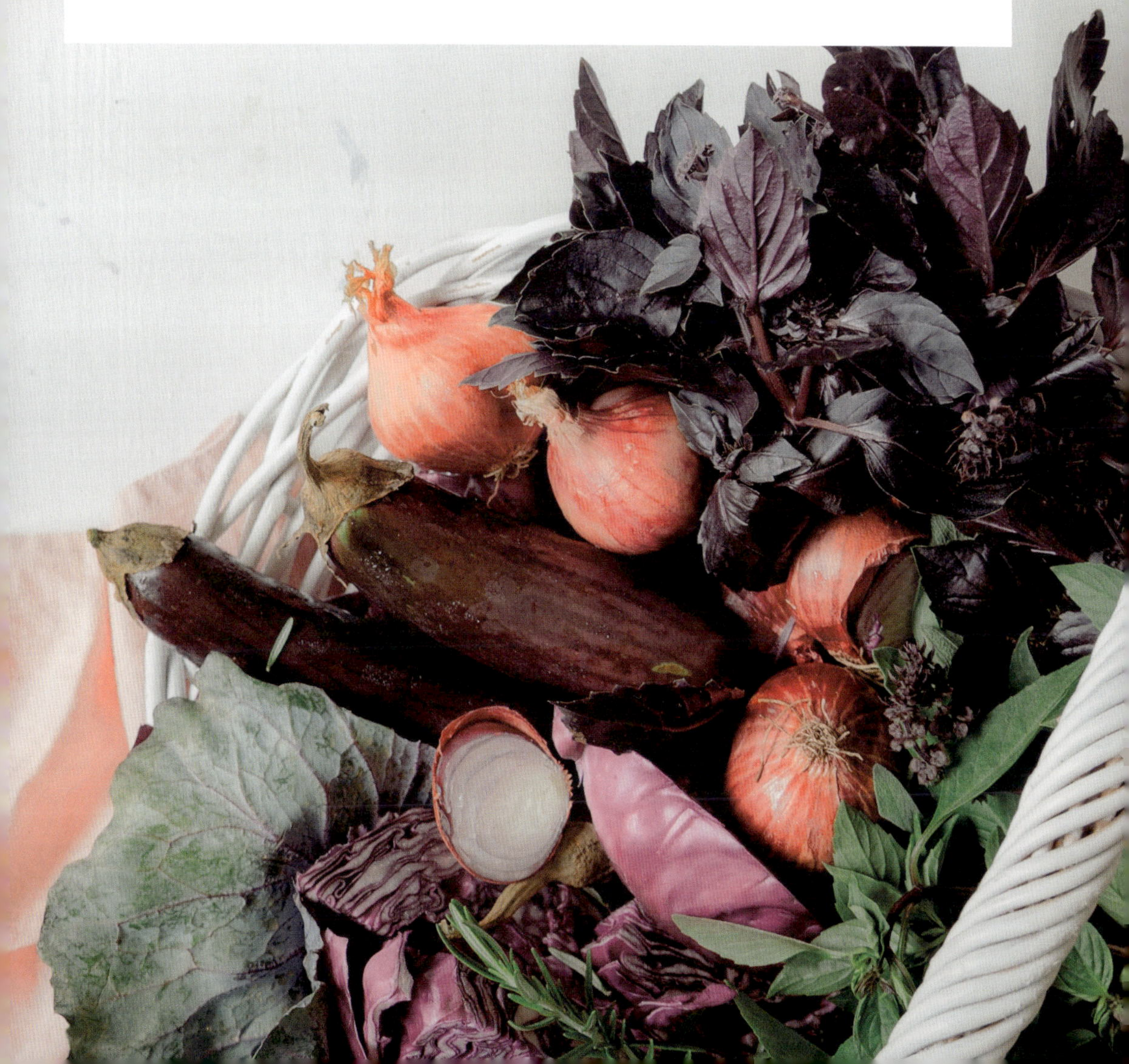

WORKSHEET

MATCH THAT NUTRIENT

Micronutrients are essential for the healthy functioning of our body systems.

Based on what you learnt in the previous article, match the micronutrient to its main function(s) in the body.

Hint – micronutrients can link to more than one function.

Multiple nutrients are needed for the optimal functioning of each body system; some directly and some indirectly. This exercise will help to familiarise you with some of the more distinct ones.

- Zinc
- Iodine
- Selenium
- Iron
- Magnesium
- Calcium
- Vitamin A
- Vitamin C
- Vitamin D
- Vitamin E
- Vitamin K
- B-complex vitamins

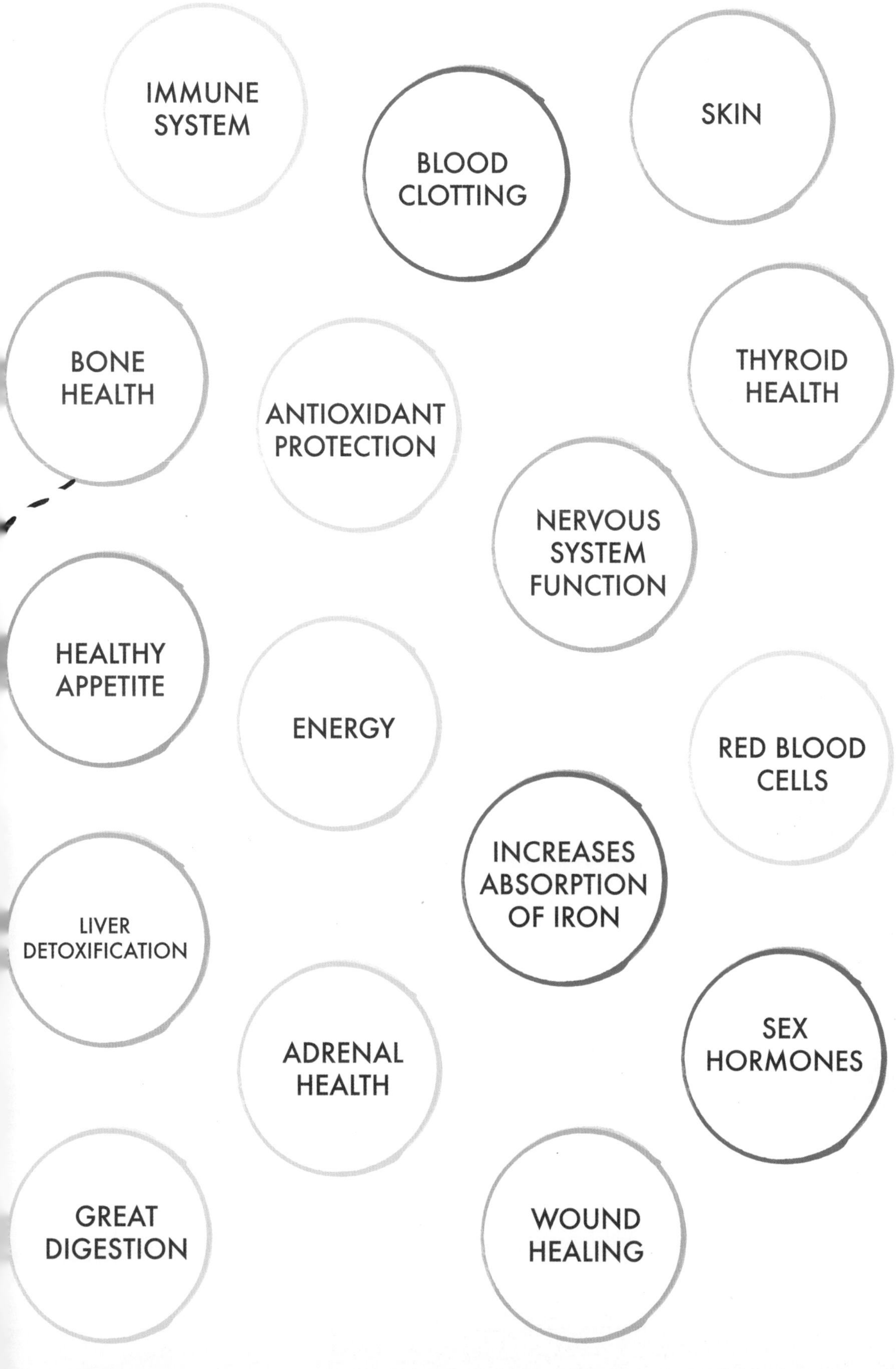
IMMUNE SYSTEM
BLOOD CLOTTING
SKIN
BONE HEALTH
ANTIOXIDANT PROTECTION
THYROID HEALTH
NERVOUS SYSTEM FUNCTION
HEALTHY APPETITE
ENERGY
RED BLOOD CELLS
INCREASES ABSORPTION OF IRON
LIVER DETOXIFICATION
ADRENAL HEALTH
SEX HORMONES
GREAT DIGESTION
WOUND HEALING

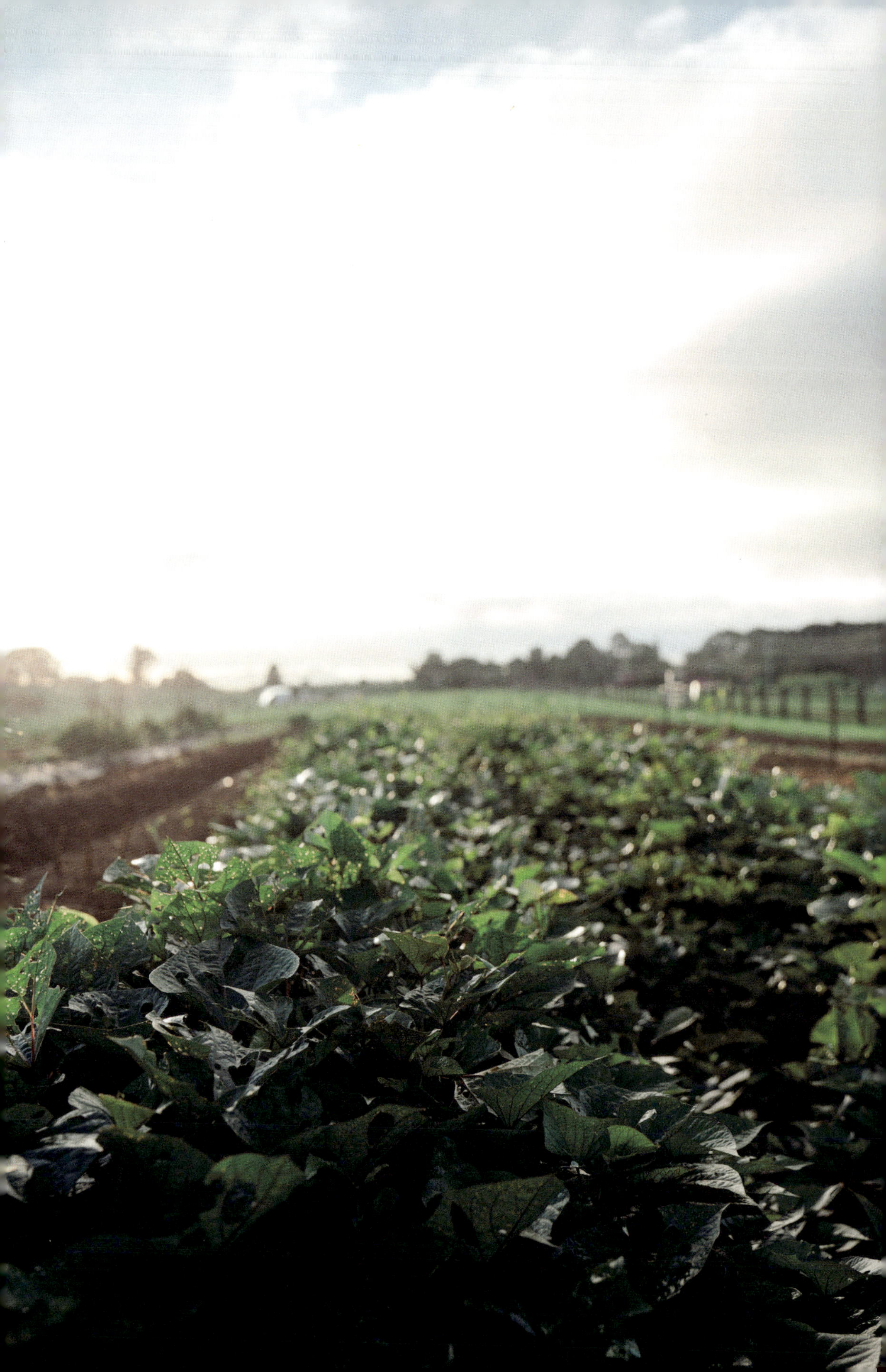

Plenty of plants

THEIR UNIQUE AND POWERFUL SUBSTANCES

Specific plant foods contain powerful substances, often referred to as *phytochemicals*, that can be highly beneficial for your health. Like antioxidants, these chemicals boost the immune system and help to slow ageing and degenerative processes. They also provide protection against free radical damage and reduce the risk of developing a range of lifestyle-related diseases.

FLAVONOIDS

Found in abundance in a wide range of fruits and vegetables, including apples, cranberries, tomatoes, celery, kale and parsley, as well as in green and black tea. Flavonoids help cool inflammation and slow oxidation — thereby helping to protect your cells from damage. Flavonoids have also been shown to support the immune system, suppress the growth of tumours, prevent blood clots and improve skin integrity — even more reason to amp up the plant content of what you eat.

ANTHOCYANINS

Part of the flavonoid group, anthocyanins are responsible for the purple colour of some plants. In fruits, the colourful skins attract the attention of animals, who upon eating the fruits then excrete and disperse the seeds. In photosynthetic tissues (such as green leaves), anthocyanins have been shown to act as a 'sunscreen', protecting cells from intense light damage by absorbing blue-green and ultraviolet light, thereby protecting the leaves from light stress. They also have powerful antioxidant qualities, and are found in most purple foods, including blueberries, bilberries, cranberries, raspberries, blackcurrants, cherries, eggplant and red cabbage, to name a few.

INDOLES

These amazing phytochemical substances are found in cruciferous vegetables, such as broccoli, cauliflower, kale, Brussels sprouts and cabbage. They behave like antioxidants, reduce inflammation, and have been shown to support healthy estrogen metabolism. Indoles are one of the reasons I adore the cruciferous family of vegetables, so whenever you can, include them in your diet.

SULFORAPHANE

Sulforaphane is a superhero component of cruciferous vegetables. Sulforaphane is an antioxidant and stimulator of natural detoxifying enzymes. It may help to reduce the risk of breast, bladder and prostate cancers. Studies show that people who regularly eat plenty of cruciferous vegetables have reduced incidences of many cancers. Found in the highest concentration in broccoli sprouts, it's also found in Brussels sprouts, cabbage, cauliflower, broccoli, bok choy, kale and watercress. Just in case you needed another reason to eat cruciferous vegetables!

CAROTENOIDS

Carotenoids are the coloured plant pigments the body can turn into vitamin A. Their colour, which ranges from yellow to bright orange to deep red, is directly linked to their structure. People consuming diets rich in carotenoids from whole foods, such as fruits and vegetables, have been shown to have a reduced risk of developing a number of chronic illnesses.

Lycopene is well known for its ability to support prostate health and is responsible for giving tomatoes their distinct red colour. It is also considered to be a carotenoid despite the fact it doesn't convert into vitamin A. Lycopene, the orange-red pigment found in tomato and watermelon, is still of value due to its potent antioxidant potential.

Antioxidants help the body reduce the inflammatory action of free radicals. Oxygen atoms like to combine in pairs. Single oxygen atoms (known as free radicals) are unstable and interact with the lipids found in cell walls, causing inflammation and damage. Sometimes your own body uses free radicals to fight infections and abnormal cells; however, when they are in excess they cause inflammation and damage to cells, such as those that line your arteries. Eating a diet rich in plant foods is one of the most effective ways to supply your body with the antioxidants it needs to prevent and repair any damage. Antioxidants donate oxygen back to the single oxygen, pairing it up so that it can no longer operate as a free radical and damage tissues.

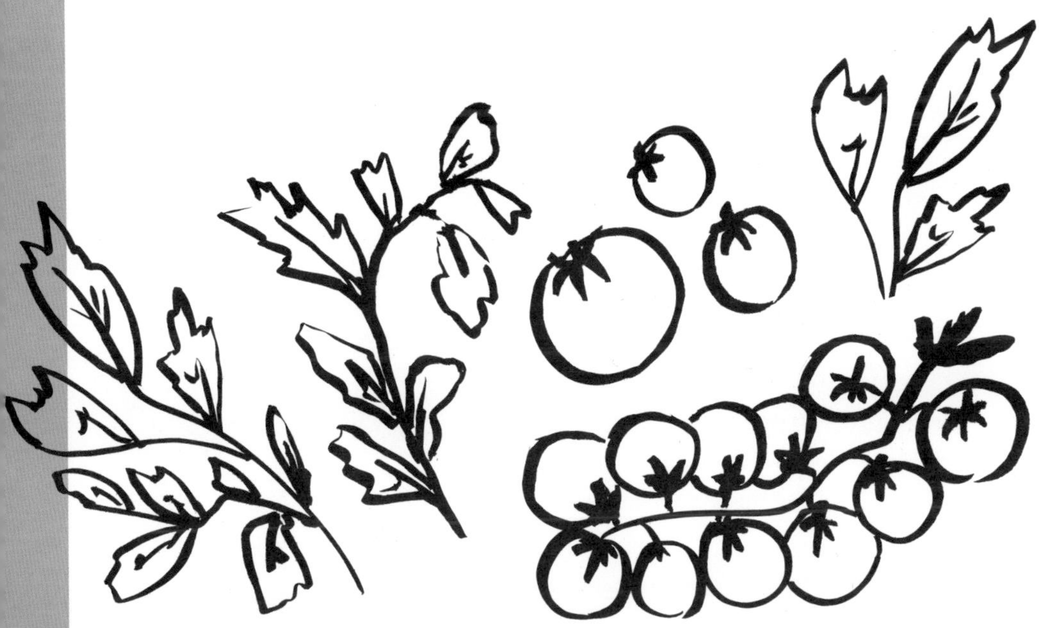

What happens to food in your body?

DIGESTING DIGESTION

When we eat real, whole foods our body obtains both macronutrients and micronutrients. As you now know, the macronutrients are protein, fat and carbohydrate (and alcohol), and the micronutrients are the vitamins and minerals.

Digestion allows us to extract and absorb these nutrients from our food, and this involves both mechanical processes (think chewing) and biochemical processes (further breakdown through the action of enzymes). Essentially, all nutrients are broken down to their smallest, microscopic parts in the gut, and then absorbed across the gut wall into the bloodstream.

Our digestive tract is a long tube that starts at our mouth and ends where the waste leaves the body. The macronutrients and micronutrients from our food are digested and absorbed at different points along this tube, with the help of other organs like the liver, gallbladder and pancreas.

Digestion starts in the mouth, with chewing. Not only does chewing begin to break down your food from a mechanical perspective, it primes your digestive tract for the chemical digestion of food. Chewing really matters and has an enormous impact on digestive function.

CARBOHYDRATES

When carbohydrates are consumed, whether they come from starchy foods or sweet foods, they are broken down into sugars (predominantly glucose, but also some other sugars such as fructose) in the digestive tract.

Chemical digestion of carbohydrates begins in the mouth.

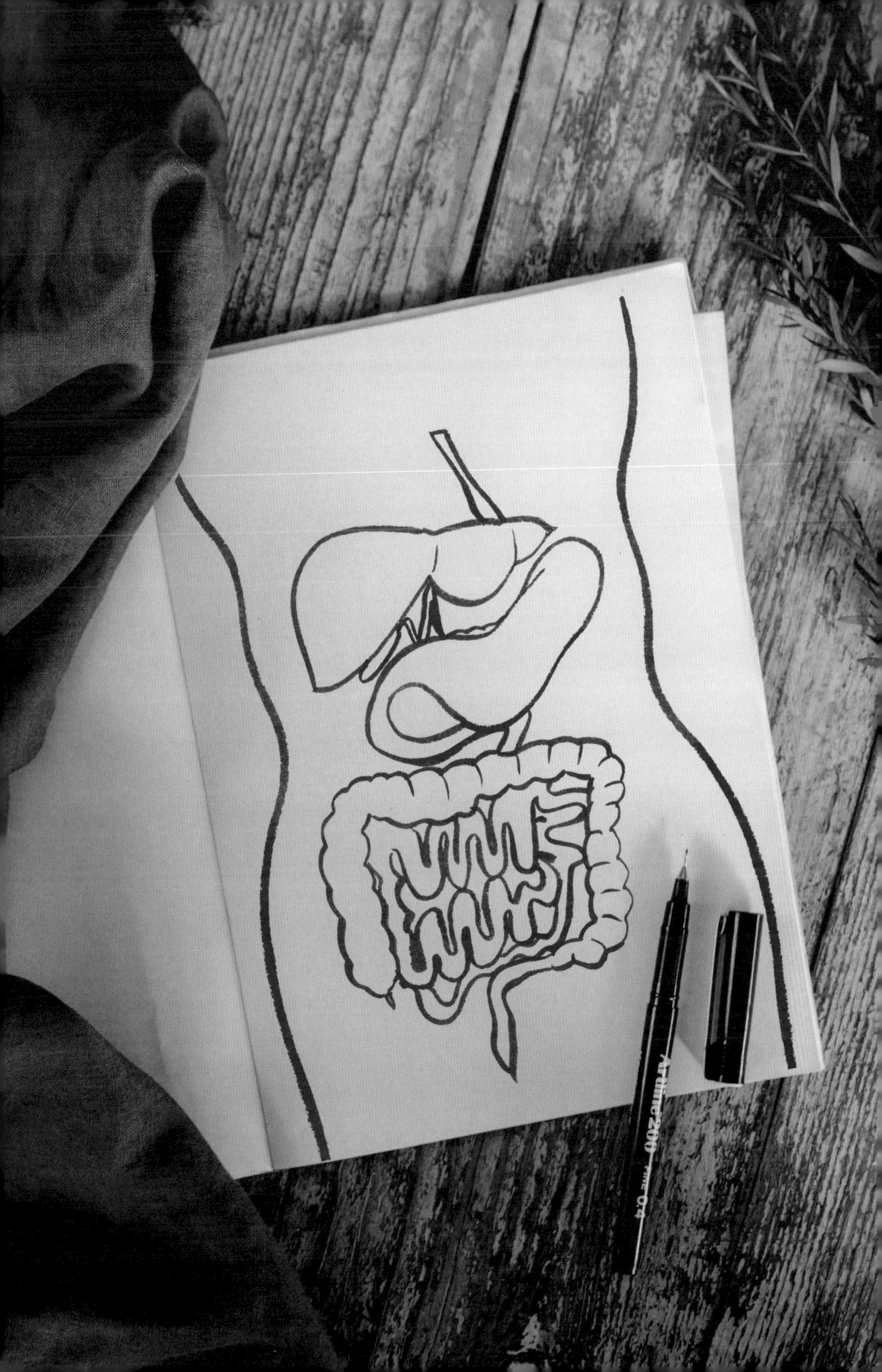
Artline 200
0.4

As we chew, food mixes with our saliva, which contains digestive enzymes that break the carbohydrates down into smaller chains of sugars.

The partially digested carbohydrates continue their journey down your oesophagus, through the stomach, and into your small intestine, where digestion continues. In the upper part of the small intestine, numerous enzymes (from the pancreas and the small intestine) are involved in breaking the carbohydrate down into its simplest form — sugars. These sugars are then absorbed across the gut wall, and are transported throughout your body in the blood.

The hormone insulin enables glucose to move from the blood into our cells where it is metabolised to yield adenosine triphosphate (ATP), the energy currency of our cells. An excess supply of glucose in the blood can lead to insulin transporting the glucose to fat cells, increasing their size; hence increasing your body fat levels.

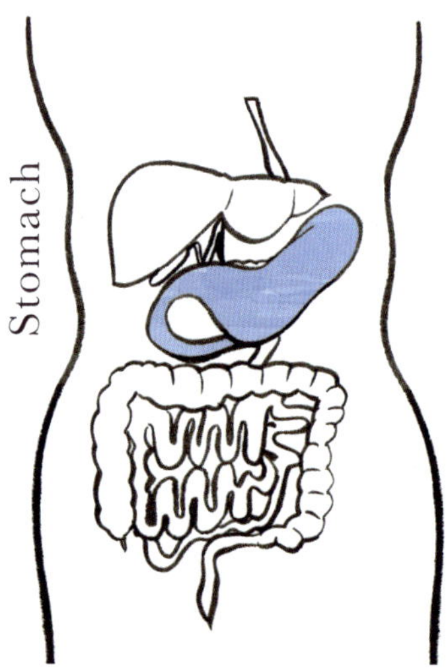

PROTEIN

Imagine a big long chain, twisted up on itself so that it looks like a big tangled ball; this is essentially what a protein is. In this analogy, each link in the chain is an amino acid (the building blocks of protein). When we digest protein, our body essentially untangles this big chain and breaks it apart until we are left with individual links (free amino acids). Our body uses the amino acids to build different proteins with different functions.

Chemical digestion of protein begins in the stomach. As you may know, the pH of the stomach is very low, making it an acidic environment, and this is no accident: stomach acid is absolutely essential for optimal protein digestion.

Acid secreted in the stomach causes the big tangled chain to unravel (in scientific terms, denaturation), which then enables further digestion of the protein by exposing all of the links in the chain. Stomach acid also activates specific enzymes in the stomach that are responsible for snipping up the unravelled chain into many shorter chains (called peptides).

Note the use of medications that increase the pH of the stomach, and therefore decrease the acidity, is extremely common in Western society. While these may be medically necessary for some people, it is important to know that these medications may affect the body's ability to digest protein optimally.

From the stomach, the partially digested protein moves into the small intestine, where it comes into contact with more digestive enzymes released from the pancreas and the small intestine. These enzymes break the remaining links in the smaller chains (peptides), releasing the single links (amino acids).

The amino acids are then absorbed across the wall of the gut into our bloodstream, and are transported to where they are required in the body. They build everything from the cells of your immune system (which defend against infection) to the neurotransmitters in your brain (which impact your mood) to the cells that form your muscles (which give you strength to carry your groceries and your children). What you eat, actually becomes a part of you.

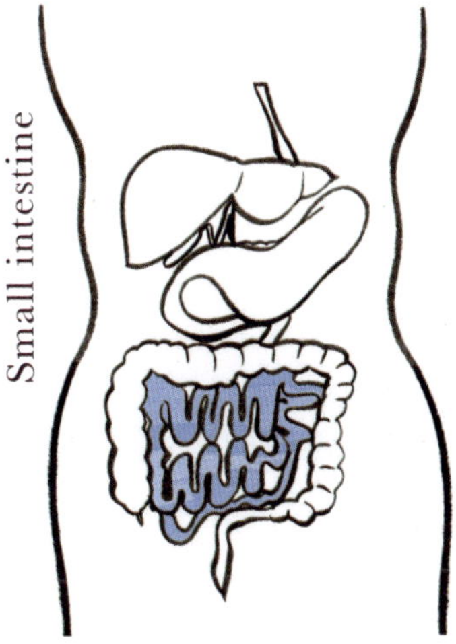

FAT

Although some fat digestion occurs in the stomach with the help of digestive enzymes, the majority takes place in the upper small intestine. When fat empties from the stomach into the small intestine, bile (produced by the liver) is released from the gallbladder and this is essential for the emulsification of dietary fats. You are probably aware that oil and water don't mix; that is, unless an emulsifier is present. The same is true in our body — remember water accounts for about 60–70 per cent of our body weight — and this is why our liver and gallbladder are essential for the digestion of dietary fats. The fats that we consume in our food are mostly in the form of triglycerides (a molecule of glycerol attached to three fatty acid chains).

Triglycerides are then broken down by enzymes released from the pancreas, and are absorbed into the cells lining our small intestine. The journey from these intestinal cells to the bloodstream differs depending on the chemical structure of the triglyceride; specifically, the length of the fatty acid chains. Short- and medium-chain fatty acids move straight from the intestinal cell into the blood, and hitch a ride on albumin (a protein in our blood) to the liver, while long-chain fatty acids are incorporated into carrier molecules that enter the lymphatic system.

These molecules drain from the lymph into the bloodstream, and deliver fats to where they are needed in the body, before returning to the liver. Most of the food you eat is long-chain, while some of the fats, such as those in coconut and butter, are medium-chain.

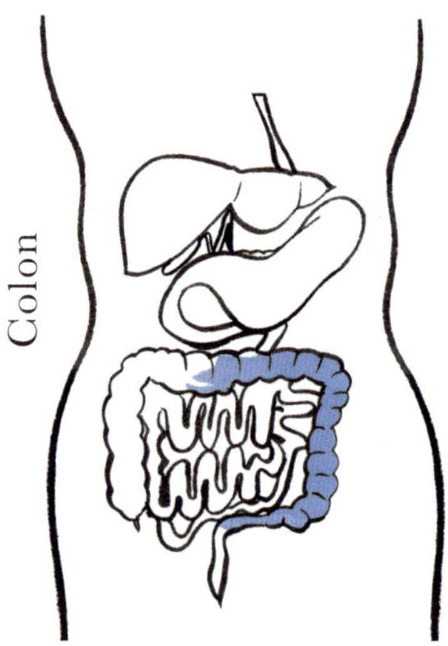

DIETARY FIBRE

Dietary fibre resists digestion in the human body, and the fibrous particles sail through our digestive tract relatively intact. This is because we lack the enzymes to break down the fibres, or the digestive enzymes we do produce are not particularly effective in breaking down the fibre. However, some dietary fibre can be digested by the bacteria residing in the colon, and this leads to the production of short-chain fatty acids that nourish the gut lining.

VITAMINS

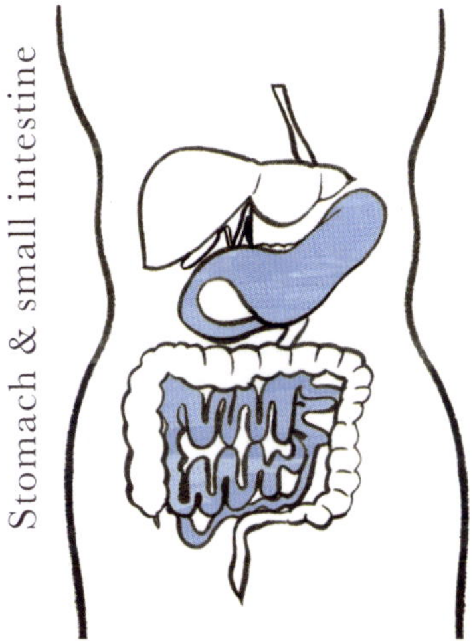

The absorption and transportation throughout the body of the two classes of vitamins depends on whether they are fat-soluble or water-soluble.

The fat-soluble vitamins (vitamins A, D, E and K) are absorbed in the same manner as fat and are therefore better absorbed when they are consumed with good quality fats. Fat-soluble vitamins are extracted from our food and incorporated, along with fats, into carrier molecules that enter the lymphatic system. These carrier molecules drain from the lymph into the bloodstream and transport the fat-soluble vitamins throughout the body to be utilised.

The water-soluble vitamins (vitamin C and B group vitamins) are extracted from our food in the stomach and small intestine and are absorbed across the wall of our small intestine into the bloodstream. Once in the bloodstream, they are transported throughout the body to cells where they can be utilised.

MINERALS

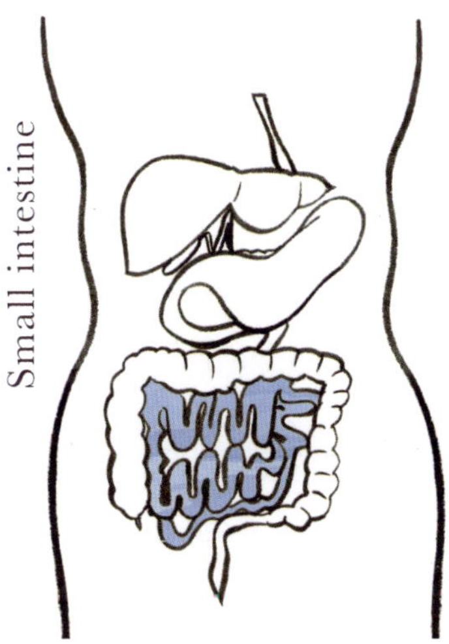

As our food is digested, minerals (chemical elements such as magnesium, calcium, iron, zinc, selenium and iodine) are released and are absorbed across the wall of the small intestine with the help of transporter molecules. Some minerals use the same transporter molecule (for example, iron and calcium), so they effectively compete for absorption. Once they are absorbed into the bloodstream, minerals are transported around the body either in their free form or bound to other carrier molecules.

What is brown fat?

NOT ALL BODY FAT IS EQUAL

When we think of 'body fat', we typically conjure up images of love handles and soft bits; we certainly don't consider this concept positively. However, not all 'body fat' is equal. We have more white fat than brown fat in our bodies but brown fat (brown adipose tissue) is different to white fat in that, under the right conditions, it actually produces heat and burns energy. In fact, when fully activated, brown fat generates significantly more heat than any other tissue in the body.

We typically find brown fat along the sides of the neck. It is also often found running along the region just above our collarbone, across the shoulder and down into the upper arms as well as between the shoulder blades of the upper back and along each side of the upper spine.

It's packed with mitochondria — the power sources for our cells — which gives it its darker colour. While regular white fat passively stores energy from our excess energy consumption, brown fat burns energy. Due to its role in helping to regulate the body's core temperature by producing heat, babies and small animals accumulate a large amount of brown fat. To produce that heat, energy has to be burnt, which is why having brown fat is actually good for us.

Over the past decade, researchers have discovered that brown fat doesn't completely disappear in adult humans, and that it may in fact play an important role in our metabolism.

Research suggests that most, if not all, adults have small pockets of brown fat.

SO HOW CAN YOU SUPPORT BROWN FAT?

The best ways are to move regularly ensuring you are building muscle and, secondly, to utilise cooler temperatures.

Cooler temperatures

Nobody feels comfortable getting very cold, but research suggests that exposing yourself to cooler temperatures helps increase brown body fat. Due to the frequent use of air conditioners and heating systems indoors, plus the double whammy of less time spent outside in Nature, a general lack of exposure to temperature variation is likely to be a contributing factor to low brown fat concentration. A simple way to expose yourself to cooler temperatures is to blast yourself with cold water at the beginning and end of your shower — it will also go a long way towards waking you up!

Movement

We know regular movement has been shown to increase the activity of brown fat — not to mention the benefits that regular movement has for your metabolism and body composition in general. Moving frequently has been shown to play a part in controlling body fat and muscle mass development by having a positive effect on the release of hormones. Think build muscle, rather than running long distances. The more muscle you build, the better.

Eating to satiety

Address any emotional or stress eating and work towards building great awareness of your internal hunger signals. Over-eating confuses the processes that control the hunger hormones, which can raise the risk for many other health problems as well as lead to additional white fat storage. Nevertheless, you don't want to under-eat either. When you aren't consuming enough energy, it may slow down brown fat activation, and this can have other negative effects on your metabolic rate. Eat until you are just full, which generally requires us to SLOW down.

Why eat real food?

WHAT DO YOU WANT YOUR FOOD TO DO FOR YOU?

There are countless theories about the best way to eat for excellent health, yet what science has firmly established is the protective benefits of a high plant diet. Whole foods contain all of the vitamins and minerals and the natural plant compounds all known to support human health. Without nutrients, we die, and we get our nutrients primarily through the foods we choose to eat.

Eating whole, real food is about all of the perks you get, such as nutrient density, but it is also about what you miss out on — the potentially harmful substances in processed food that can disrupt your body's natural rhythms, biochemistry, communication systems and hormonal systems.

> “When you eat mostly real food, you omit or minimise the artificial colours, flavours, sweeteners, preservatives and additives that can be present in processed foods.”

When you eat mostly real food, you omit or minimise the artificial colours, flavours, sweeteners, preservatives and additives that can be present in processed foods. You also miss out on ingredients that have been bleached and/or pummelled so that any nutrients that may have been in the original food have to be added back synthetically for that food to even have any goodness. And yet, most people eat these foods daily without giving any thought to what they might be doing to their insides. Whatever goes on, on the inside, becomes visible in some way on the outside. You cannot fill up on stimulants, such as too much caffeine and refined sugars, and live on a diet that is virtually devoid of nutrients and still expect to have great health and energy long term.

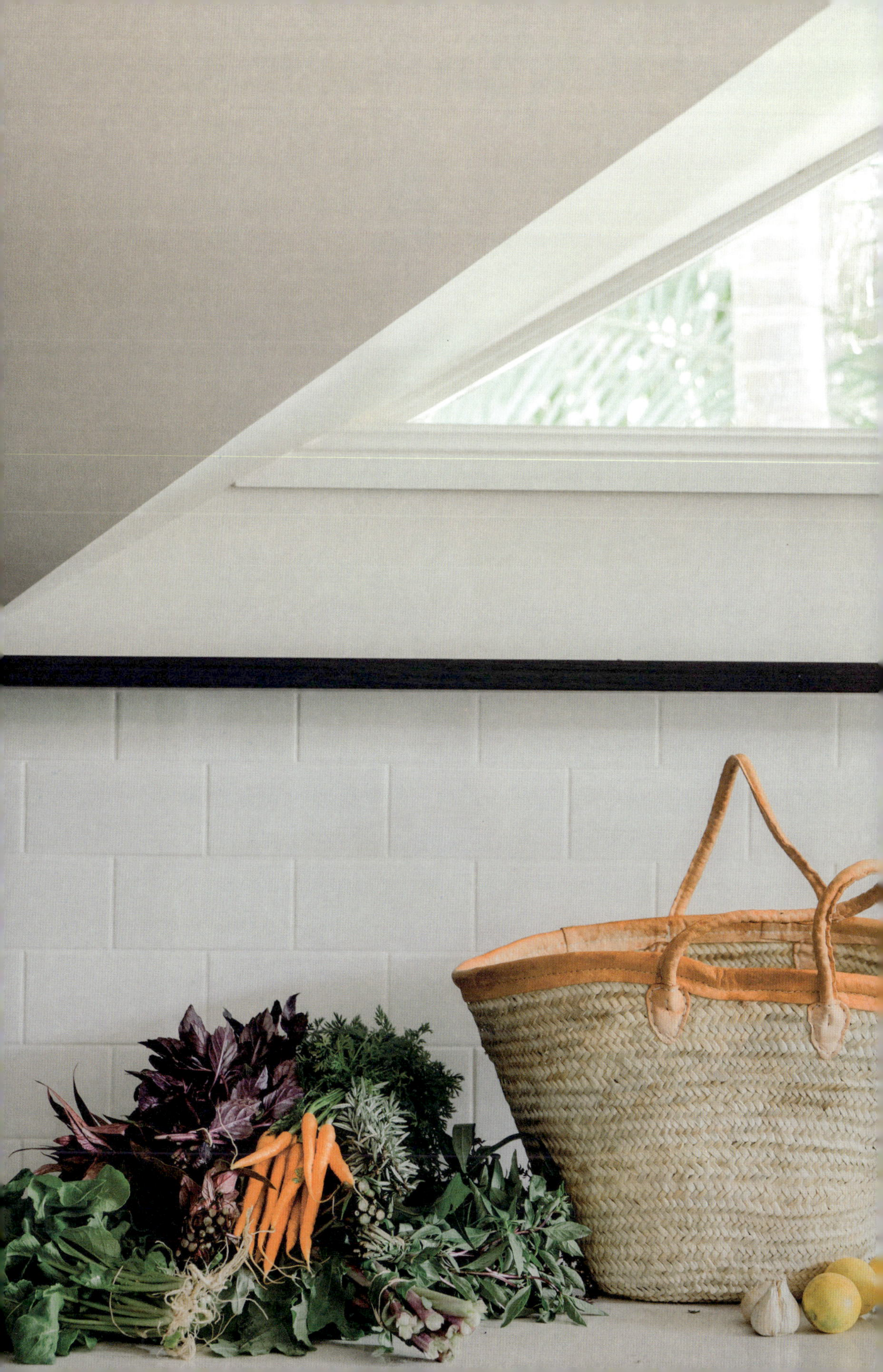

Consider again, do too many people live too short and die too long?

Let's say you eat 35 times a week, three main meals and two snacks each day. And let's say that currently seven of those 35 meals meet the criteria for a health-enhancing, nutrient dense meal. If you simply add one real food meal, snack or smoothie each week for the next two months, your real food intake will then be at 15 out of your 35 meals. And you will have more than doubled the amount of nutrients in your diet in eight tiny weeks out of your very long life!

The above is an example of how you can enhance your nutritional intake in a practical way.

For most of you, a shift like this will feel simple and much more manageable than a complete overhaul of your pantry and essentially your life. Unless a radical approach works for you (and if it does — go for it!), gradual changes will be far more sustainable for you and/or your family.

What do you want your food to do for you, or give you?

- Provide higher nutrient density.
- Decrease your overall synthetic chemical load.
- Enhance and support the detoxification processes through consuming fewer 'liver-loaders' and supplying the nutrients necessary to optimise these functions.
- Support the energy systems of the body through optimal nutrient intake, while lowering the intake of substances that can interfere with the creation of, and your experience of, energy.

A health-enhancing diet is one based on plant foods. Incorporating more plant foods into your diet is the quickest and easiest way to increase nutrient density and variety. Plant foods are good sources of soluble and insoluble fibre. Insoluble fibre helps provide bulk to our stools to keep our bowels regular, and is used to help feed our gut bacteria. Feeding the good bacteria is an essential component of keeping the balance between the good and not-so-good bacteria in the gut. A healthy digestive system is the foundation of great health, including a robust immune response.

Nutritionally, leafy greens are legends. They not only contain vitamins and minerals, but they enhance the quality of your blood. The power of greens is well demonstrated by the way gorillas live, and, given that they have similar DNA to humans (but have not been influenced by marketing), we can perhaps learn a lot from their innate food choices. The diet of gorillas is over 50 per cent piths, shoots and green leaves and yet they have one of the highest muscle masses of any living creature. They eat small amounts of animal protein, which they obtain mostly from insects, but the ratio of greens to animal is enormously in favour of a high plant diet.

Our bodies thrive on being supplied with living foods, so the more plants we incorporate into our diet, the better we feel. One of the main reasons plants accumulate nutrients is to develop future seeds so they can reproduce and the species can survive. Seeds require a high density of nutrients to fulfil their reproductive functions. Even once they have germinated, they need a significant amount of energy and nutrition to sprout and survive. Sprouts are nutrient-packed powerhouses and make for a great addition to your diet.

Plants accumulate nutrients long before they create their seeds, and there is no better place for accumulating and storing nutrients than in the leaves. Hence, greens leaves are one of the most nutritious foods on Earth. Seeds, too, are rich in nutrients, but plants don't want their offspring to be eaten, so many plants also add protective mechanisms to their seeds by endowing them with a range of inhibitors, alkaloids and other substances that may be harmful to predators. Nature is truly amazing.

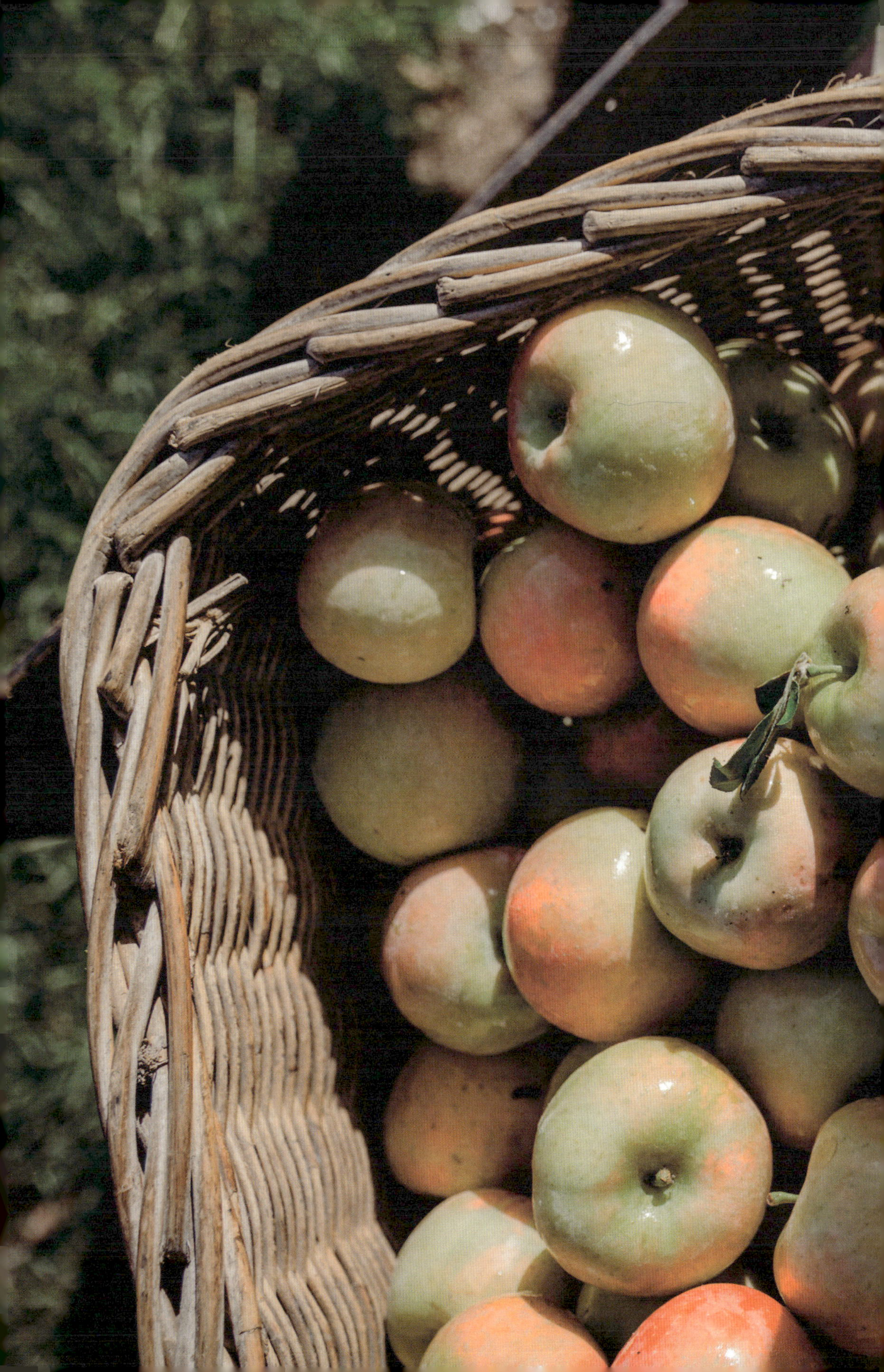

If you grow greens or herbs yourself, the best time to harvest them is before the formation of seeds. This is when the green leaves have the highest concentration of nutrients. After a plant blossoms, nutrients begin to accumulate inside the seeds, and once the seeds are gone there is almost no nutrition left in the leaves. They tend to turn yellow, and dry out and fall off — think of a parsley plant after it has gone to seed — so that the remaining nutrients return to the soil and the plant can rest until the next growing season. Seasons and cycles in Nature all serve a purpose, and human health relies on these cycles to nourish and sustain our life.

DECREASING THE SYNTHETIC CHEMICAL LOAD

Decreasing the synthetic chemical load is another important aim of optimal nourishment. Choosing to eat less processed food goes some way toward this, as you start to ingest fewer artificial substances, such as artificial sweeteners, preservatives and other additives.

Eating more organically or biodynamically grown food, or simply choosing spray-free options, can play a major role in achieving this.

Plants have innate mechanisms designed to help protect themselves from pests. When a plant is left to grow of its own accord and is not sprayed with pesticides, the plant creates substances within itself to help ward off pests. These substances don't just have the ability to help protect the plant, they also often behave as antioxidants when humans consume them. If the plants are sprayed with pesticides or herbicides, they no longer have to (and don't) produce these substances that enhance human health and help slow down ageing and degeneration. So eating organic food is not just about what you miss out on — pesticides — but also what you get — more antioxidants.

Pesticides and other synthetic chemicals, such as artificial sweeteners, preservatives and many of the numbers (additives) you see on packeted food ingredient lists typically have to be altered inside the body before they can be excreted. The liver is one organ involved in this process. The liver has to prioritise detoxification processes, and if there are more "liver-loaders" present than available pathways for this to occur, these foreign substances are usually stored in the fatty tissue of your body. Hence when any weight loss process is undertaken, liver support is of immense importance.

ESTROGEN-LIKE COMPOUNDS

Some herbicides contain compounds that can mimic estrogen in the human body, in both males and females of all ages. This is of great concern. For estrogen or estrogen-like compounds to exert their effects, they have to bind to estrogen receptors, and when they do, the lovely, or not so lovely, effects of estrogen are experienced. Given that children today are exposed to herbicides for their entire lifetimes, it is likely that their exposure to estrogen-like compounds, in addition to what the body produces itself (mostly from puberty onwards), is contributing to the earlier age of menarche being reported across the Western world. Please pause and consider the ramifications of this. On another note, body fat cells also produce estrogen in boys and girls, men and women. So with the sky-rocketing childhood obesity challenges comes even more estrogen production.

> "Eating organic food is not just about what you miss out on, pesticides, but also what you get, more antioxidants."

If the prospect of decreasing the synthetic chemical load as a goal of what you want your food to do for you is overwhelming, then don't start here. Start small. Come back to this when you are ready or grow these practices slowly.

In the meantime, focus on enhancing your detoxification processes, discussed below, to upregulate your body's ability to excrete these substances.

ENHANCING AND SUPPORTING DETOXIFICATION PROCESSES

Another reason to eat whole, real food is to enhance the body's ability to detoxify itself. Detoxification is a process that is often misunderstood. It goes on inside of us, all day, every day. We wouldn't be alive without it. However, the lifestyle choices we make influence how efficiently our body detoxifies.

The liver plays a major role in detoxification, which is essentially a transformation process. The body takes substances that would harm you if they were to accumulate and changes them into substances that are less harmful so that you can excrete them.

Substances that either require detoxification, or impact on this process, include alcohol, caffeine, synthetic substances (such as medications, pesticides, and ingredients in skincare products), trans fats (damaged fats usually found in bought cakes and biscuits, muesli bars and deep-fried food), and some sugars, such as refined sugars. These are the substances I refer to as 'liver loaders'. The liver also has to detoxify substances your body makes itself, such as estrogen and cholesterol, which can have their own impact on your health.

When I am guiding people with what foods serve their health, one element that is firmly in my mind is minimising (or, in some cases, eliminating) 'liver-loaders', as this allows the body to pull toxins out of 'storage' to be processed and excreted. Your health and energy are enhanced when you have fewer stored problematic substances.

Food is designed to supply the body with the nutrients necessary for the detoxification processes in the body to work efficiently. For example, the first stage of detoxification by the liver requires B vitamins for that process to occur.

Our best food sources of B vitamins are wholegrains and yet many people have cut them out, or at least back, in their diet. Many people feel better without grains (or with less or only specific types, for example gluten-free grains) in their diet and I am by no means suggesting that you suddenly go back and eat bucket-loads of grains to get your B vitamins if you feel better without them. All I want to point out is that, unknowingly, people can miss out on nutrients crucial to the inner workings of their body and their optimal health.

The second stage of liver detoxification requires sulphur, which we get from eggs, garlic, onion, shallots and the brassica family of vegetables. This phase also requires amino acids that we obtain from protein-containing foods.

Choosing a wide variety of whole foods — and perhaps trying some gluten-free grains, such as brown rice, if gluten-containing grains disrupt your digestive system — may assist these vital cleaning systems in your body. Eating real food also tends to help with regular bowel motions and this too enhances the detoxification processes as the liver no longer has to pick up the shortfall of digestion. The liver loves, and is stimulated by, bitter foods and there is no better way to stimulate the bitter taste buds than with green leafy vegies. And given the workload of the liver in our modern lives, it was a huge reason why I created Bio Blends Liver Love.

SUPPORTING THE ENERGY SYSTEMS OF THE BODY

When I ask people how they are these days, I most often hear *exhausted, stressed, busy, frantic, broken* and *tired*. I don't want this for you. I want you to feel amazing; I want you to feel energised, vital and alive. Without energy, it is difficult to take care of the basics, let alone make your own dreams come true and contribute to those around you.

> *How do you wake up in the morning? Do you bounce out of bed, grateful that a new day has dawned that you are fortunate to be part of? Or do you press the snooze button five times, wondering how on earth it can be morning already?*

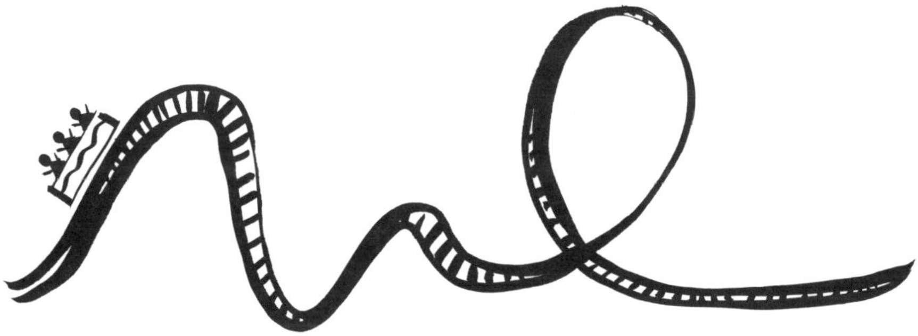

Mostly I hear the latter.

What is your energy like over the course of a day? Do you feel like your blood glucose is less like the even flow of a river, and more akin to a roller coaster, with dramatic highs and lows in your moods and also your energy levels? When you have a burst of energy, does your temper explode? Or are you someone who simply wishes you could spend the next year in bed? My point? Your energy levels significantly influence the quality of your life.

Food is designed to energise us in a lovely, even way. If what you have been eating (or drinking) wires you — amps you up with intensity, and you overreact to small things — or perhaps it makes you feel sleepy, then it may not have been serving you. Eating real food helps support the energy systems in your body, because we have all of the equipment inside of ourselves to break real food down and extract and utilise the energy it offers us. There is growing concern that there are substances in some processed foods that we have no ability to break down. Given your food is the only way you get physical energy, why would you want to mess with that?

The way energy is created within the body involves a series of biochemical pathways that nutrients drive. I won't bore you by going into detail here, although I am tempted to blow your mind at just how astonishing your body is and to show you the immense power of nutrients to drive your biochemistry and to remind you that life truly is miraculous! For now know that by increasing the nutrient density of your diet, you help enhance your energy systems, which can lead not only to a healthier life, but a much happier one.

WORKSHEET

Think about your upcoming week and the eating occasions that will be present. Pick one meal, or snack, each day for the next seven days and work out what you could swap or incorporate into each meal to begin to increase more whole, real foods into your diet.

I CURRENTLY CHOOSE:	INSTEAD I COULD CHOOSE:

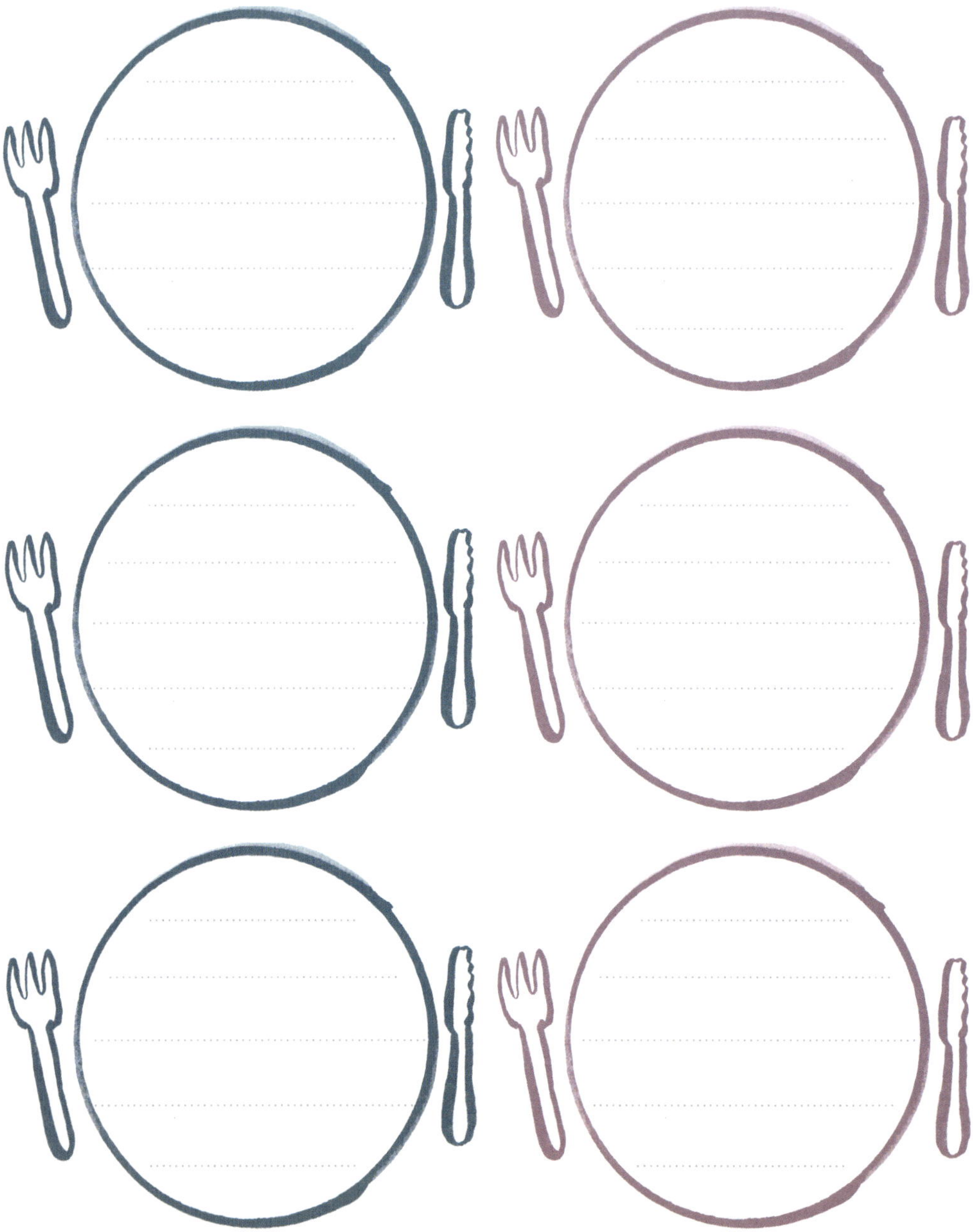

I CURRENTLY CHOOSE:

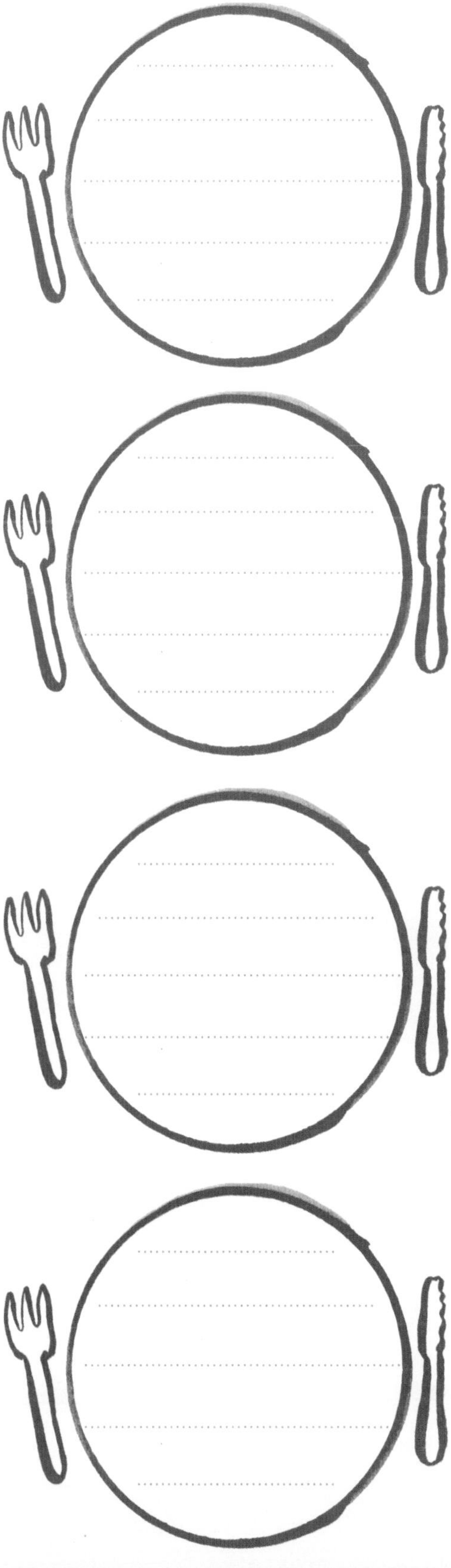

INSTEAD I COULD CHOOSE:

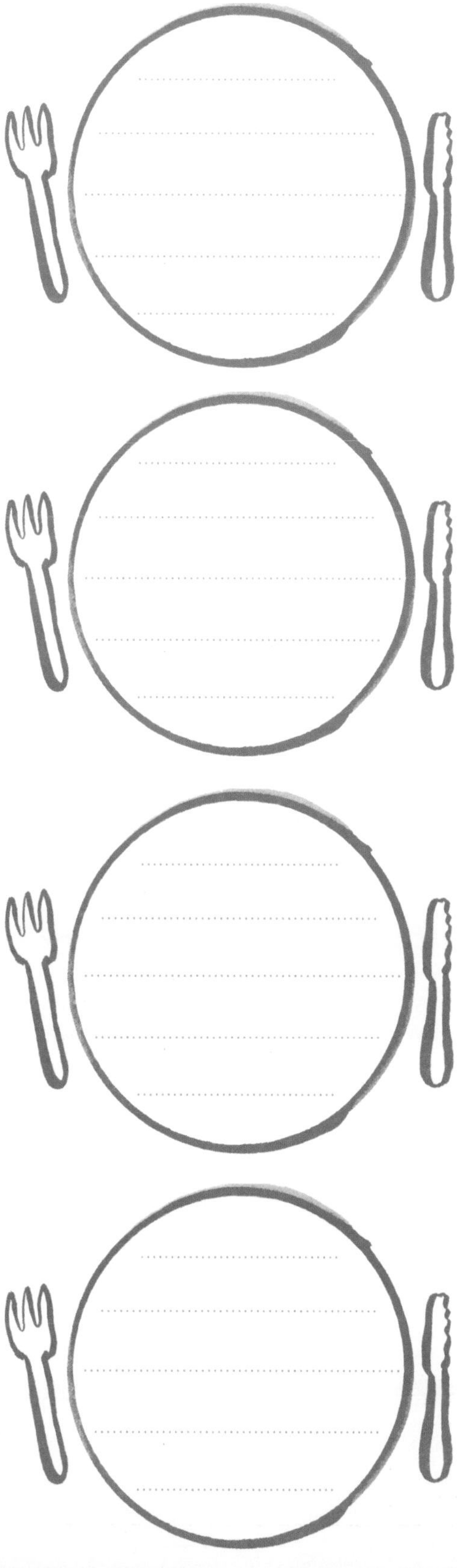

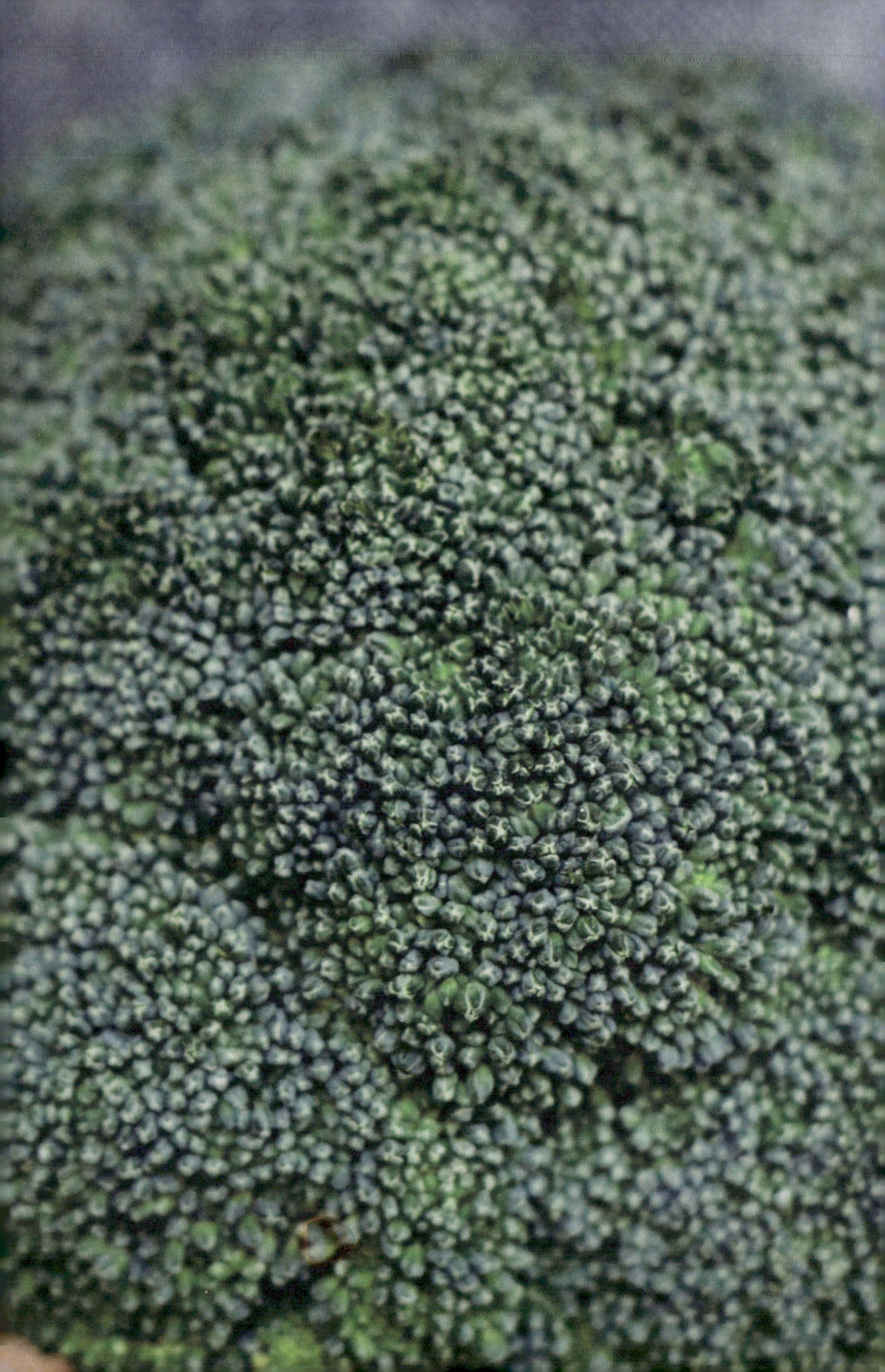

When something bites your broccoli

THE LOW-DOWN ON PESTICIDES

The use of synthetic pesticides on food to be consumed by humans and other animals became widespread and accelerated in the 1940s. Prior to then, plant- or animal-derived compounds or, later, by-products of the petrochemical industry and even arsenic and mercury, were used to keep pests at bay. Sometimes with dire consequences. The use of synthetic pesticides is therefore relatively new to the food chain when you consider that science suggests that humans have been on the planet for about 150,000 years. Today, food grown without the use of these pesticides (and that meets additional standards) is referred to as 'organic food', which 70-odd years ago was simply called 'food'.

Produce can only be labelled 'certified organic' if it has been packaged, harvested, raised or grown without any use of possibly harmful chemicals including antibiotics, pesticides, fertilisers, insecticides or growth hormones. 'Certified organic' also means that the produce has not been genetically modified. Everyone benefits from us choosing organic. It not only protects the health of our biochemical pathways and body systems, it's better for the soil and the health of the planet.

Growing our own produce is the ideal way to get organic food; however, if that's not a viable solution for you, try your local farmers' market.

The impact that conventional farming practices is having on soil fertility is getting a lot of attention on the worldwide stage. People are beginning to take notice of ecologists' warnings about how poor quality soil is affecting all life.

Additionally, more and more people are discovering for themselves that the sustainability of the food supply is intrinsically linked to the maintenance of soil fertility.

When soils are used over and over and over again without nutrient dense replenishment or crop rotation, the way it is in conventional farming practices, it diminishes its nutritional value. Nutrients are drawn out of the soil every time a crop or vegetables — anything — is grown. The nutrients are used by the plant to grow and we then get the benefits when we consume that food. Add to this that farmers then periodically saturate their crops with unnatural chemical fertilisers. I refer to them as "unnatural" for many reasons, one of which is that they don't contain the range of nutrients essential for life. The chemical fertilisers used in conventional farming are primarily made up of only three nutrients: nitrogen, phosphorus and potassium.

> “Poor soil health creates poor plant health which in turn leaves plants without the ability to defend themselves, and so the pests come.”

Sadly, there are still further consequences of conventional farming methods. Poor soil health creates poor plant health which in turn leaves plants without the ability to defend themselves — and so the pests come.

That's one of the ways and reasons pesticides have infiltrated our food supply. It all starts with the health of the soil which leads to the food supply being contaminated with substances that are potentially problematic to human health. Additionally, the poor soil health means that the food is deficient in nutrients — so our bodies can end up toxic *and* deficient.

What does this feel like? In the short term, these nutrient

deficiencies most often manifest as lousy energy, body aches, joint pain, failing eyesight and thousands of other scenarios that people are encouraged to simply accept as part of 'ageing'. Long term, nutrient deficiencies contribute to major illnesses, such as numerous cancers, heart disease and type 2 diabetes, to name a few.

SO WHERE DO WE GO FROM HERE?

In 1962, Rachel Carson insightfully wrote: "If we are going to live so intimately with these chemicals…taking them into the very marrow of our bones — we had better know something about their nature and their power." Where we stand now, over five decades later, there is much more we know about their power, but much more still, that we are yet to learn.

On 20 March 2015, scientists from 11 countries, who were convened by the World Health Organization's (WHO) International Agency for Research on Cancer, made available their unanimous conclusions about glyphosate, the world's most used herbicide (Roundup is the most well-known version of glyphosate).

These experts, who published their findings in one of the most prestigious medical journals in the world, *The Lancet Oncology*, established that this commonly used herbicide is "probably carcinogenic to humans". Their work suggests that glyphosate probably plays a role in humans developing cancer. In 1992 this herbicide was barely used on US farmland yet by 2012 it is estimated that around 250 million pounds (about 113 million kilograms) was being used.

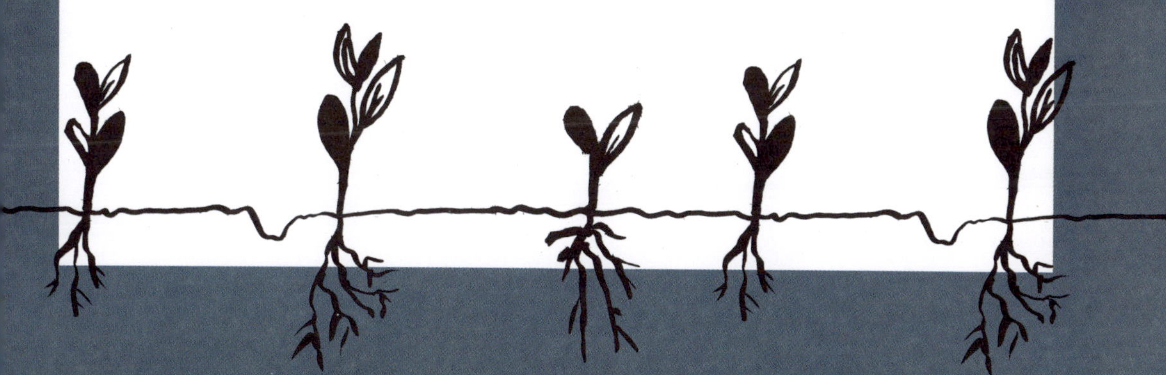

Further to these considerations are results from additional studies led by a team at the University of Canterbury in New Zealand, who found antibiotic resistance in bacteria, including resistance to ciprofloxacin (which is commonly used in human medicine), as a result of exposure to some formulations of glyphosate and other common herbicides.

Sometimes, it takes a health crisis to wake you up, and to make changes to lifestyle choices, or at least to investigate them. When it comes to exposure to potentially problematic substances, that's what I see more and more people doing.

This is deeply concerning, so I would like you to consider where and how you can begin to decrease your exposure to these potentially problematic substances. It became so important to me that, across a bunch of years where funds were very tight, I didn't buy new clothes or shoes for more than four years, unless they cost less than five dollars (op-shop), so that I had funds to buy organic food. That's how much eating organic food meant to me.

> "Consider where and how you can begin to decrease your exposure to potentially problematic substances."

When I talk about problematic substances I am referring to the pesticides and herbicides that conventional produce is sprayed with, and the synthetic chemicals with which people clean their homes and wash their clothes, as well as put on their skin.

We are so very fortunate to live in a world where we have access to alternatives.

Despite all of our accomplishments in the world, we owe our existence to a 30-centimetre layer of topsoil and the fact that it rains. Soil is eroding seven times faster than it is being built up naturally and it is estimated that more than three billion tonnes of topsoil is eroded from US farmlands each year. In organic farming, soil is the foundation of the food chain. This is another reason why it is critically important to support organic and sustainable agriculture sooner rather than later, for the health of people and the planet.

YOUR CHOICES

The reason your apple looks so perfect is because it has been sprayed to make it look that way. The reason there are no bugs in your broccoli is because it's been sprayed to ensure they don't want to eat it. Finding bugs in your broccoli or imperfections in your apples can be a sign that your produce has been grown with as little interference as possible — and often without the use of chemicals. We've simply been conditioned to think that our produce is supposed to look a certain way and shouldn't be sheltering any slimy friends.

We cannot see or taste the chemicals on our food, but they are there. We really are guinea pigs with regards to the long-term consumption of substances such as pesticides. There *are* requirements to test pesticides before they can be used on food for human consumption. However, I do not believe you can compare the results from, say, a six-month period, to being exposed to them over an entire lifetime. We also cannot test what takes place when all of the chemicals are mixed and then combined inside our bodies every day — the way they are when we eat conventionally grown produce day after day, year after year.

Fresh food the way it comes in Nature is an incredibly important part of our diets and I want to encourage you to choose organic produce whenever you can.

If choosing to switch to completely organic feels like too big an ask, think about the way you eat the food. We don't eat the skin of an orange. It may have been sprayed, but how much gets

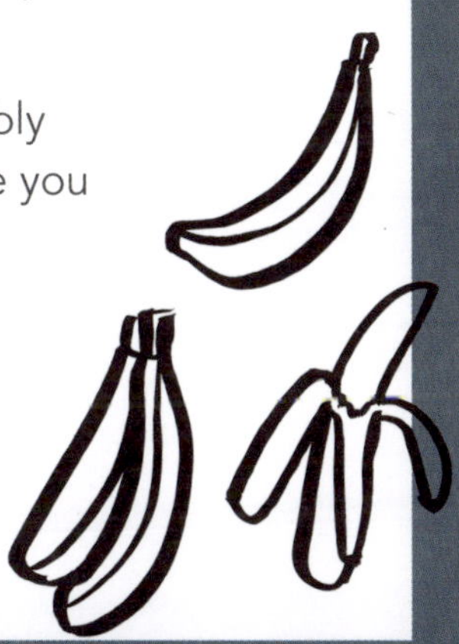

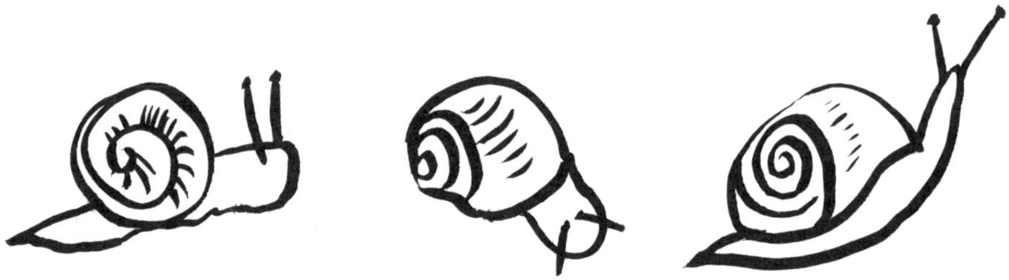

through the skin? We actually don't know. But it makes sense that there would be less chemical residue in the flesh (inside) of an orange than on the skin. So perhaps choosing a conventionally grown orange is not too bad. Yet if you think about a pear, we usually eat the whole thing so it would probably be best to choose an organic (or biodynamically grown) pear wherever possible.

Really contemplate this: organic food is the true cost of food. I've shared this tale in other books but it contains a powerful message, one worth mentioning again here. I once opened and ran an organic café. My supplier was a local farmer who delivered fresh greens he'd picked that morning from his biodynamic farm to me once a week. He always had wonderful tales to tell of his life on the farm so I always set aside some time on delivery day to chat with him. One day, when I asked him how he was, his reply was along the lines of "not so good".

He went on to tell me that snails had invaded his broccoli patch, virtually overnight, and when I paused to consider this, I realised that, if they took hold, a portion of this man's meagre livelihood would be lost. So, given that his farming principles do not involve spraying the patch to get rid of the invaders (which would have taken less than 30 minutes to do), I asked him how he deals with snails on his broccoli. My farmer friend went on to tell me that snails lose their 'stick', their ability to suction on to things, in salty water so he made up a bottle of salt and water, and he spent two days, crouched down on all fours, crawling between his broccoli plants, squirting saline water up under the fronds.

Not only that, he didn't kill the snails, but collected them in a bucket and fed them to the chickens "to keep them in the food chain", as he so delightfully put it.

Think about each of these scenarios. Spraying your patch in under 30 minutes versus crawling around on your haunches for two days. For me, that illustrates precisely why organic and biodynamic food costs more — it reflects the real cost of food. Plus it has a greater nutritional value; not to mention what's left out.

The more we demand organic and say no to pesticides, the more organics will have to be supplied. The more of us who choose it, the cheaper it will become. I know I'm on my soapbox and I really do want to remain real and practical with the advice I offer. So, in simple terms, choose organic food whenever you can.

If organic food is too costly for you to buy, or perhaps just unavailable in your area, try this solution to remove pesticides. To clean food of both dirt and pesticides at the same time, fill your sink with three parts water to one part vinegar, wash your fruits and vegetables, then rinse them in fresh water, pat them dry and store them for use. Pesticides tend to be fat-soluble, and so general washing to get rid of dirt and germs does not remove them.

Do what is practical for you. And then stretch a little further.

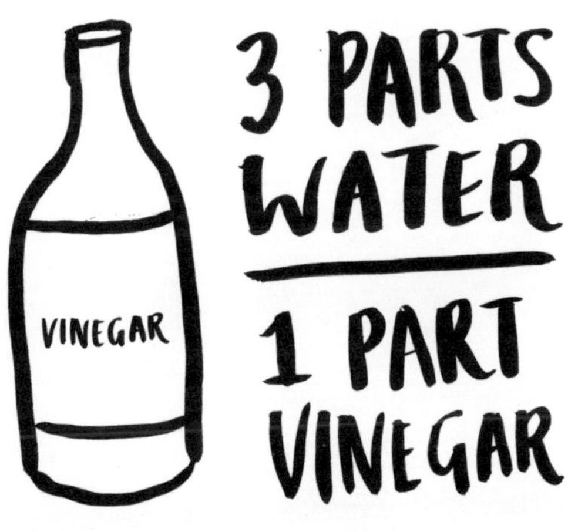

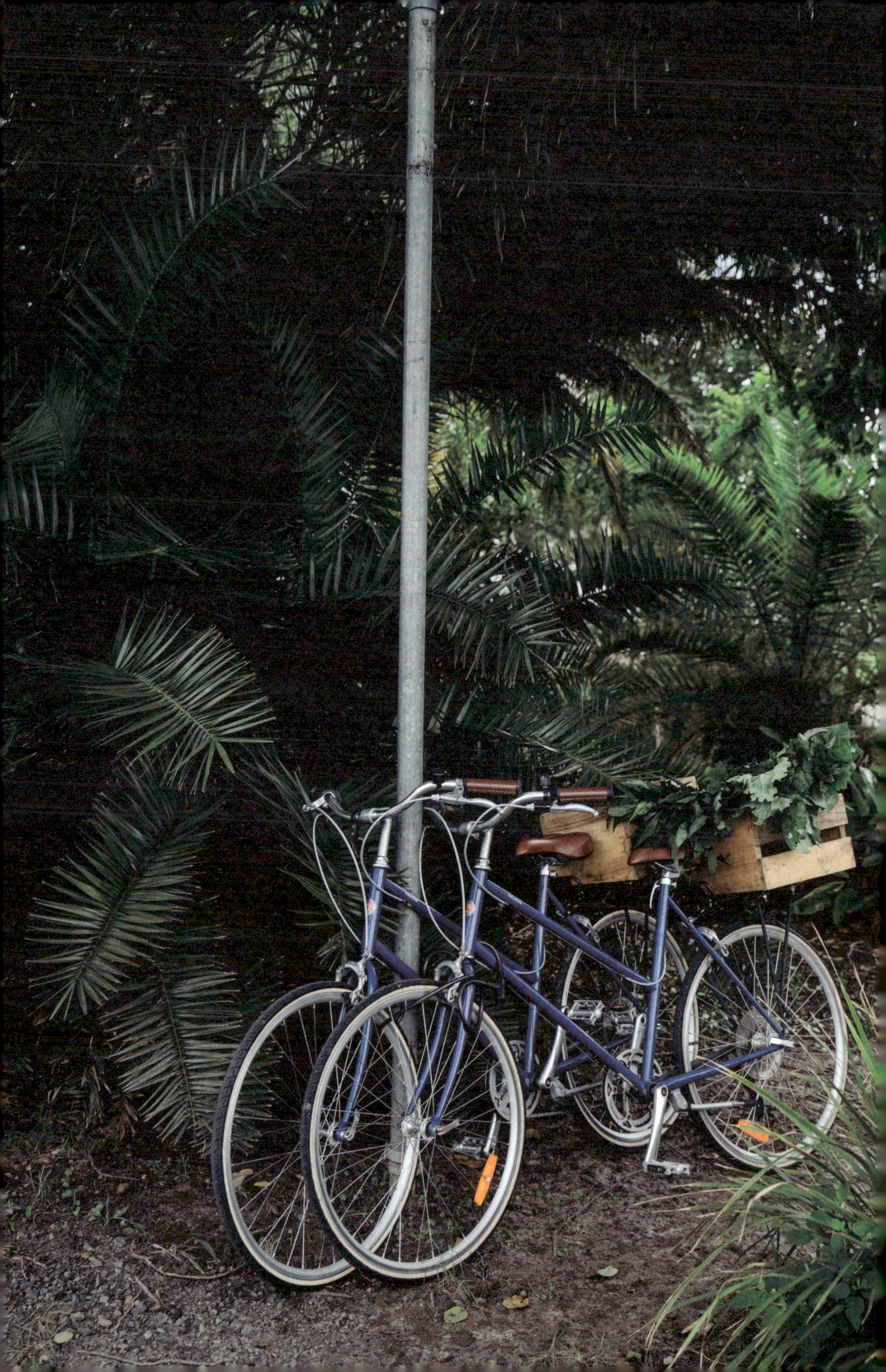

Finding your food language

THE WORDS YOU USE MATTER

There are many reasons why you might be confused about what to eat. You can walk into a bookstore and find a book that says "eat carbohydrates as they are important for energy", while right beside it you will likely find a book that says "don't eat carbs, as they will make you fat and tired". Not only that, there are additional challenges consumers face when trying to make food choices that meet their needs and these relate to the language we use to describe food.

How many times have you been encouraged to eat something because it is healthy? Again, you could read an article that tells you low-fat cheese is healthy, while another will that say low-fat cheese is not heathy, but kale is healthy. What people perceive to be 'healthy' varies. Yet there is another word that more aptly describes whether a food will most likely benefit you or not: nutritious.

> *Consider this: food is not heathy. People are. Or they aren't. Food is nutritious. Or it isn't. And the more nutritious food you eat, the healthier you will tend to be. It can be that simple.*

That alone can be a wonderful guiding light for you in your myriad choices.

Asking the question, "Will this nourish me?" before you eat anything can help you discern whether it is the right choice for you. Is it a whole, real food? If so, the answer is more likely to be 'yes', as these foods contain the substances — micronutrients and phytochemicals — essential for outstanding health. If the food is in a packet and has been highly processed, the answer is likely to be 'no'.

With the popularity of the low-fat era and to a certain extent dieting language, it has been easy for too many people to consider food nothing more than the calories that it supplies. Yet obviously food is so much more than that: the food you eat literally becomes part of you, and it is the vitamins and minerals in nutritious foods that keep you alive. Really think about that.

> Yet there are also times when you will do well when you ask the question "Will this nourish me?" with reference to your soul.

For example, you arrive at your girlfriend's house on a Friday night, and she has had her heart broken. She pulls out a bottle of bubbles and takeaway food and over the evening you both polish off the lot. The last thing you want is to sit there over the course of that evening stressing about your food and drink intake. You are there to be with her, help her laugh, share stories and support your mate. Mostly you make your food choices about the physical nourishment of your 'Earth suit' — providing it with the nutrients it needs to drive all of the biochemical reactions that essentially create your health. But sometimes you need soul food, which is catching up with your friend and supporting her. Probably just don't hang out with her every day if she's going to pull out champagne and takeaways every time you visit...

You get my drift. And please don't use a night like this as an excuse to 'fall off the wagon', or be under the false belief that you've 'ruined' something (refer to page 248 for more on this).

The concept of whether or not a food is 'good for us' has become far too confusing as we have more and more, often-conflicting but well-meaning voices in the health and nutrition world.

A great way to strip nutrition or health information back and make sense of it all is to bring it back to the fundamentals of good health, which most health professionals agree on regardless of their background.

These include:

- eat more vegetables
- decrease or omit refined sugars
- avoid or minimise processed meats
- stay hydrated
- base meals and snacks on real, whole foods
- sleep well
- sit less
- move more
- maintain (or preferably build) muscle mass.

I think it's also incredibly important to remember that, while there are some core nutrition fundamentals that benefit most people, there is no one-size-fits-all when it comes to how we nourish our bodies. Your body is your best barometer: notice how certain foods make you feel and pay attention to any patterns. Food is supposed to energise you; if what you are eating is consistently making you tired, it may not be serving your health. Your own body knows what is best for it. Make nutritious food choices to support your health.

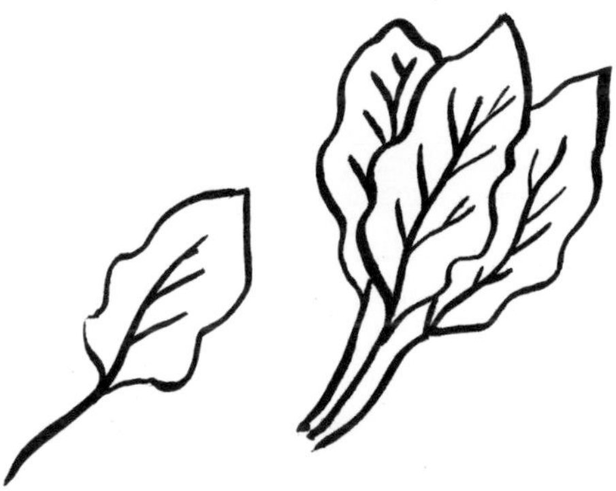

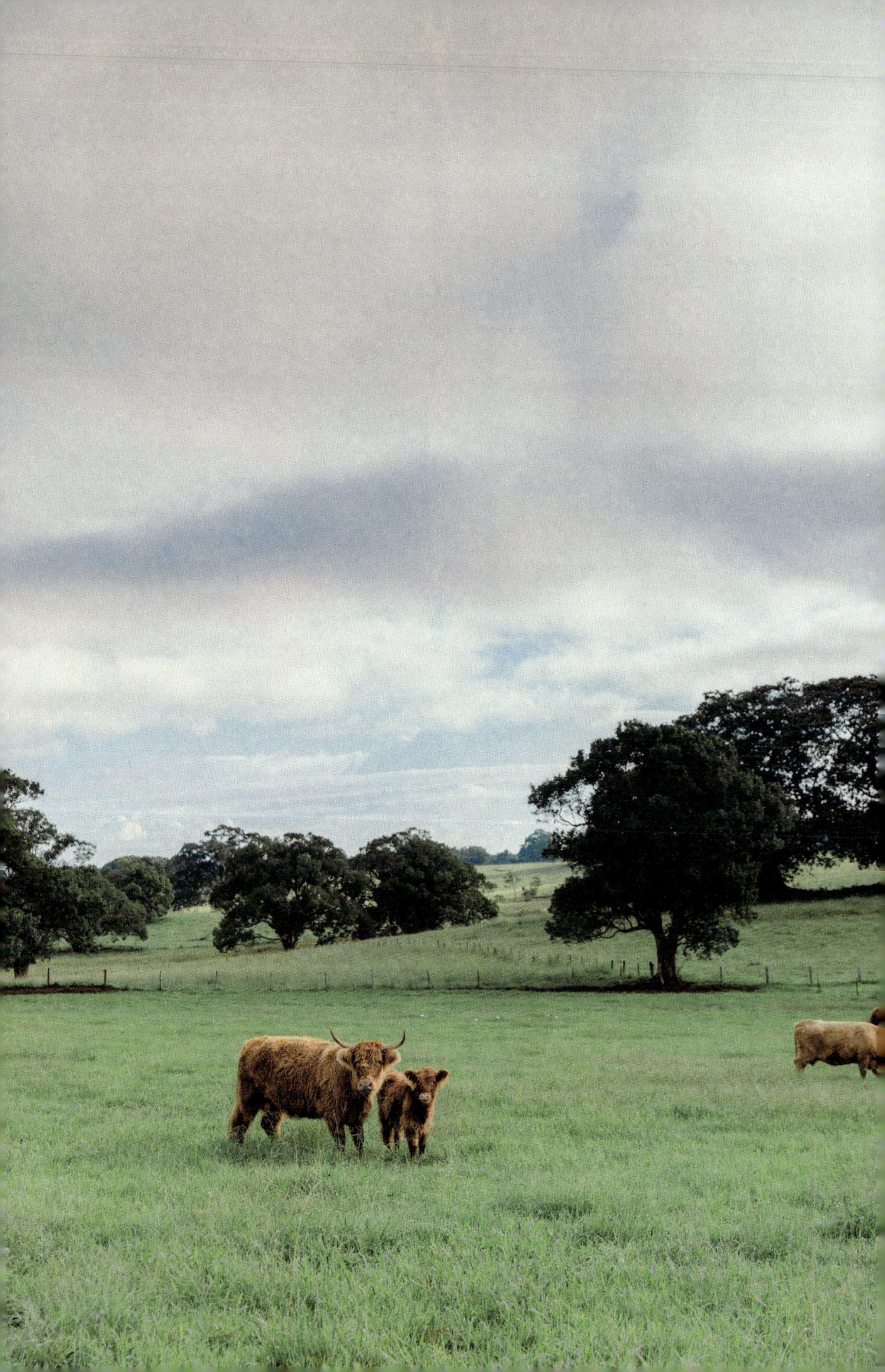

Ethical eating

CONSIDERING THE SUPPLY CHAIN

Do you ever stop to consider where your food comes from? From the farmer who commits their life to feeding you through to the entire chain of production that takes place before something ends up in your shopping basket? We are incredibly fortunate in the Western world to have an abundance of food available to us that we don't have to grow, harvest or hunt for ourselves.

But on the other side of that fortune lies a disconnection to the supply chain that means we often forget the impact that our choices have on the world around us. I raise this, neither to elicit guilt, nor to make a political statement, but because I think it's important we all ask more questions.

The way that we source our food today is far removed from how our ancestors did. In ancient times we were, of course, hunters and gatherers, subsisting directly from the land. While those days may have been whittled back to a distant memory, it's only been since around the middle of last century that our food-sourcing habits took a major change.

Not long after the end of World War II, the industry of food began to boom. A little behind other Western countries on the other side of the world, both Australia and New Zealand saw the beginnings of the supermarket in the 1950s. Before supermarkets really took off, most households still did their shopping at the local butcher and greengrocer. Some may have even had their meat and milk delivered by the milkman. The 1950s was the decade that birthed 'faster' food, as processed and pre-made foods became more popular and widely available.

In the past few decades, we have seen that drive for convenience continue to grow and massive supermarket corporations take the lion's share of the marketplace; making it increasingly difficult for independent stores to stay competitive through the sheer force of the corporations' combined buying power.

And while in some ways this does help the consumer to have access to affordable food options, it does come at a cost.

Those often the most impacted are the farmers themselves. Big retailers promise their customers to keep prices down, with the consequence that farmers of fresh produce sometimes struggle to cover the costs of production. Another reason to shop at your local farmers' market where you can support the farmer directly! The industrialisation of food has also had a significant impact on both the environment and animal welfare.

Conventional farming practices are impacting on soil fertility, certain pesticides have been linked to masses of bee colonies dying out and it's hard to go a month without hearing about the poor conditions that livestock live in through factory farming.

> Unless we're prompted to, we don't often stop to think about where our food comes from before it gets into our shopping basket.

Unless we're prompted to, we don't often stop to think about where our food comes from before it gets into our shopping basket. When we go to the supermarket we're more regularly thinking about things that happened that day, or what we might cook for dinner, or how we're going to get our children to eat the vegetables they so often snub their nose at. We're usually not thinking about whether the farmer who grew the carrots takes adequate care to rotate his crops, or whether the plastic-wrapped chicken breast in our hands came from a chicken who had plenty of freedom to forage around outside in the sun.

I have already discussed how important I think it is that you choose organic produce and products where possible. I'm passionate about increasing your nutrient intake and the benefits that this has on your health.

But I'm also incredibly passionate about sustainability and the impact that we all have on our planet and its inhabitants.

Although we aren't given a lot of information about the production methods that everything we buy passes through before it gets to us, we still have more power than we realise. With every purchase you make, you are communicating to producers and manufacturers where you stand on the quality, sustainability and integrity of the products available on the market.

Maybe cost prohibits you from switching to organic or sustainable products. It's true that these kinds of products are more expensive — because the costs of production are so much greater. It stuns and saddens me that we live in a world where the true cost of food and products is not affordable for all. And we all need to do what we can to help change this. It costs nothing to ask questions. It costs nothing to take a more conscious approach to shopping by omitting something from your shopping basket because you've found out that it was produced in a factory with unsafe working conditions for employees, for example.

Most of us are pretty well educated about how to eat for our health, but as consumers who mostly buy food from supermarkets (where we are served by people who very likely don't even know where the food has come from), we have little opportunity to connect with what took place to get our food to us.

Nevertheless, there are loads of resources available — documentaries, books, research papers — all of which can help to build your knowledge if you are keen to learn more about how you can be a more ethical consumer. My personal favourite is the book *The Ethical Carnivore* by Louise Gray.

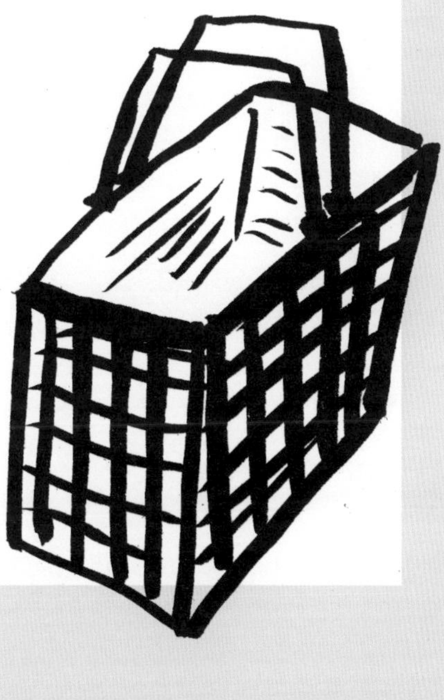

But even if the thought of reading a book of that nature feels like hard work, simply by buying from small, local producers and suppliers, or as mentioned before from farmers' markets, you are able to chat with the people who have either purchased or grown the food.

I encourage you to ask them about their farming practices or where they source their food from and commit to purchasing the more ethical produce.

These choices in themselves communicate to producers and manufacturers that you want more nutritious, sustainable and ethical products on offer. We all have a part to play in shaping the world around us and shifting some of the practices we feel at times powerless to change, but that are unacceptable to us.

I encourage you all to act on what you care about.

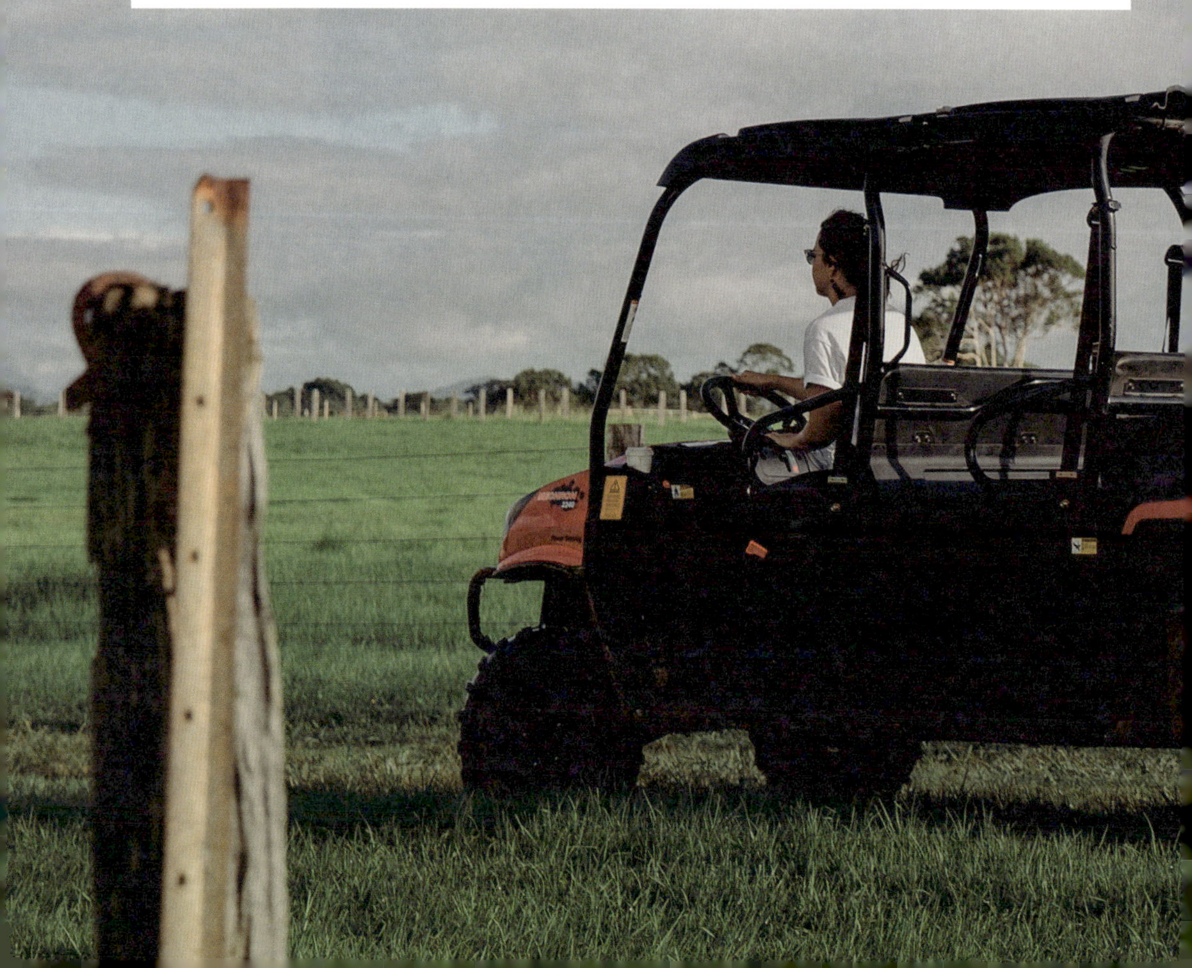

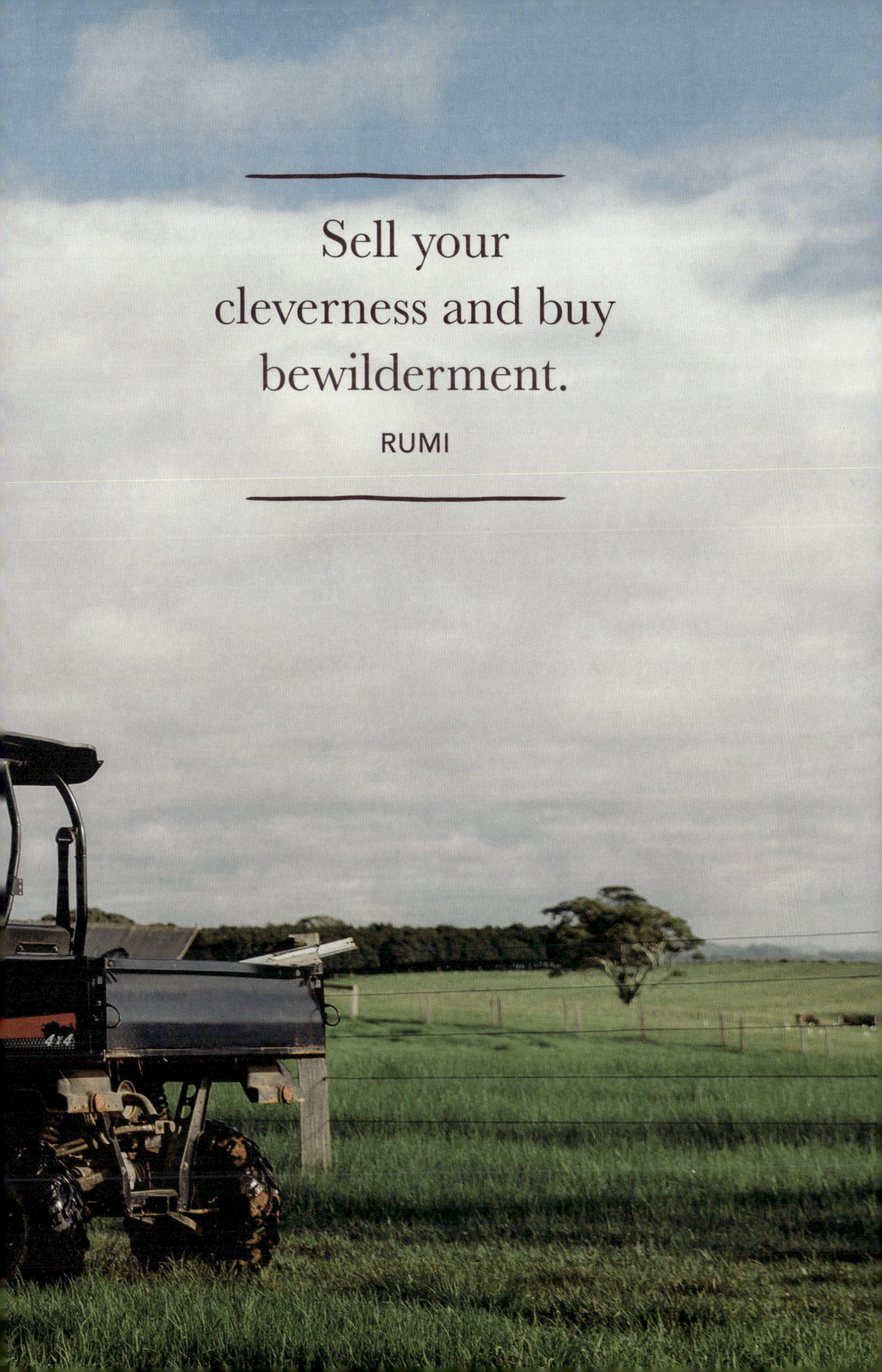

Sell your cleverness and buy bewilderment.

RUMI

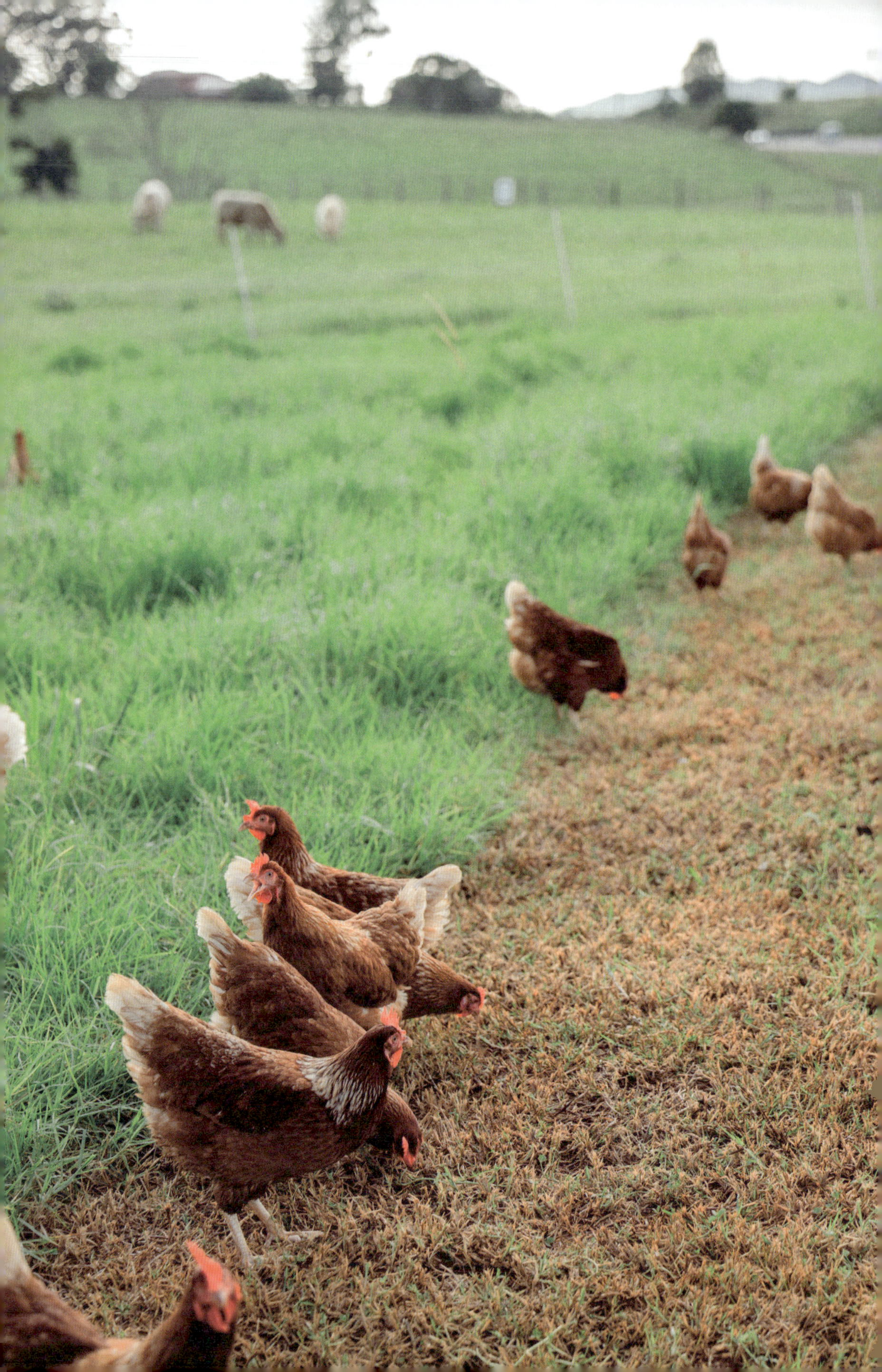

Reducing rigidity

NUTRITION POLARISES PEOPLE

Significantly increasing the plant content of your diet is a powerful way to boost the nutrient density essential to great health, vitality and shine. So what about meat and fish? Nutrition polarises people. We all eat and therefore we all have our own opinions about what makes up a healthy diet. I always encourage people to eat in a way that nourishes their body, mind and soul, and for some this means following a vegetarian or vegan diet.

However, many people choose to eat meat and/or fish and describe feeling more nourished when they include it in their diet. My message to you is simple: eat the real food that nourishes you. Be rigid with your eating if, and only if, that serves you and/or the planet, depending on your beliefs (or a health condition). For example, if you feel deep in your heart that living a vegan lifestyle is right for you, then be true to that. Be sure, however, that you are getting optimum amounts of vitamin B_{12}, iron and zinc in particular (refer to chapter on Micro-nourishment on page 69 for more about this).

A concept that might assist you to find a high quality yet flexible way of eating is what I call having a "flexitarian" approach. I want to guide you to be in touch with what your body needs, not what your head tells you you want, or what a rule you created for yourself, possibly years ago, dictates, if this rule no longer serves you or the planet. A flexible approach enables you to nourish your body with what it needs, when it needs it. For example, there will be days when you feel that a meal that includes potato will nourish you beautifully, whereas there may be other days when you feel that potato won't serve you; you may feel like you will feel tired after eating it. But if you have a rule that says, for example, carbs after 3pm are bad, then you won't eat potato for dinner, no matter how much your body needs what they offer.

I find more and more people also define themselves using how they eat as a descriptor: "I'm a vegan", for example. And I have met countless people who judge others for how they choose to eat, if it is different from their own way. Yet judgement does not serve your health, or the planet, or anyone you meet, in any way. Eat in a way that feels right for you and allow others to do the same.

> If you eat meat, opt for grass-fed, free-range and organic.

If you eat meat, opt for grass-fed, free-range and organic. I appreciate that these options may cost more. However, in my opinion, and based on my observation of people's diets over the past two decades, many people would benefit from reducing their portion sizes of meat. A fist-sized portion is a rough guide for a main meal. Organic lamb, for example, provides protein and vitamin B_{12}, as well as the minerals iron and zinc in highly bioavailable forms, which means the body is able to utilise the minerals easily.

When it comes to seafood we experience a great divide in opinions again. Understandably, there is reason for concern about including seafood in your diet, as more information is emerging about heavy-metal contamination. Reducing your exposure to mercury is essential. If you eat fish, it is best to choose small, white fish, which have a lower risk of mercury contamination. Small fish are also a better choice because they have had less exposure and time to accumulate mercury. However, remember that having good zinc levels in your body is critical for your body to be able to detoxify and excrete any heavy metals that you are exposed to, such as through air pollution from cars' exhaust fumes.

Fish is an example of a nutrient dense food. Besides containing protein and nutrients such as selenium and vitamin D, fish also contains the anti-inflammatory omega-3 fatty acids. Clinically, omega-3 fatty acids have been shown to reduce the risk of developing many degenerative diseases, including heart disease. Fish can also supply the body with DHA, an omega-3 fatty acid that is beneficial for brain development, so it is particularly important for pregnant women and breastfeeding mothers. Flaxseeds (linseeds) are high in another omega-3 fatty acid known as ALA. The human body can convert ALA into EPA and DHA, a process that is upregulated during pregnancy. Again, I encourage you to eat what nourishes you. Just be sure to include some omega-3-rich foods.

Note that the way some fish and seafood are farmed now is having detrimental impacts on the environment, so again I encourage you to seek out wild and sustainable seafood. The more questions you ask, the better.

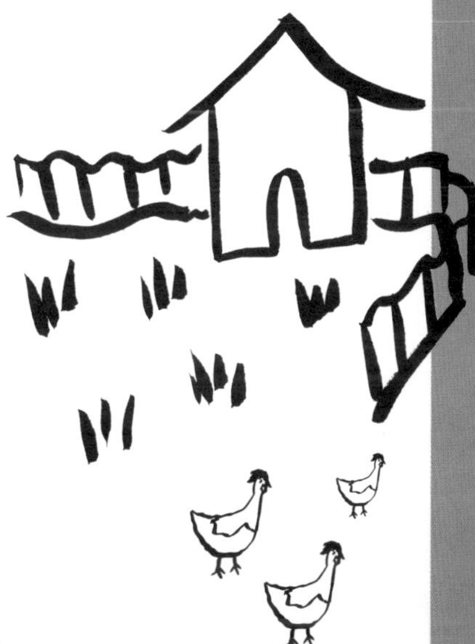

If you eat chicken, purchasing organic chicken is highly recommended. Organically grown chickens have been fed an organic diet and have been raised without the use of antibiotics. Free-range chickens have been allowed access to the outdoors, as opposed to being confined to the henhouse, with some producers also feeding them an organic diet. Chicken is a good source of protein and also contains niacin (vitamin B_3), which helps the body convert food into fuel (energy). Additionally, niacin is involved in the production of the sex and stress hormones in the adrenal glands. It also contains methionine, an amino acid involved in mood regulation and the maintenance of our DNA.

If yours has been a "meat with every meal" household up until now, consider starting "meatless Mondays", and eat only plant-based foods that day.

Once you and/or family members/housemates experience the taste sensation of a vegetable-based meal you like (try some from the *Real Food Chef, Real Food Kitchen* or *The Energy Guide*), you may find that three vegetarian meals per week becomes an easy option. Keep in mind too, the recommendations from the most respected source of cancer prevention research and information, the World Cancer Research Fund (WCRF), states "limit your intake of red meat to no more than 500 grams per week, and avoid processed meat".

See the piece Nutrition Conundrums on page 217 for more about this. Don't go meatless if it is not your thing and if meat nourishes you, which it does for many. Have consideration for how the animals were raised though, both their nourishment and how they were cared for. Butchers will know about this much more than a supermarket, or read the labels on the meat in the supermarket.

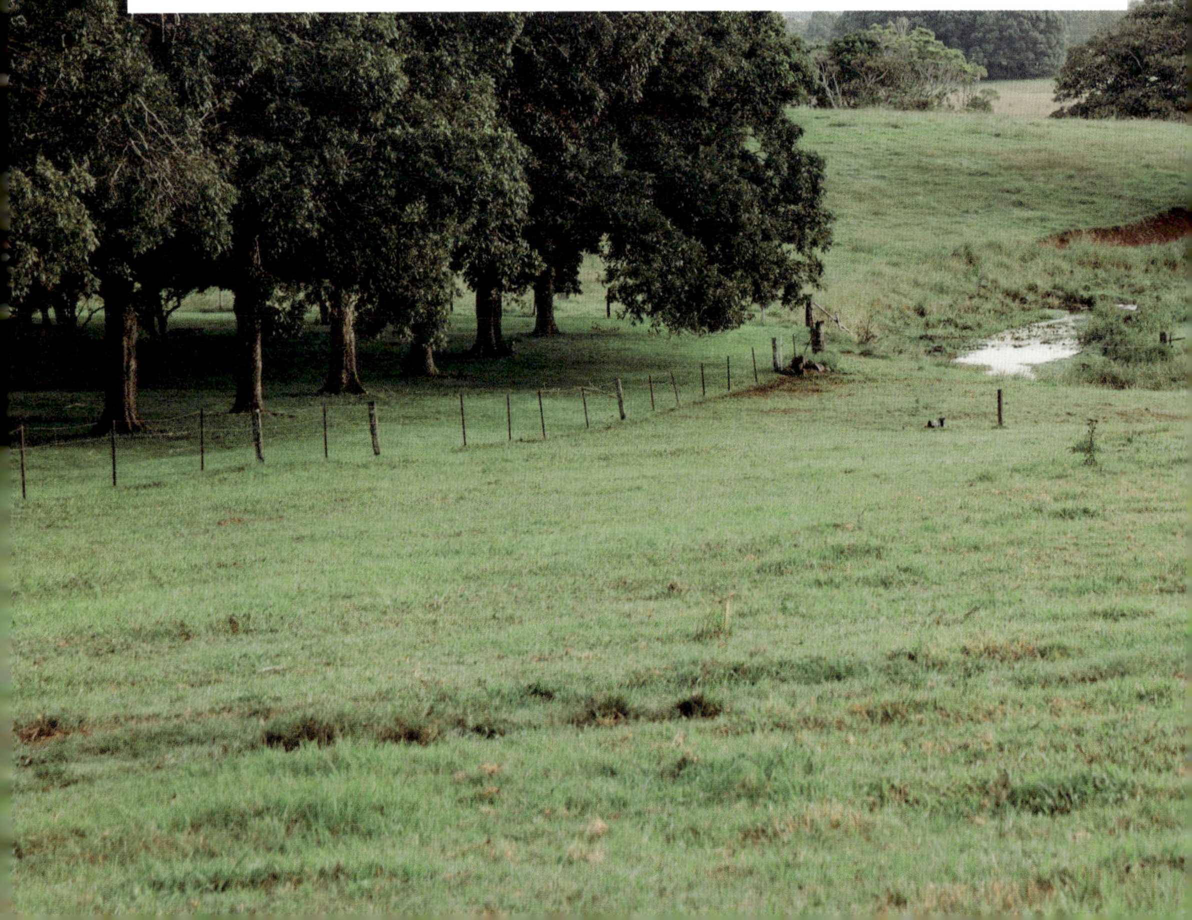

No act of kindness,
no matter how small,
is ever wasted.

AESOP

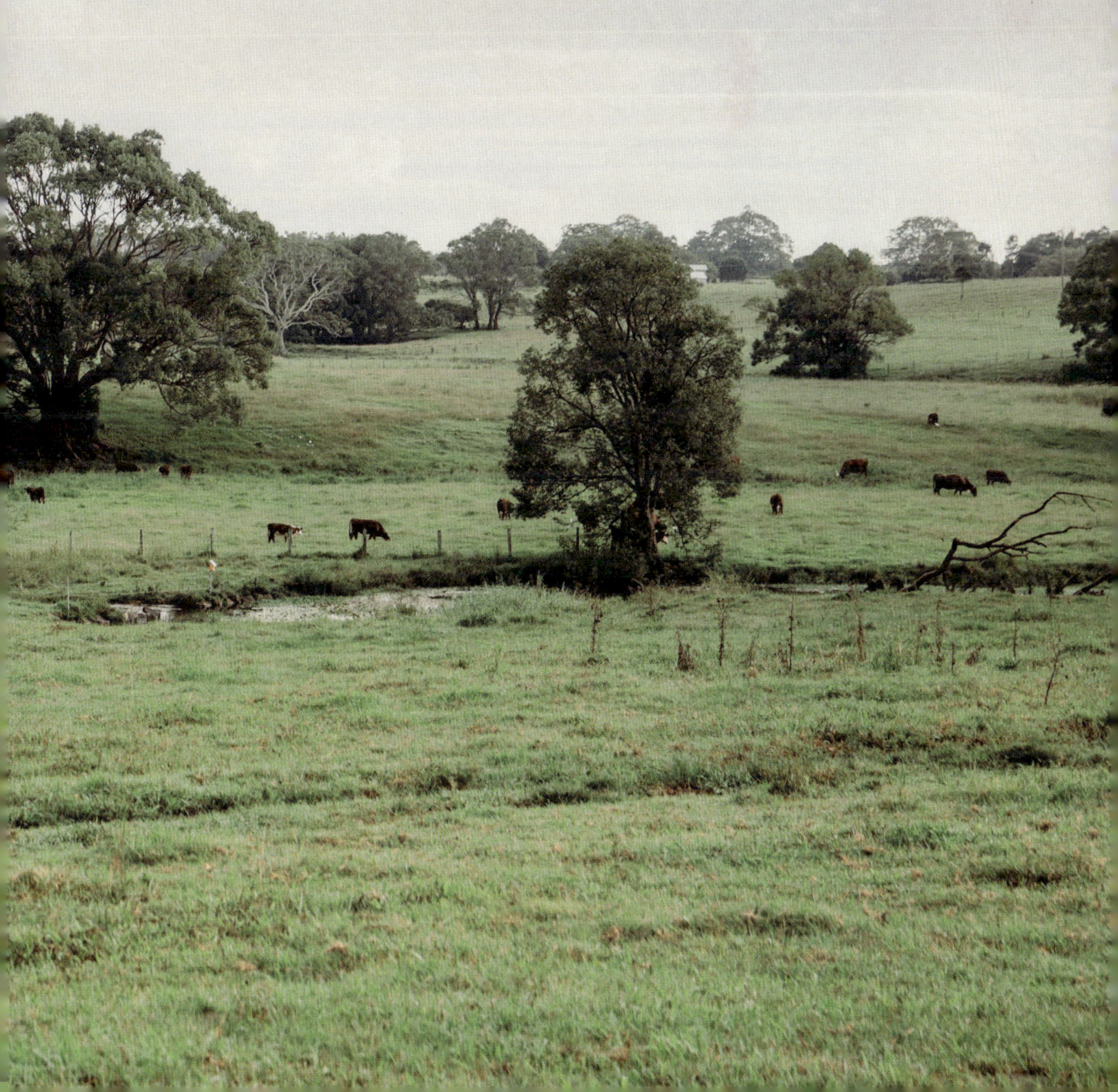

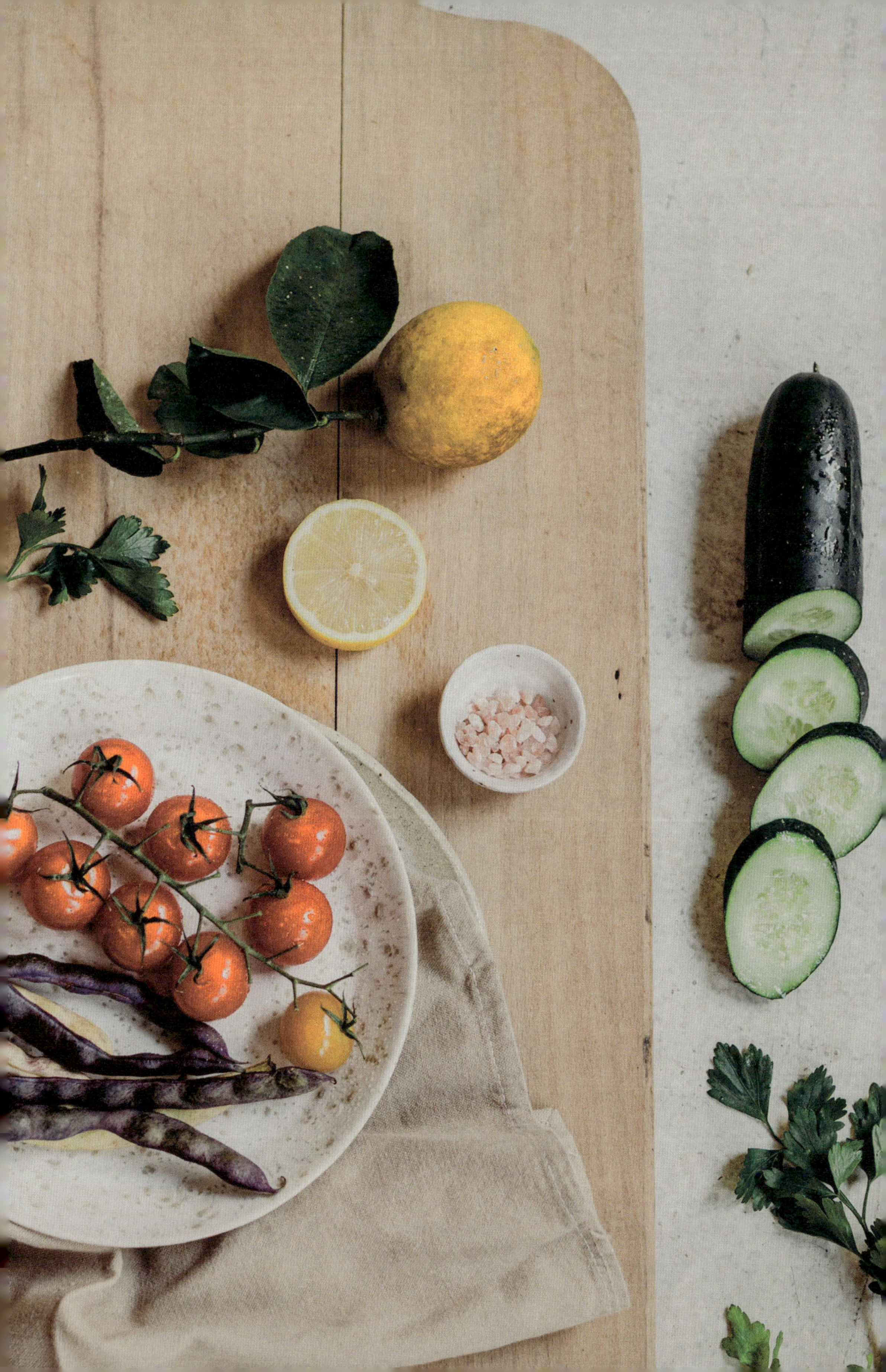

Superfoods: nutritious or trends?

WHEN FASHION GUIDES YOUR FOOD

Every week, you can read about a new food being touted as the latest 'superfood'. Everything from goji berries to açaí berries, from soy (yes, it was once referred to as a 'superfood') to spirulina, have had their names up in lights. Essentially all real, whole foods have superstar properties, offering you vitamins, minerals and substances unique to those foods that the body needs to thrive.

The problems with labelling certain foods as superfoods include that too many people falsely believe they can eat as much of these foods as they like, such as is occurring with the daily açaí bowl craze at the moment. Beyond that, though, consider that when something becomes labelled as a 'superfood' in the West, indigenous communities can suffer. For example, when quinoa surged in popularity, some South American populations were left without one of their staple traditional foods and prices soared. Many farmers were also not paid what they deserved and a host of sad situations arose. We need to think beyond our own desires and lives when we are making repetitive food choices to consider how our choices impact others.

For me, all whole and real foods are super. Humble parsley, lemons, spinach...the list is almost endless.

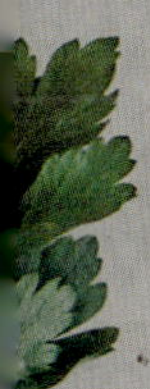

Food is nourishment

WHERE ARE YOU GETTING YOUR NUTRIENTS FROM?

Our food is the only way our body gets the nutrients it needs to keep us alive. Pause for a moment and really consider that it is nutrients that fuel the millions of biochemical processes inside of us that keep us healthy. From providing us with energy to healing that tiny cut on our finger, our food choices impact everything our body does.

This table is to remind you why it is good to choose a wide variety of whole, real foods — as opposed to processed foods, which often have very few nutrients.

In order to get back in touch with your body's innate wisdom that knows what you need to eat for your health, begin making more of your food choices based on the signs and symptoms your body is giving you. This table helps by listing the nutrients found in an array of whole foods, so you can choose what to focus on based on what it provides your body. For example, if you suffer with cramps, you might like to increase your food sources of magnesium, so you might choose to have some almonds, kale and spinach across your day.

This list is not exhaustive. Some of the foods listed here have additional nutrients and health benefits, and of course there are thousands of other nutrient dense whole real foods that are not listed here. Simply use this as a guide to assist your food choices.

Almonds

CONTAINS

Vitamin E, calcium, magnesium
B-group vitamins

ASSISTS YOUR BODY

Antioxidants, skin health, bone health, heart health, energy

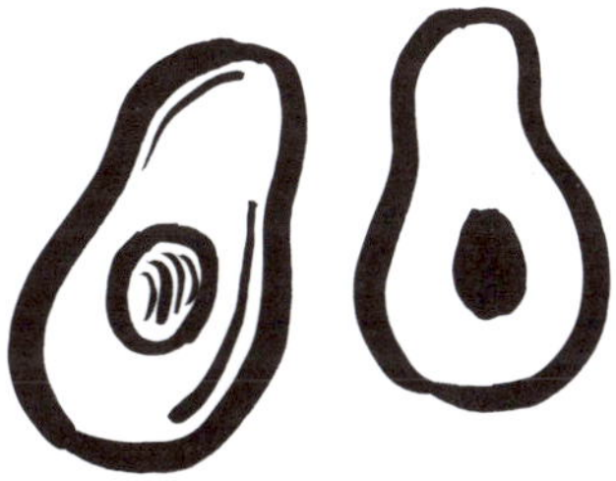

Avocado

CONTAINS

Vitamin E, monounsaturated fats, B-group vitamins, fibre

ASSISTS YOUR BODY

Antioxidants, skin health, energy, gut health

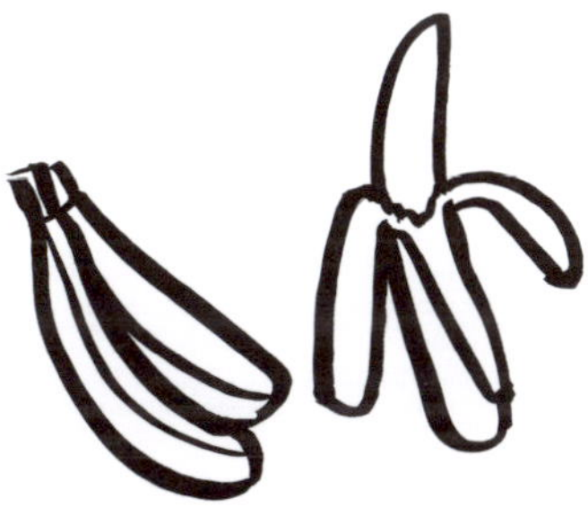

Bananas

CONTAINS

B-group vitamins, vitamin C, potassium, magnesium

ASSISTS YOUR BODY

Energy, antioxidants, fluid/electrolyte balance, neurotransmitter production

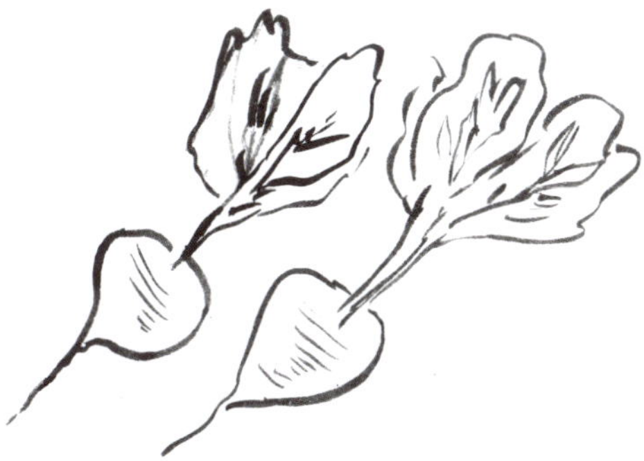

Beetroot

CONTAINS

Nitrates, folate, phytonutrients (betalains)

ASSISTS YOUR BODY

Improves physical performance, lowers blood pressure, antioxidants, healthy cell production

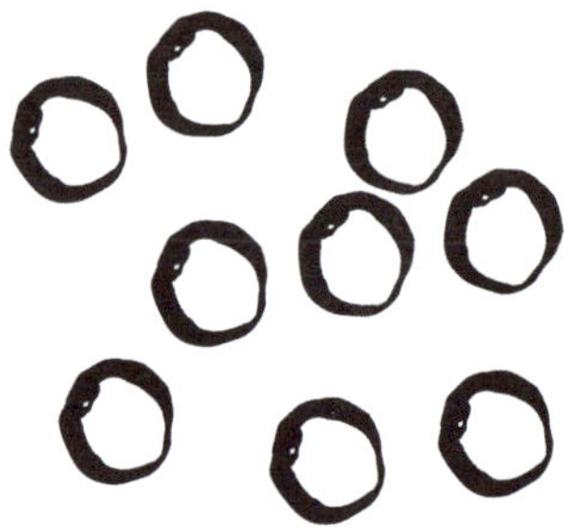

Berries

CONTAINS

Vitamin C, flavonoids

ASSISTS YOUR BODY

Antioxidants, anti-inflammatory actions

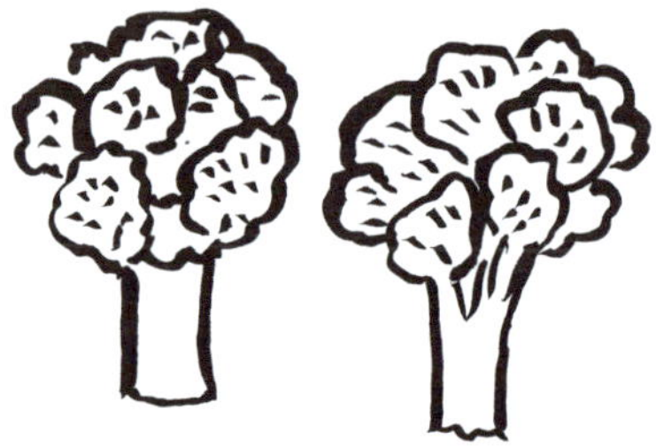

Broccoli

CONTAINS

Vitamin C, calcium, B-group vitamins, sulforaphane, indoles

ASSISTS YOUR BODY

Antioxidants, bone health, energy, liver detoxification, anti-inflammatory actions, healthy estrogen metabolism

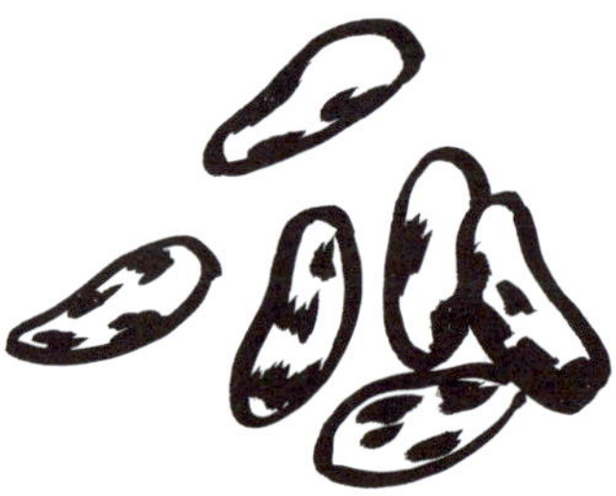

Brazil nuts

CONTAINS

Selenium, nourishing fats

ASSISTS YOUR BODY

Healthy thyroid function, antioxidants, immune function

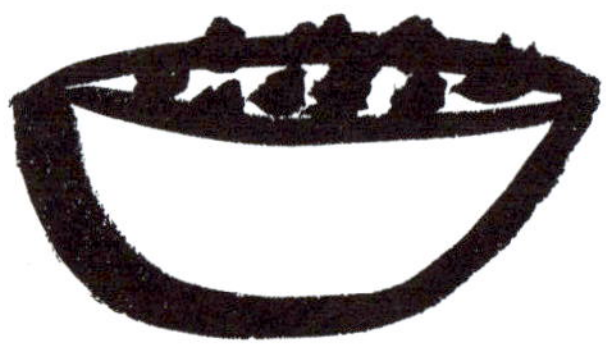

Brown rice

CONTAINS

B-group vitamins, magnesium, vitamin E

ASSISTS YOUR BODY

Energy, electrolyte balance, antioxidants

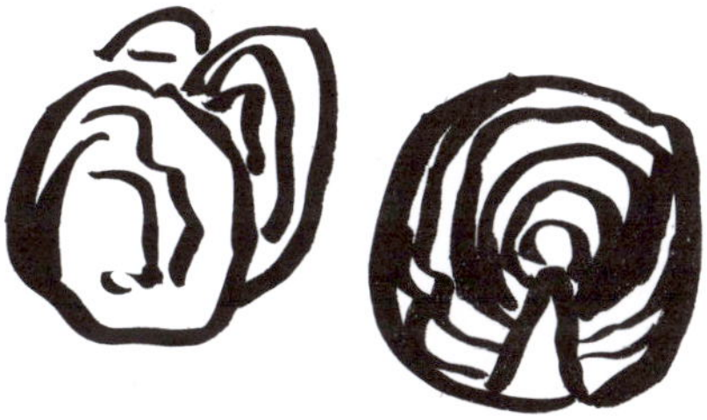

Cabbage

CONTAINS

Sulforaphane, vitamin C, vitamin K, carotenoids

ASSISTS YOUR BODY

Liver detoxification, antioxidants, blood clotting

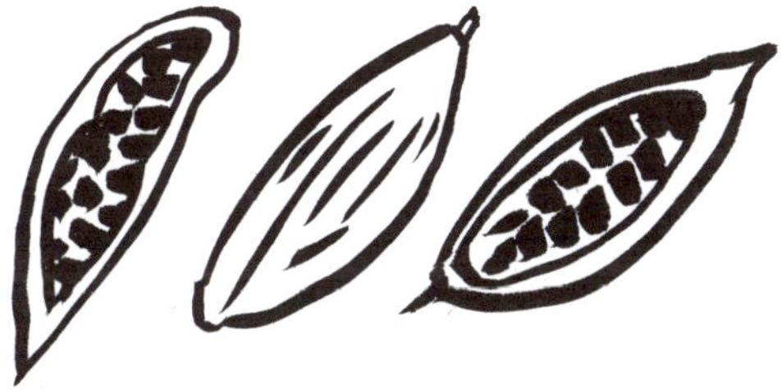

Cacao

CONTAINS

Magnesium, flavonoids

ASSISTS YOUR BODY

Muscle relaxation, healthy nervous system function, antioxidants, heart health

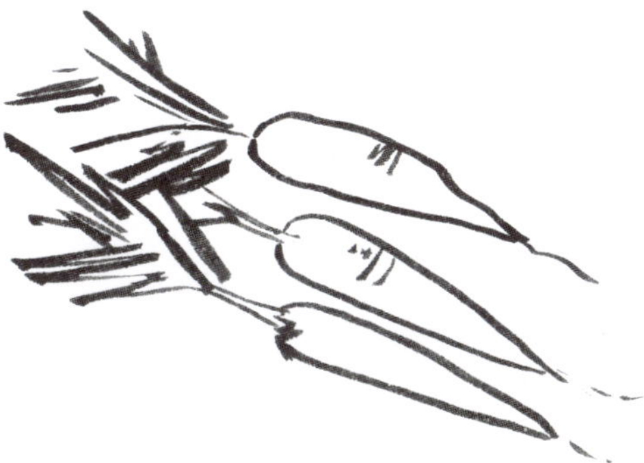

Carrots

CONTAINS

Beta-carotene (vitamin A), potassium

ASSISTS YOUR BODY

Eye health, antioxidants, electrolyte balance

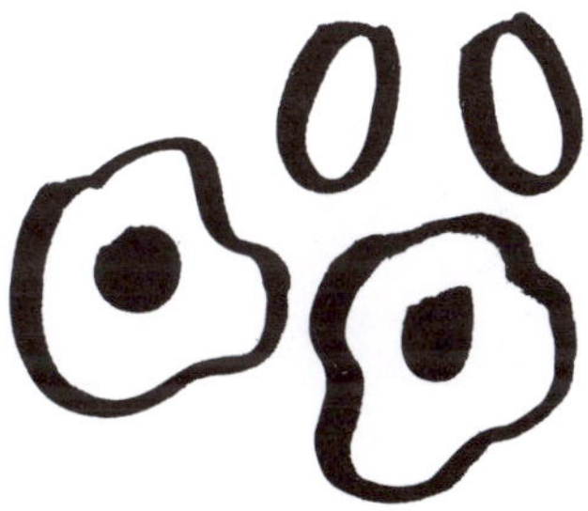

Eggs

CONTAINS

B-group vitamins (including B_{12}), iron, vitamin A, vitamin E, selenium, carotenoids (lutein, zeaxanthin), protein

ASSISTS YOUR BODY

Energy, blood oxygenation, antioxidants, eye health, skin health, healthy thyroid function

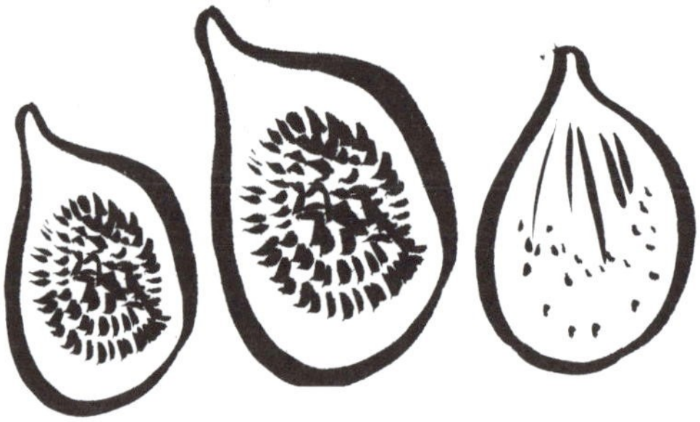

Figs

CONTAINS

Calcium, magnesium, fibre

ASSISTS YOUR BODY

Bone health, electrolyte balance, gut health

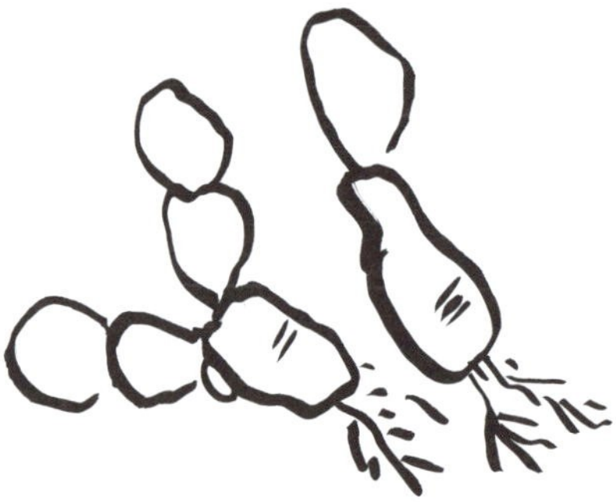

Ginger

CONTAINS

Phytonutrients

ASSISTS YOUR BODY

Antioxidants, anti-inflammatory actions, immune function, eases nausea

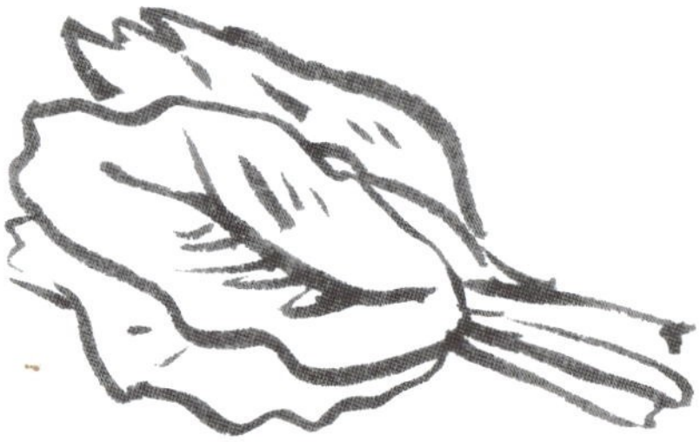

Kale

CONTAINS

Sulforaphane, vitamin C, vitamin K, B-group vitamins, iron, calcium, magnesium, carotenoids (lutein, zeaxanthin)

ASSISTS YOUR BODY

Liver detoxification, antioxidants, blood clotting, energy, blood oxygenation, bone health, eye health

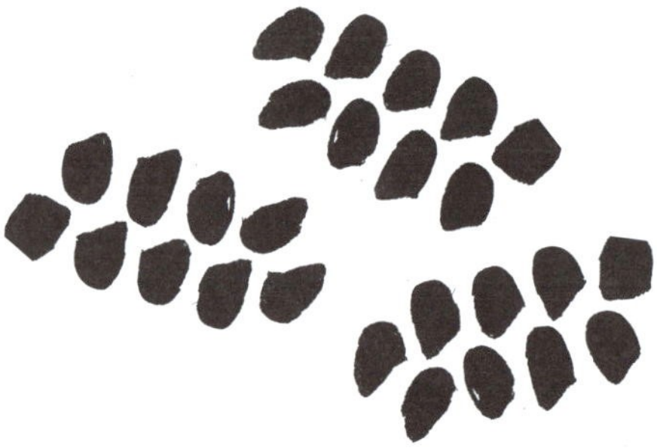

Legumes
(e.g. black beans/chickpeas)

CONTAINS

Iron, folate, fibre, B-group vitamins, magnesium, protein

ASSISTS YOUR BODY

Blood oxygenation, protects against DNA damage, healthy gut flora, energy

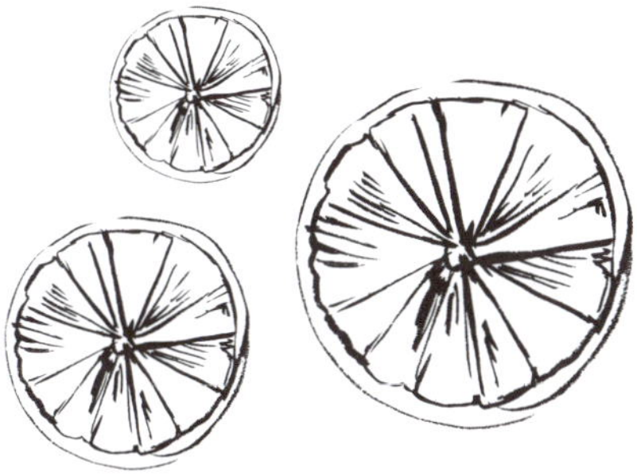

Lemons

CONTAINS

Vitamin C, citric acid

ASSISTS YOUR BODY

Antioxidants, enhances iron absorption, stomach acid production

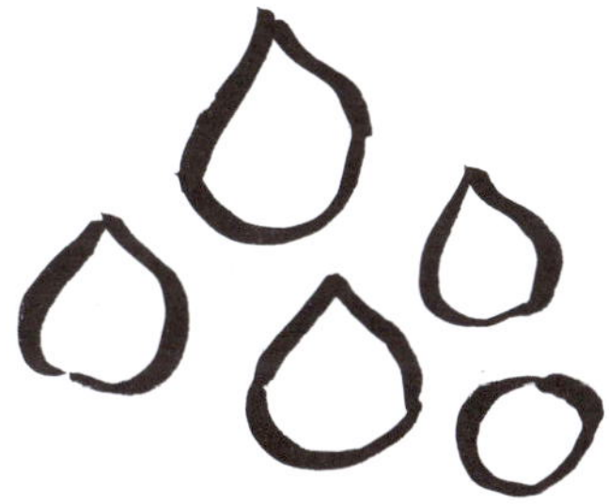

Macadamia nuts

CONTAINS

Monounsaturated fats, vitamin E, magnesium

ASSISTS YOUR BODY

Skin health, heart health, antioxidants

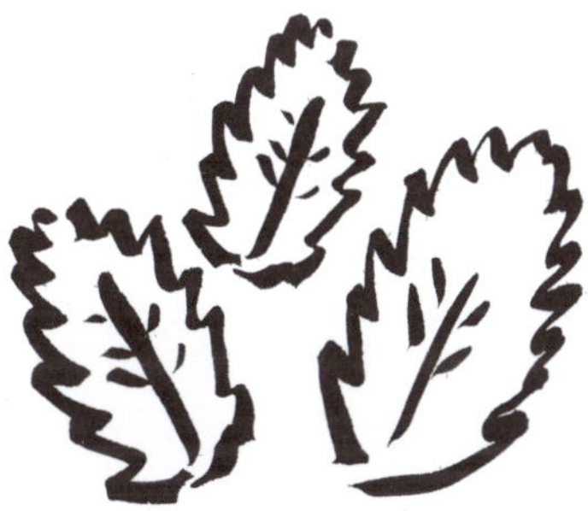

Mint

CONTAINS

Vitamin C, carotenoids, flavonoids

ASSISTS YOUR BODY

Antioxidants, eases digestive discomfort

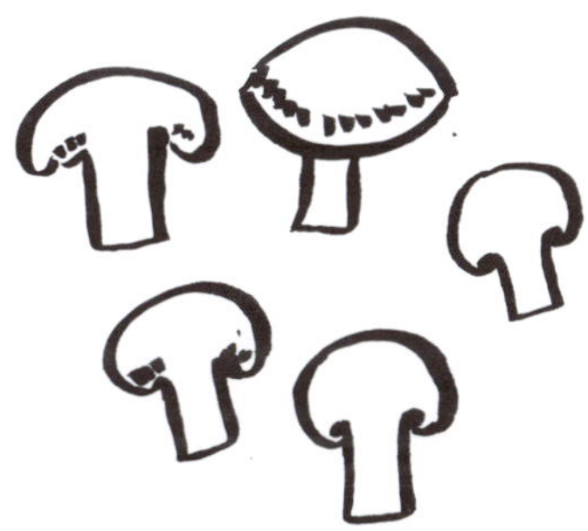

Mushrooms

CONTAINS

Vitamin D (if exposed to sun), B-group vitamins

ASSISTS YOUR BODY

Immune function, bone health, energy

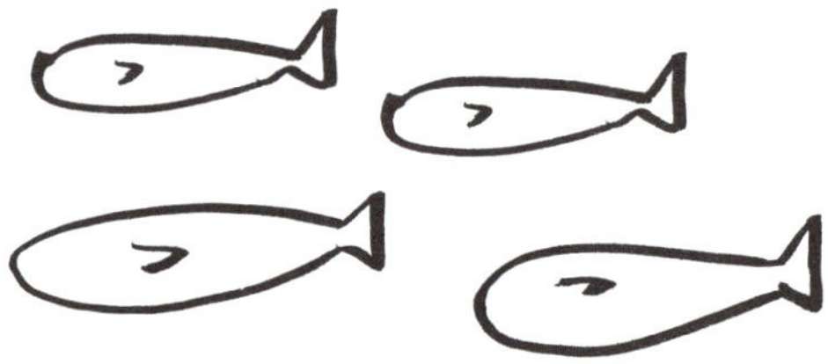

Oily fresh fish

CONTAINS

Omega-3 fatty acids (DHA), selenium, iodine, protein

ASSISTS YOUR BODY

Anti-inflammatory actions, heart health, brain health, antioxidants, healthy thyroid function

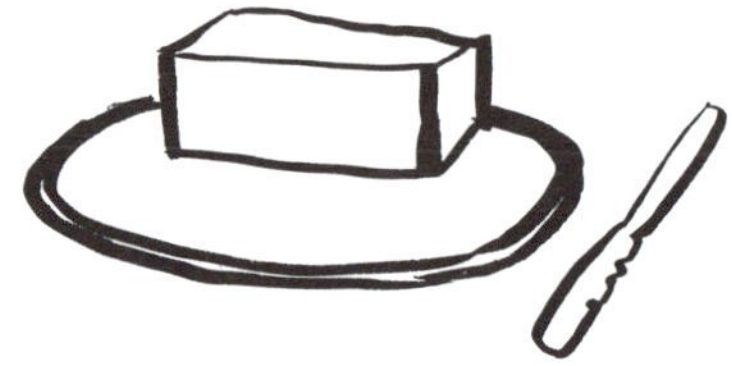

Organic butter

CONTAINS

Lauric acid, vitamin A, medium chain triglycerides (MCTs), conjugated linoleic acid (CLA)

ASSISTS YOUR BODY

Antibacterial and antifungal action, anti-inflammatory actions, antioxidants, satiety

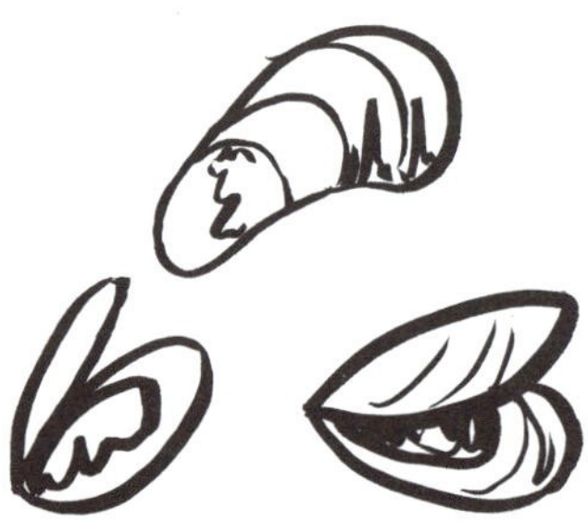

Oysters

CONTAINS

Zinc, omega-3 fatty acids, iodine, selenium, iron

ASSISTS YOUR BODY

Sex hormone production, anti-inflammatory actions, healthy thyroid function, blood oxygenation

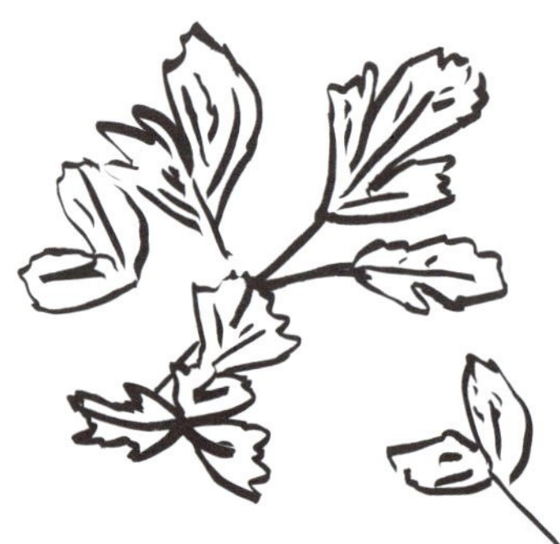

Parsley

CONTAINS

Vitamin C, iron, carotenoids, vitamin K

ASSISTS YOUR BODY

Antioxidants, anti-inflammatory actions, blood oxygenation, eye health, blood clotting

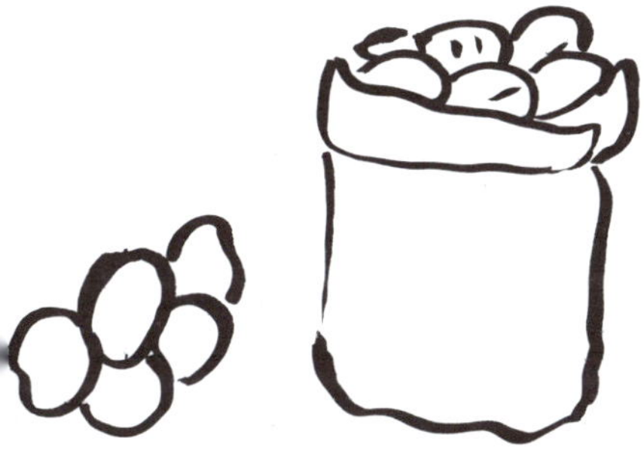

Potatoes

CONTAINS

Vitamin C, potassium

ASSISTS YOUR BODY

Antioxidants,
fluid/electrolyte balance

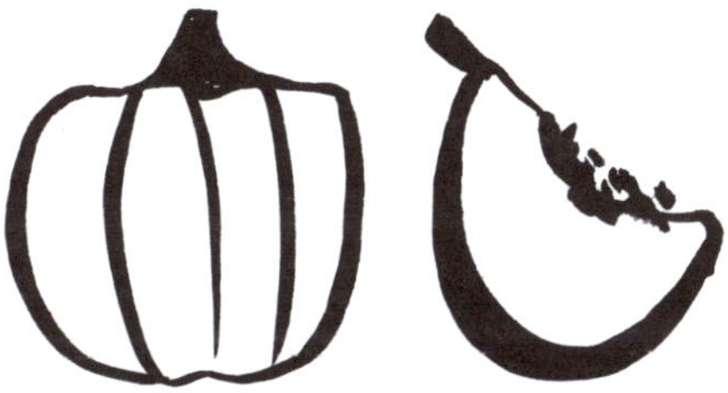

Pumpkin

CONTAINS

Beta-carotene (vitamin A), lutein, zeaxanthin, B-group vitamins

ASSISTS YOUR BODY

Eye health, energy, antioxidants

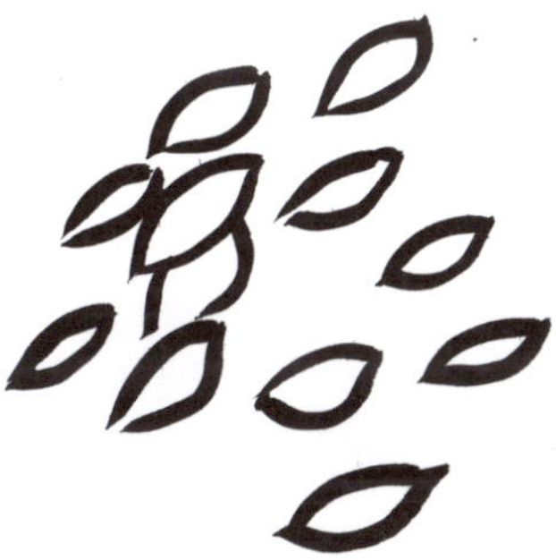

Pumpkin seeds

CONTAINS

Zinc, nourishing fats, magnesium

ASSISTS YOUR BODY

Healthy skin, sex hormone production, nervous system function

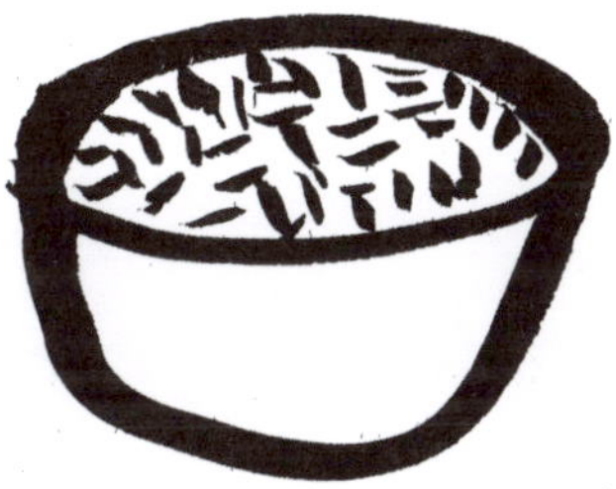

Quinoa

CONTAINS

B-group vitamins, plant-based protein, fibre

ASSISTS YOUR BODY

Energy, gut health

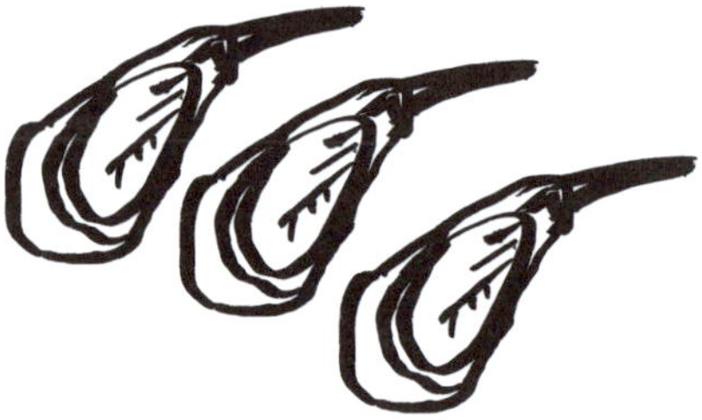

Red meat

CONTAINS

Iron, zinc, vitamin B_{12}, protein

ASSISTS YOUR BODY

Blood oxygenation, healthy reproductive function, muscle maintenance

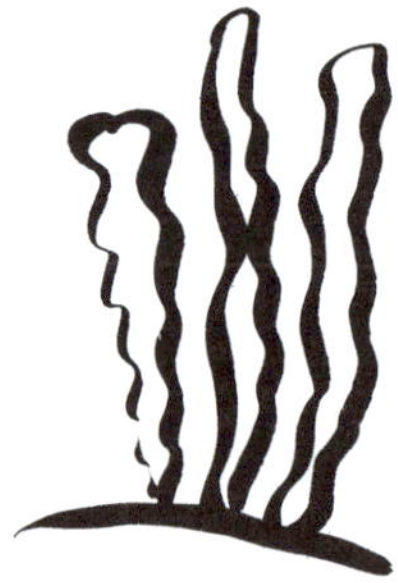

Seaweed

CONTAINS

Iodine, magnesium

ASSISTS YOUR BODY

Healthy thyroid function, fertility, nervous system function

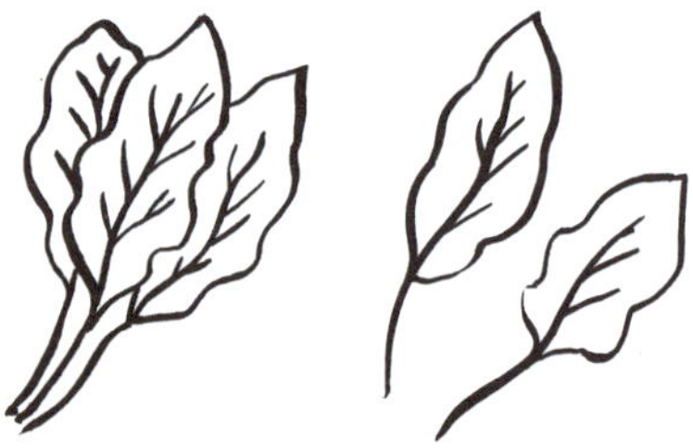

Spinach

CONTAINS

Folate, calcium, magnesium, phosphorus, vitamin C, carotenoids (vitamin A), B-group vitamins

ASSISTS YOUR BODY

Antioxidants, protects against DNA damage, energy, bone health, eye health

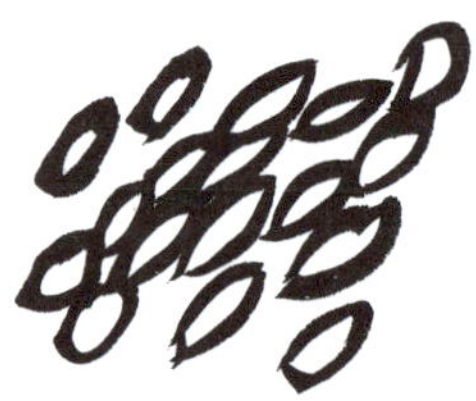

Sunflower seeds

CONTAINS

Vitamin E, zinc, magnesium

ASSISTS YOUR BODY

Protects skin, antioxidants, electrolyte balance, immune function, wound healing

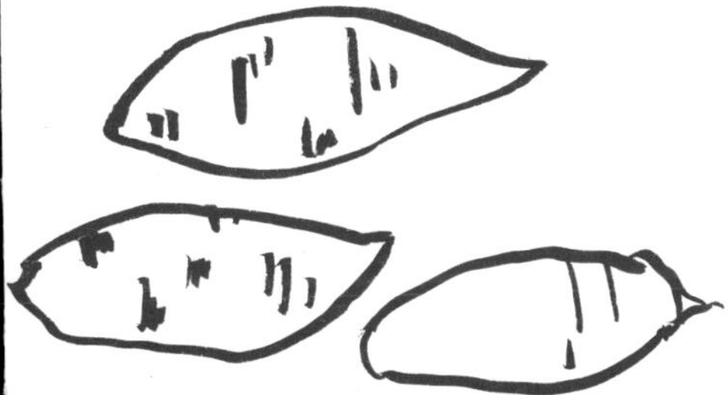

Sweet potatoes

CONTAINS

Beta-carotene (vitamin A), vitamin C, potassium

ASSISTS YOUR BODY

Antioxidants, eye health, electrolyte balance

Tomatoes

CONTAINS

Lycopene, carotenoids (vitamin A), vitamin C

ASSISTS YOUR BODY

Antioxidants, heart health, skin health

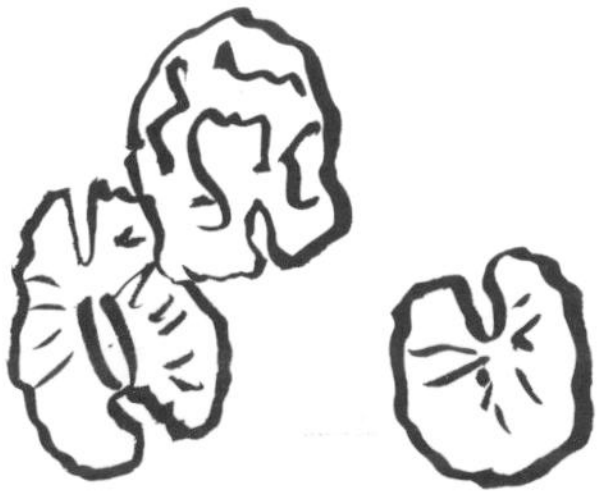

Walnuts

CONTAINS

Omega-3 fatty acids, vitamin E, magnesium, B-group vitamins

ASSISTS YOUR BODY

Anti-inflammatory actions, antioxidants, heart health, nervous system function, energy

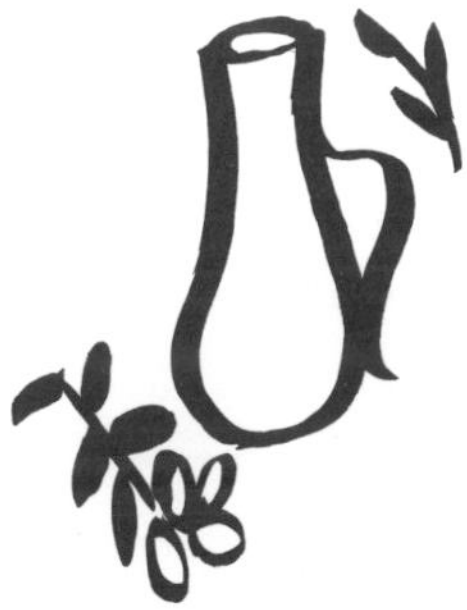

Extra Virgin Olive Oil

CONTAINS

Vitamin E, nourishing fats, phytonutrients

ASSISTS YOUR BODY

Antioxidants, anti-inflammatory actions, heart health, skin health, increases absorption of fat soluble vitamins

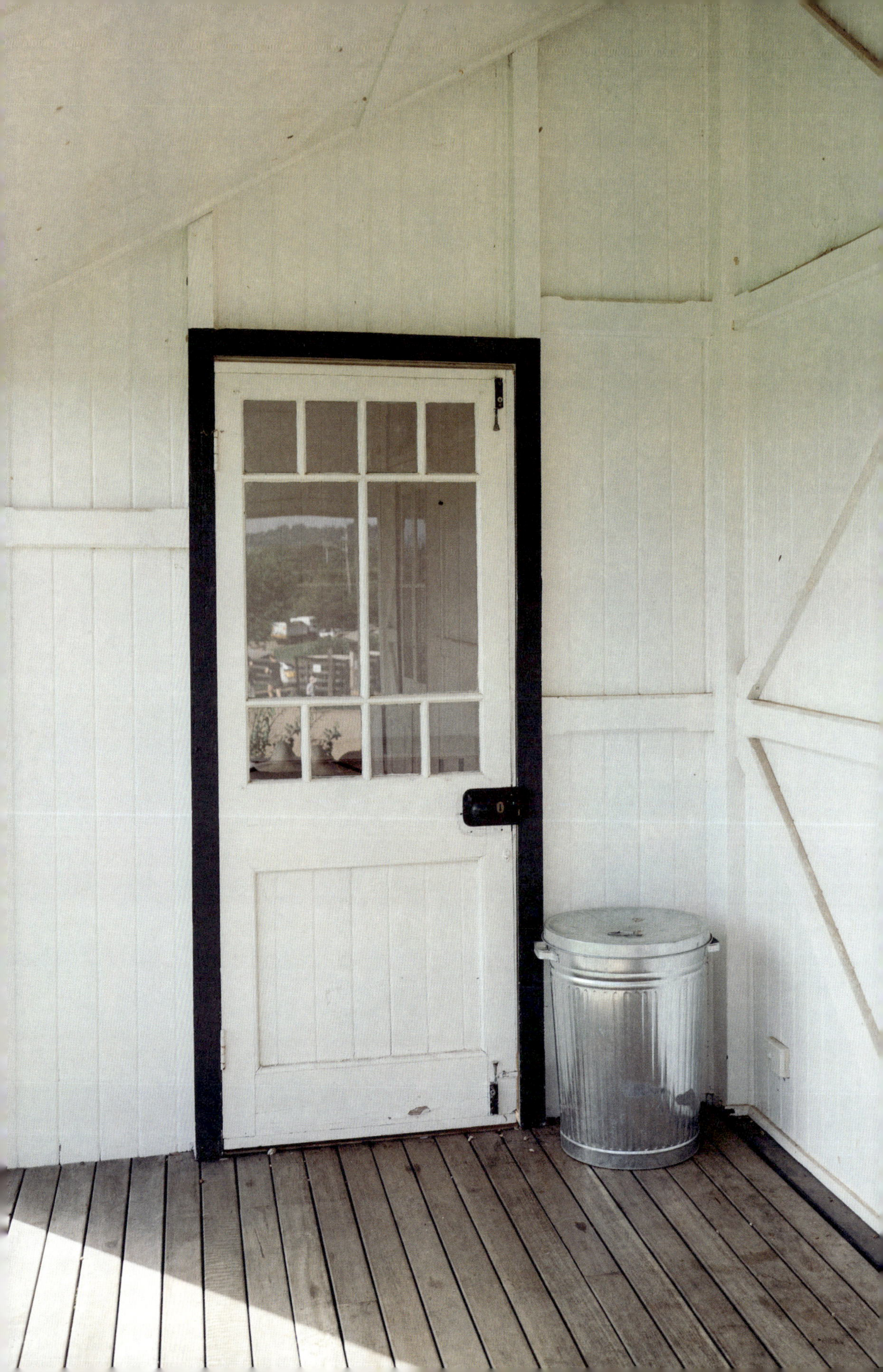

Don't be misled

GETTING WISE TO HIDDEN RUBBISH

My focus in guiding someone back into the driver's seat of making their own food choices is always on what to include, what to eat more of: whole, real food. However, for those for whom making nutritious food choices is somewhat new, I have included a list of ingredients — notice I didn't say foods — that are best minimised, in how you eat. It's not an "avoid" list. It is not a wagon to fall off. It is simply to increase your awareness of some of the poorer quality items that can end up in the food supply that are better off minimised.

On a food label, the first ingredient is in the highest concentration in the product. Ingredients are then listed in descending order.

It is best to eat whole, real food. Yet there are also some better or sometimes even nutritious choices that can be made from packaged foods. For example, you might buy hummus. Most of them contain preservatives; few, however, don't — choose those brands.

Do you think preservatives are added to food to assist your health in any way? No. They are there to extend shelf life. So how do preservatives do that? By preventing bacterial growth.

Yet you have three to four kilograms of bacteria living in your large intestine, which are essential to every aspect of your health, including your immune function, your mood, your sleep, not to mention your digestion. As we don't know the long-term effects on our gut bacteria of eating foods that contain preservatives, they are likely best avoided.

Added sugars that are best minimised:

- agave nectar
- agave syrup
- Barbados sugar
- barley malt
- barley malt syrup
- beet sugar
- blackstrap molasses*
- brown sugar
- brown rice sugar
- buttered syrup
- cane juice
- cane juice crystals
- cane sugar
- caramel
- carob syrup
- castor sugar
- coconut palm sugar*
- coconut sugar*
- coffee sugar
- coffee crystals
- confectioner's sugar
- corn sweetener
- corn syrup
- corn syrup solids
- date sugar
- dehydrated cane juice
- demerara sugar
- dextrin
- dextrose
- evaporated cane juice
- free-flowing brown sugars
- fructose
- fruit juice
- fruit juice concentrate
- glucose
- glucose solids
- golden sugar
- golden syrup
- grape sugar
- HFCS (high-fructose corn syrup)
- honey*
- icing sugar
- invert sugar
- lactose
- loaf sugar
- malt syrup
- maltodextrin
- maltol
- maltose
- mannose
- maple syrup*
- molasses*
- muscovado
- palm sugar
- panocha
- powdered sugar
- raw sugar
- refiner's syrup
- rice syrup
- rice malt syrup
- saccharose
- sorghum syrup
- sucrose
- sugar (granulated)
- sweet sorghum
- syrup
- treacle
- turbinado sugar
- white sugar
- yellow sugar

These choices above contain some nutrients — and are therefore somewhat better choices. It is still best to minimise how much of these you consume.

~~950~~ ~~220~~

~~212~~ ~~952~~

~~682~~

Ingredients best minimised:

- hydrolysed soy protein, soy isolates
- hydrolysed whey
- palm oil
- nitrites
- canola oil (also called rapeseed oil)
- thickeners
- concentrated fruit juice
- pesticides
- trans fat — found in processed cakes, biscuits, muesli bars, pastries and take-away foods
- preservatives (many of these are listed as numbers in the 200s)
- additives
- MSG (number 621)
- poor quality salt
- tinned tomatoes (due to acid stripping the lining of the tin, and the lining is plastic) — it is better to buy them in glass jars, usually called "tomato passata"
- artificial sweeteners
- unspecified "vegetable" fats.

OTHER THINGS TO CONSIDER MINIMISING INCLUDE:

- anything you can't pronounce
- numbers in general
- foods that are designed/ manufactured to live for a long time
- foods that make your body feel uncomfortable after you eat them
- too much fruit: don't be a fruit bat, or if you are craving lots of fruit look at what this might be about — the nutrients in certain fruits or sugar craving
- cold, raw food during winter
- fads and diets or mono-eating — living off five foods
- food heated in plastic
- lollies
- food that you know in your heart don't serve you
- eating because you "should" (no matter the day/time/occasion)
- foods that repeat on you, no matter how 'nutritious' they are
- food that is not in season
- food that has travelled a long way; consider the carbon miles, and the age from picking, which leads to a decrease in nutrients
- meat, if you don't know how it was grown or what it was fed or how the animals were treated.

EXCLUSIONARY OR MINIMISING DIETS

However, beyond minimising processed foods due to the lack of nutrients they typically contain and substances some of them contain that we are not able to break down (or may even harm us if we consume them regularly and long term), some people need to avoid some whole and real foods. Or they may need to avoid certain substances that are naturally present in whole, real foods.

There are chemicals naturally present in foods — that is how they have flavour. The names of some food chemicals include phenolic compounds (high in sulphur) and amines (typically in aged foods).

LOW FODMAP DIET

Research has shown that some people with IBS benefit from what is known as a low FODMAP way of eating, which minimises the intake of substances that will ferment in the gut. FODMAP is an acronym for Fermentable Oligosaccharides (such as fructans), Disaccharides (such as lactose), Monosaccharides (such as fructose) and Polyols (such as xylitol). These are substances that in some people are poorly absorbed and if so, they can lead to some of the symptoms of IBS. In my experience, for some people this needs to be low in all of the FODMAP components, while for others, for example, they only need to avoid onion, garlic and apples. An experienced nutrition professional can guide you with the details of this if it is something you feel you need to explore.

SUGAR

Table sugar comes from sugar cane, but it is refined (processed) 14 times before it gets to your table or into your food. All of the nutrients that were originally in the sugar cane juice — B vitamins and magnesium, for example — are destroyed in that process, leaving zero nutrition in sugar.

Refined sugars don't serve anyone's health. If you haven't done so already, I suggest you get them really low or omit them from how you eat. It's essential to every body system inside you.

GLUTEN AND DAIRY

Some people feel better without including gluten-containing grains in what they eat, or even all grains. Others feel better without dairy foods. Some both. How do you work this out?

Having worked with people one on one for two decades, here are the clues that I use to guide me to guide you...

A gluten-free way of eating may be trialled for four to eight weeks if you have:

- an autoimmune disease or elevated autoantibodies

- Irish heritage
- gut-based symptoms or a gut-central disease, or
- unexplained fatigue, dry skin, hair and nails, and a tendency to constipation.

A dairy-free way of eating may be trialled for four to eight weeks if you:

- have a history of recurrent (or current) Streptococcus-based infections, such as tonsillitis, ear infections, chest infections, bronchitis
- have a history of (or current) eczema
- have chronic sinus problems
- clear your throat constantly
- have recurring excessive flatulence with an offensive odour, or
- mostly breathe through your mouth.

Considering these guidelines, is there a dietary trial you are keen to undertake to see how you feel and what symptoms may resolve as a result?

You need to keep in mind that the trial is only four to eight weeks out of your very long life and it may offer you great insight into your health, or not. If you continue with this way of eating beyond eight weeks, it is essential that you consult an experienced nutrition professional to ensure you are meeting your nutritional requirements.

When you arise in the morning,
think of what a precious privilege
it is to be alive – to breathe,
to think, to enjoy, to love.

MARCUS AURELIUS

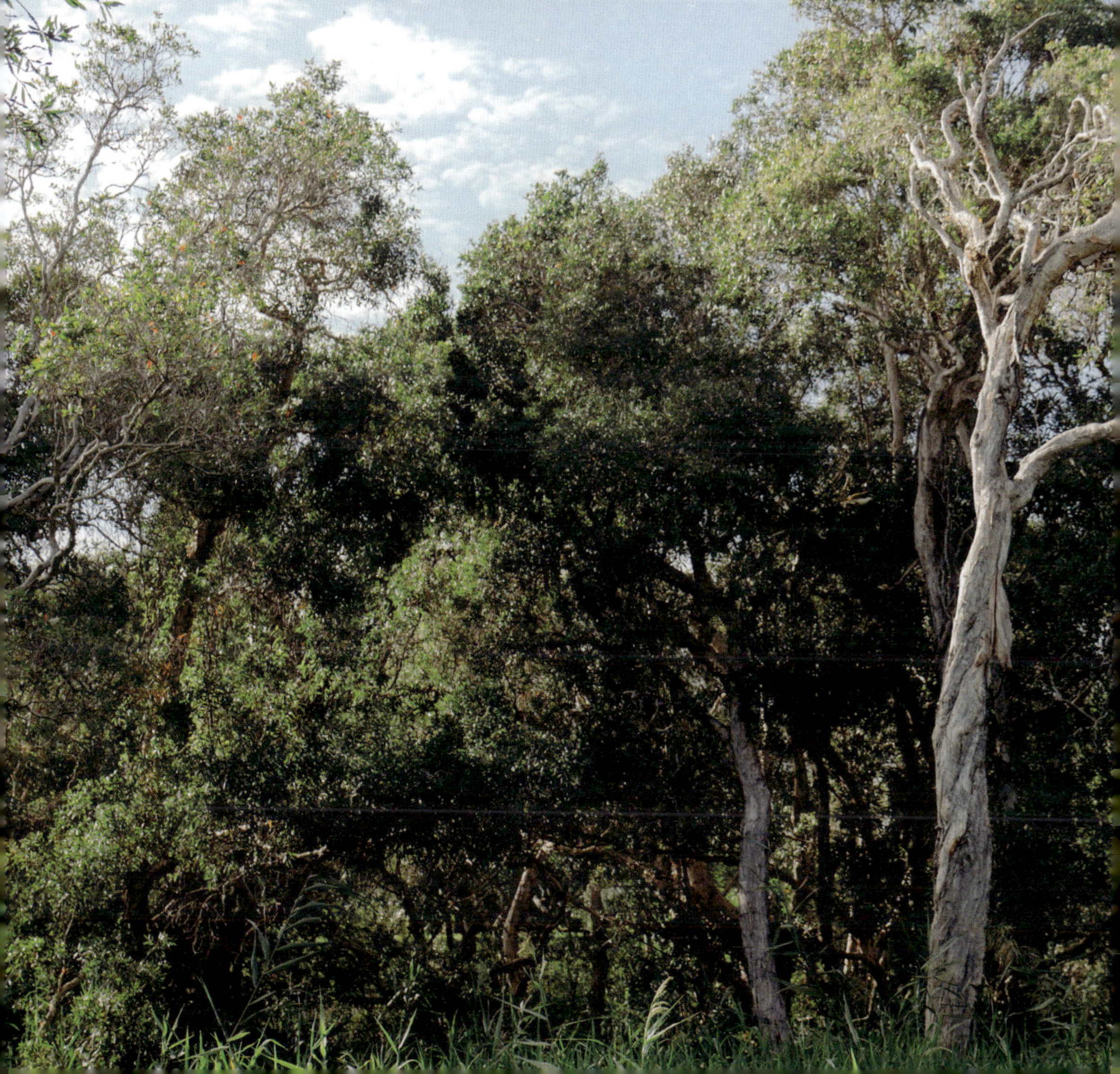

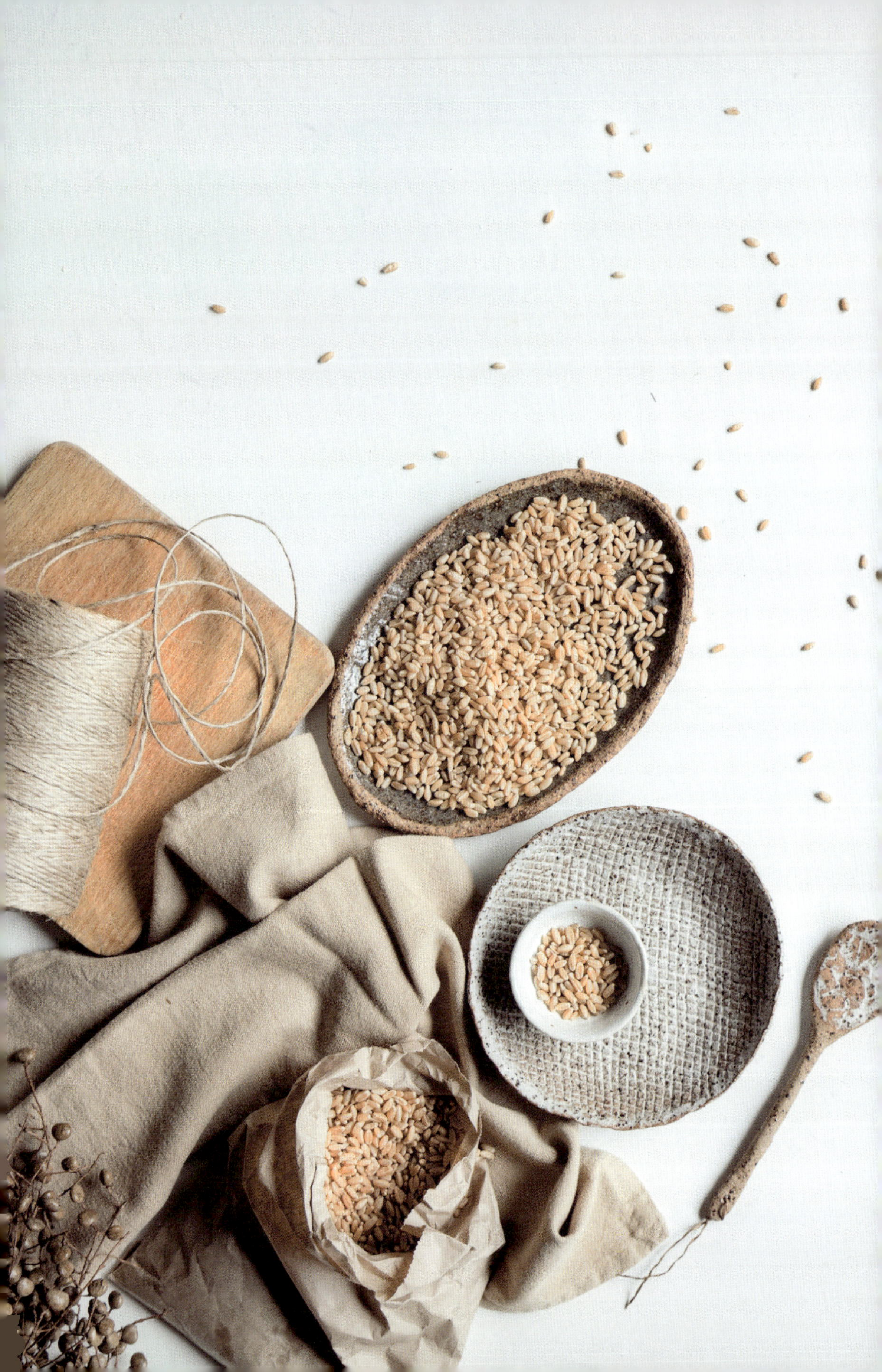

A guide to gluten

UNDERSTANDING GRAINS

People diagnosed with coeliac disease cannot eat gluten-containing foods. Yet there are others who, despite not testing positive to coeliac disease, have numerous symptoms that resolve through the same dietary changes. My take on this is that science isn't finished yet. What if there are 50 more mechanisms through which the human body reacts to gluten and coeliac disease is only the main one we currently know about? I will refer to 'all of the others' as 'gluten-intolerant' for the purpose of this chapter.

Gluten is the name given to a protein in wheat, rye, barley and oats that affects people with coeliac disease.

Gluten is a composite name representing:

- gliadin in wheat
- hordein in barley
- secalin in rye
- avenin in oats.

There are current gluten tests that can measure gliadin, hordein and secalin, but not avenin, because it is a slightly different protein. In the same way that gliadin is an essential component of wheat, avenin is an essential part of oats. As such, oats will never be gluten free (i.e. avenin free) — even if they are described as gluten free according to current testing standards.

While some people with coeliac disease and those who are gluten-intolerant can tolerate oats, others can't. Statistics from Coeliac Australia suggest that approximately one in five (20 per cent) of people with coeliac disease react to pure uncontaminated oats. That is, they react to oat avenin. It is therefore unwise to ever 'recommend' oats, as I would not want to recommend that 20 per cent of coeliacs get sick. Since it is impossible to predict who is part of the 20 per cent, and we know that damage can occur even in the absence of symptoms, it is best that oats are not consumed by someone with coeliac disease without a biopsy prior to and during consumption.

The practicalities of doing so may prove either challenging or worthwhile. So, when people discuss gluten-free oats (and laboratories advise that oats are gluten-free), a more accurate statement would be that they are free from wheat (and rye, barley) gliadin. In other words, that there is no measurable contamination. But they still contain avenin.

WHERE IS GLUTEN?

If you feel drawn to trial a gluten-free way of eating for four to eight weeks, based on what you have learnt, the following table highlights foods that contain gluten and those that don't. Most gluten containing foods are highly processed and so are therefore not a nutritious choice anyway.

The term glutinous on a food label refers to the "stickiness" of the product, and is unrelated to the gluten content.

If the word thickener is used on an ingredients list, the source of the thickener is often included in brackets after the word. If you are not sure of the gluten content of any food, use the general rule: when in doubt, leave it out. Food labels constantly change so it is a good idea to read food labels regularly.

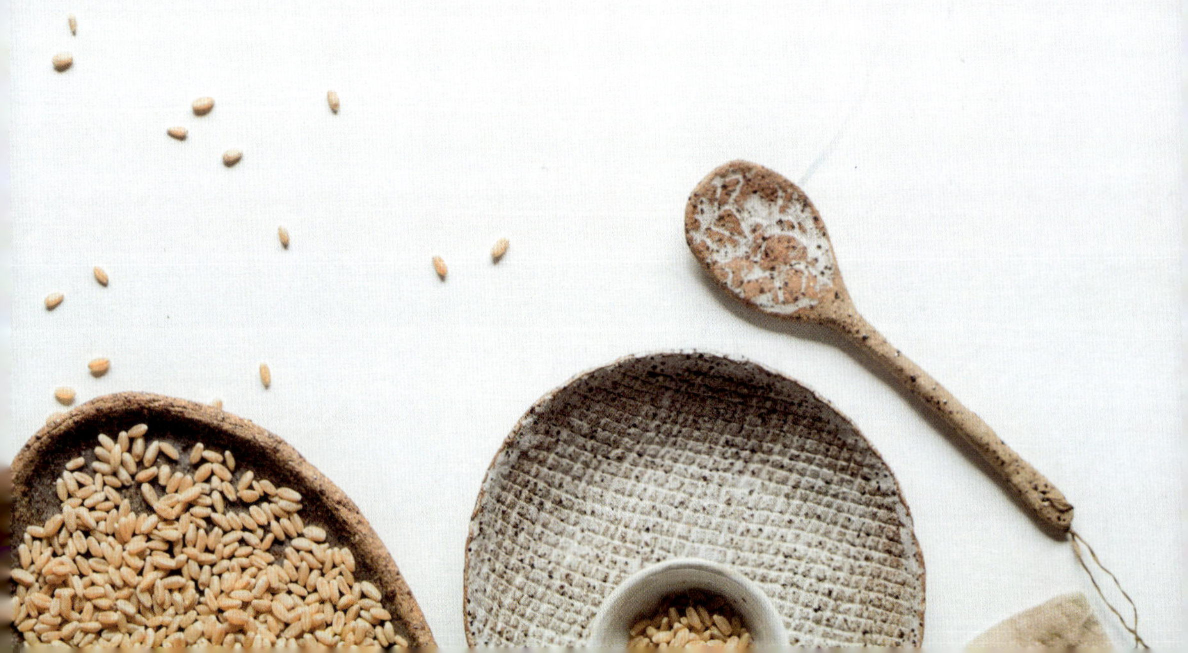

CONTAIN GLUTEN		**DON'T** CONTAIN GLUTEN
• wheat • rye • barley • oats • semolina • couscous • triticale • pasta • noodles • crumbs • wheat vermicelli • farina • burghul • spelt • durum • hydrolysed vegetable grain • soy sauce • maltodextrin*	• dextrin* • pre-gel starch* • stock* • thickeners (with a 1400s code)* • beverage whitener • hydrolysed vegetable protein • cornflour* • wheaten cornflour • wheat starch • malt • malt extract • starch* • modified starch • malt vinegar	• rice • sago • tapioca • millet • buckwheat • sorghum • arrowroot • quinoa • amaranth • besan (chickpea) • dhal • seeds • psyllium • corn/maize • cider/wine vinegar

** These ingredients may be derived from wheat, and therefore may contain trace amounts of gluten.*

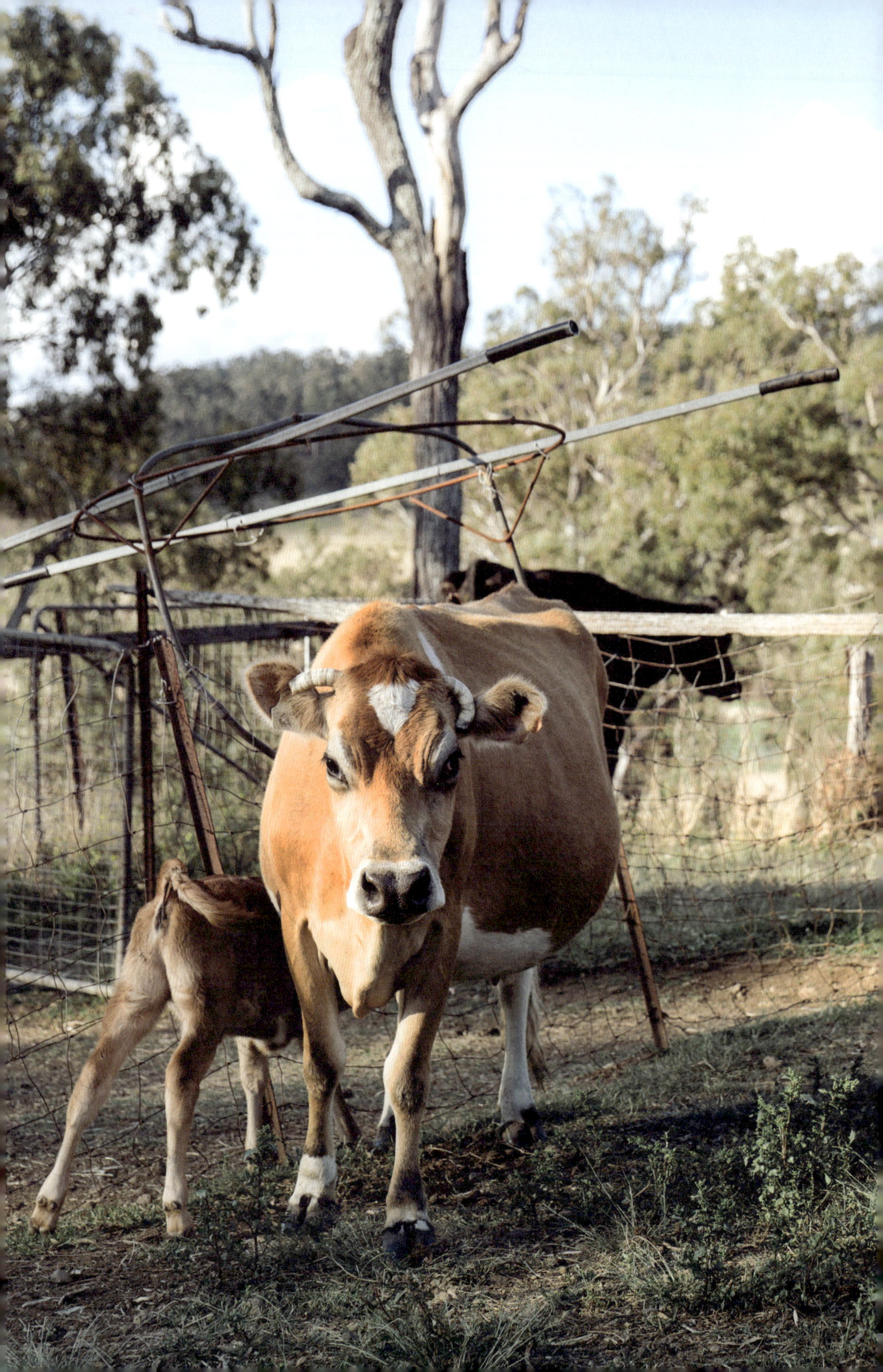

Deciding about dairy

IS IT GOOD FOR YOU?

Dairy foods contain the three macronutrients — protein, fats and carbohydrates. If someone has an adverse reaction to dairy foods, it is usually to the carbohydrates, such as lactose — or the proteins. There are numerous proteins found in cow's milk that can be divided into two main categories: the caseins and the whey proteins. Examples of caseins include beta-A1-casein and beta-A2-casein, while whey proteins include alpha-lactalbumin and beta-lactoglobulin. The fats are typically well tolerated.

Therefore, in a dietary trial to determine if someone's health challenges are related to dairy products, the proteins and the carbohydrates must be removed initially. Butter is mostly dairy fats but traces of the potentially reactive substances can be found in it, making it suitable for some people but not all. It is still best to remove butter within the dietary trial period, just to be sure.

With some new food understanding, if you feel drawn to do a dairy-free diet trial for four to eight weeks, here is some additional information to assist you. If you continue for longer than the trial period, it is best to consult with an experienced nutrition professional to ensure you are not missing out on essential nutrients.

A dairy-free diet trial for four to eight weeks:

- must be strict for the trial period
- takes into account the words that mean "dairy", as listed below
- must be followed with an assessment of how you feel.

Following a dairy-free diet is not simply eliminating dairy products, such as milk, yoghurt and cheese. The following foods are commonly included as ingredients in other foods.

Here are some of the words or items that denote dairy in ingredients lists to avoid:

- dairy
- milk, milk powder, milk protein, milk solids, non-fat milk solids
- skim milk solids, skim milk powder, skim milk protein
- casein or sodium caseinate
- whey protein, whey powder
- cheese, cheese powder
- yoghurt
- cream
- sour cream
- ice cream
- butter, margarine
- chocolate
- lactose (milk sugar)
- beverage whitener.

MILK SUBSTITUTES

Suitable for children and adults

DAIRY FOOD	ALTERNATIVE
Milk	Rice milk, macadamia milk, almond milk, quinoa milk, coconut milk (unsweetened versions, or make your own)
Dairy yoghurt	Plant-based yoghurt, such as coconut yoghurt
Ice cream	Plant-based ice cream (ensure no refined sugars)
Margarine	Avocado, tahini, olive oil, coconut oil
Cheese	Cashew cheese (bought, or make your own)

After the initial trial period, you may decide to trial some dairy foods again and observe how you feel after eating them. The first one to trial is organic butter. After that, you may like to trial goat's cheese and/or sheep's cheese and/or unsweetened full-fat yoghurt from these animals.

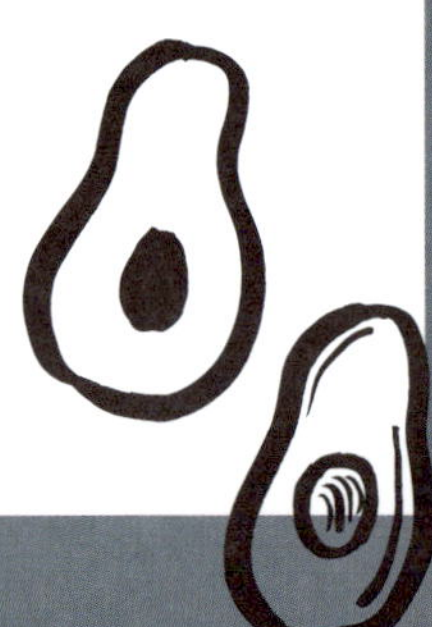

Look deep into nature,
and then you will understand
everything better.

ALBERT EINSTEIN

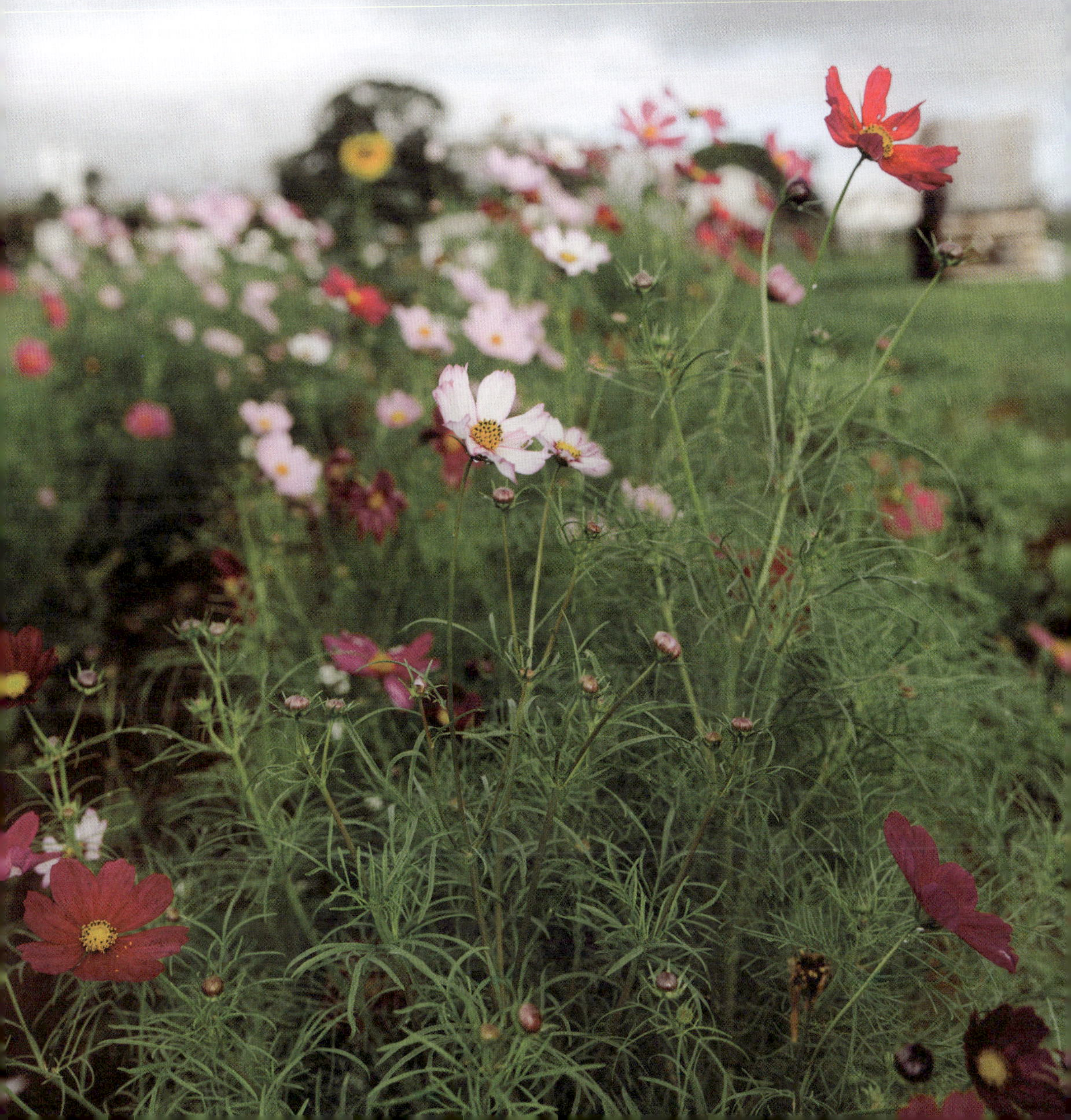

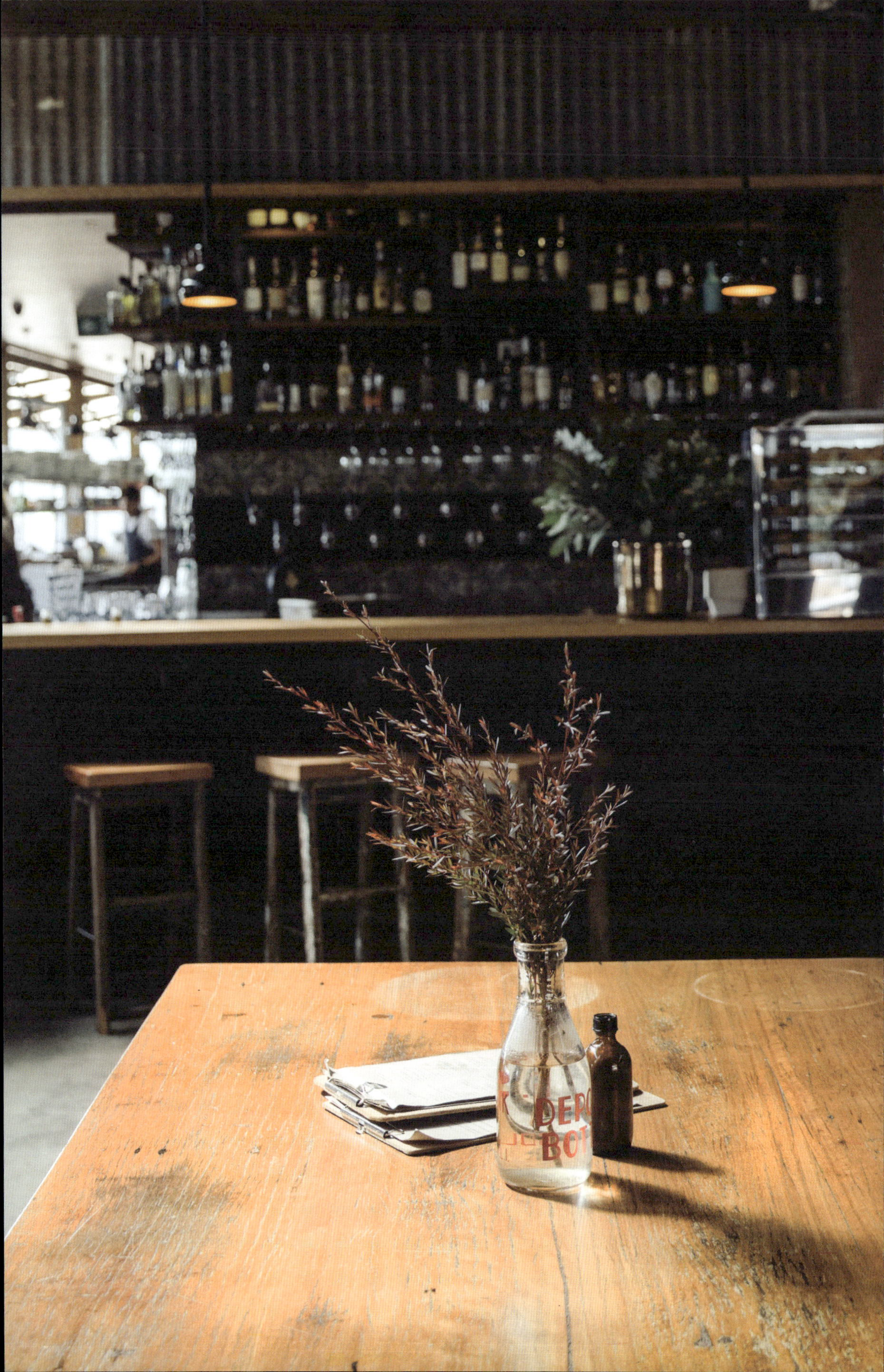

Too much of a good thing?

UNDERSTANDING ANTI-NUTRIENTS

Foods don't just contain nutrients; some foods also contain what can be called *anti-nutrients* when eaten in excessive amounts. Some common ones are phytic acid, oxalates and lectins. Alcohol and caffeine also have anti-nutrient properties.

PHYTIC ACID

Phytic acid is found in wholegrains, nuts, seeds and beans and represents a potential absorptive roadblock. Phytic acid is the principal storage form of phosphorus in many plant tissues, especially the bran portion of grains and other seeds. It contains the mineral phosphorus tightly bound in a molecule.

For humans, the phosphorus in this molecule is not readily available. In addition to blocking the availability of phosphorus, other components of the phytic acid molecule readily bind with other minerals, such as calcium, magnesium, iron and zinc, making them form a complex we are unable to absorb.

Phytic acid or *phytates* are considered anti-nutrients, but they exist in plants because they are part of the process of life. They perform many important functions for the plant, including protection against insects, maintaining the freshness of seeds for germination and protection against fungi or mould. Soaking wholegrains, beans, nuts and seeds overnight is one of the most effective ways to reduce their phytic acid content. Soaking allows enzymes, lactobacilli and other helpful organisms to break down and begin to neutralise a large portion of phytic acid in grains. Soaking in warm water also begins to neutralise the enzyme inhibitors present in all seeds and encourages the production of numerous beneficial enzymes.

OXALATES

Oxalates are naturally occurring substances that belong to a group of molecules called *organic acids* which are found in and routinely made by plants, animals and humans. The body always contains oxalates, and our cells routinely convert other substances into oxalates. For example, vitamin C is one of the substances that our cells can routinely convert into oxalates. In addition to the oxalates that are made inside the body, oxalates can enter the body from the outside as specific foods contain them.

Leafy green vegetables, nuts, seeds, most berries, certain other fruits, soy and soy products, meat and dairy products all contain small amounts of oxalates. Large amounts of oxalic acid are harmful, but are typically found in parts of foods we don't eat, such as the leaves of the rhubarb plant.

The main area of concern for oxalic acid in food is whether or not it contributes to the formation of kidney stones. Approximately 80 per cent of kidney stones are composed of calcium oxalate. Oxalic acid binds with other minerals such as calcium, which under certain conditions form a salt known as an oxalate. Oxalic acid interferes with the absorption of calcium in foods because it can bind to it, making it unusable by the body. Some individuals are more prone to problems with oxalates than others.

> *Anything consumed in excess can be harmful. However, when you review the literature, it clearly demonstrates that most people aren't consuming enough vegetables and in particular leafy greens.*

Although juices and smoothies are nutrient dense, they don't suit all people, or some people need to be conscious of how often they have them. We are all different in our makeup. Sure, I have seen the addition of these drinks improve the quality of people's health. But some people don't feel satisfied by them, or they feel really cold when they consume them, despite the weather. Plus, with juices, you don't chew, so they don't tend to stimulate stomach acid production well. You know your body best, and if smoothies or juices don't work for you I encourage you to use soups or stir-fries, or simply add greens to slow-cooked meals to still receive the benefits of a high plant way of eating.

LECTINS

Lectins are proteins found in animals and plants, particularly in grains, legumes (especially soy), nuts and seeds. They have many protective functions in the human body, from recognising pathogens to helping regulate protein levels in the blood. However, lectins can confuse the immune system in some people, and drive it to create antibodies.

> Anything consumed in excess can be harmful.

Unfortunately, lectins can also mimic other proteins that are typically present in your blood. It is not uncommon to have antibodies to some dietary lectins which means that responses to lectin-containing food can be highly variable from person to person. If the gut is injured after an immune system challenge or via any other mechanism, specific foods may lead to symptoms of intolerance. An immune system response can be stimulated by the presence of particular lectins, perpetuating immune and digestive system dysfunction.

It is possible that the gut lining becomes more sensitive to food lectins if someone has ulcerative colitis, Crohn's disease or in some cases of IBS. The mechanism/s responsible for this are not fully understood; however, it may be due to the rapid replacement of cells that line the gut (known as high cell turnover), which leads to a larger number of immature gut cells being present at one time. As immature cells have more areas where lectins can attach, this can lead to symptoms arising from lectin-containing foods.

They can also damage the walls of your intestines, in part supporting a "leaky gut", so that other large particles can cross the intestinal barrier, enter your bloodstream and begin other immune cascades.

Eating a variety of foods, rather than large amounts of one type, reduces the impact of dietary lectins. Some people also benefit from incorporating more fermented foods, such as sauerkraut and kombucha. Cooking, sprouting or soaking your grains, legumes, nuts and seeds all help to decrease the lectins. It's always better to soak or sprout your nuts and seeds.

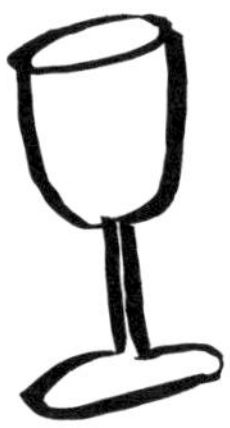

ALCOHOL

Alcohol is considered a macronutrient as it supplies the body with calories. It does not, however, contain micronutrients. Alcohol also affects the absorption of nutrients in a number of ways. It interferes with normal digestion by damaging cells in the stomach and intestine and by interfering with the release of important digestive enzymes. Alcohol also acts as a diuretic, which promotes excretion of stored minerals, such as calcium and magnesium, as well as B vitamins. Even moderate drinking has been shown to decrease vitamin B_{12} levels. The regular overconsumption of alcohol also depletes vitamin B_1, which can have mental health effects that alter the personality. Be honest with yourself about how alcohol affects you and those around you.

You don't need a health professional to tell you that you are drinking too much; you already know that somewhere inside yourself. If that is the case, bring curiosity (not judgement) to why you continue to drink in a way that is harmful to you. It is never about the alcohol, in this case.

A psychologist may assist you to dig deeper in this area if that appeals and if making some changes on your own feels too confronting. If you drink alcohol, don't drink in a way that harms you or others.

CAFFEINE

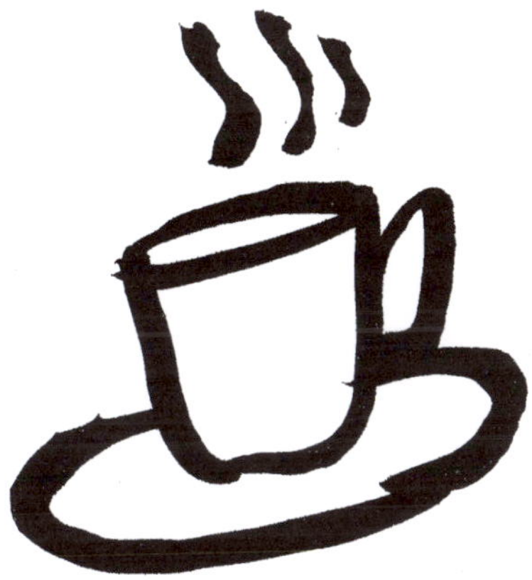

Similarly to alcohol, caffeine can promote the excretion of water, vitamins and minerals, particularly calcium and magnesium from the bones. Caffeine also blocks the absorption of calcium from the milk that you might add to your tea or coffee. In excessive amounts, tannins (a type of plant compound) found in many caffeinated drinks can also inhibit the absorption of calcium, iron, magnesium and B group vitamins.

Caffeine also leads the body to make adrenalin, the hormone behind most anxious feelings. To create adrenalin, the body utilises B vitamins and magnesium in particular, so your requirements for these are also greater if you consume caffeine. Limit your consumption of caffeine (or eliminate it) to improve your digestion, absorption and availability of nutrients.

Applying TCM principles

ANCIENT WISDOM IN TODAY'S WORLD

In Traditional Chinese Medicine (TCM), food recommendations are based on energy principles that encourage balance and an effectively functioning body that is full of energy and free of disease. Proper TCM dietary therapy identifies and treats any underlying patterns of imbalance that may be creating symptoms with a complex integrative system. However, all human bodies have a number of common fundamental requirements and TCM dietary therapy begins by addressing these.

DAMP-PRODUCING FOODS

In Western culture, we have recently come to understand the concept of eating for balance. The principle of "balance" has been a way of life for thousands of years for the Chinese and inherently shapes what they eat and when they eat it. Ingredients are selected for taste and nutrition as well as medicinal properties. For examples, the Chinese have long known that ginger is an aid to digestion, and in TCM barley is commonly believed to drain "dampness". Dampness isn't a term that most Westerners would be familiar with, but another aim of the Chinese diet is draining dampness.

Dampness

In TCM, dampness is the resultant effect of consuming foods that interrupt the flow of energy through your body. Common culprits in its creation include popular foods such as sugar, yoghurt, cheese and white flour. The main problem with dampness is that it creates stagnation, which builds blockages in the body that contribute to processes breaking down and results in pain and disease.

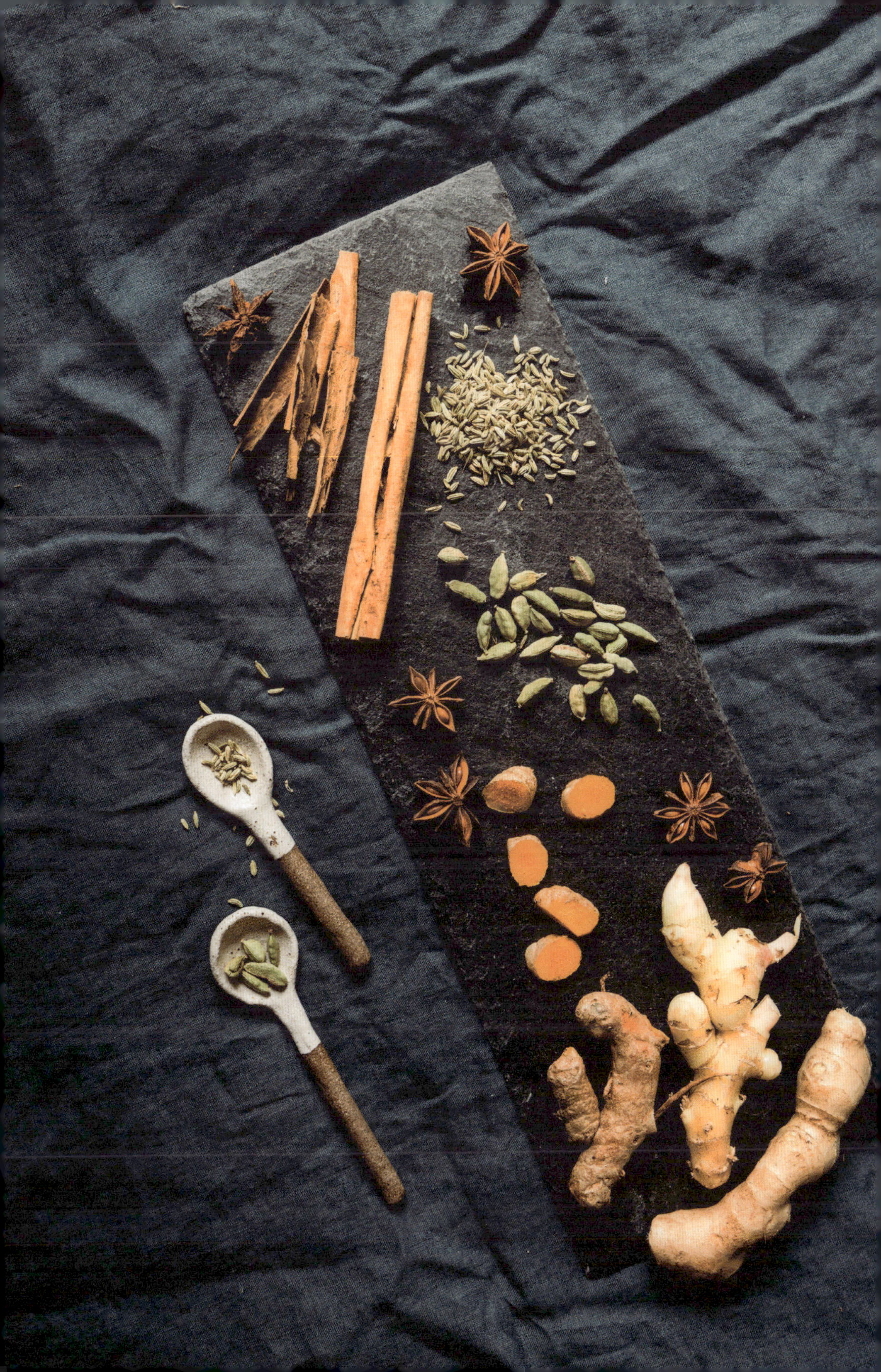

Symptoms of accumulated dampness include joint swelling, excess weight, mucus in the nose or lungs and digestive problems, such as loose stools and constipation. Arthritis and some chronic allergies are some common Western diseases that are associated with dampness.

YOUR DIGESTIVE SYSTEM IN TCM

Through TCM, the Chinese have collected data on the digestive system for over 2000 years and have declared good digestion to be the keystone of TCM and something that is fundamental to excellent health. According to TCM principles, the accumulation of dampness begins in the digestive system.

Once you have swallowed food, it enters your stomach and moves through your intestines. Nutrients are extracted from the food and any waste products are expelled via your colon. The nutrients are the food 'energy'. They become your essential life force as they are converted into the fuel you need to get through each day. Digestion is supposed to be an unremarkable event and your digestive system is ideally quiet. However, if your system becomes congested, your digestive system is not able to adequately draw the energy from the food and even though you may still excrete wastes, a residue (considered to be 'dampness' in TCM) remains within various places in your body and affects functions in numerous ways depending on where it sticks.

> "Some common Western diseases that are associated with dampness include chronic allergies and arthritis."

When dampness accumulates in the digestive tract it can create bowel challenges and indigestion. When it accumulates in the lungs, it can cause conditions like asthma. If it is not addressed, over time dampness can become a foundation for diseases involving inflammation — for example, high cholesterol, type 2 diabetes, and high blood pressure. One of the keys in TCM to treating disease is addressing and understanding dampness. Once it has accumulated it becomes much more difficult to remove so it's important that we don't allow this dampness to develop initially.

TCM WAY OF EATING

Warm and cooked foods

According to TCM, it requires extra energy for your body to process cold and raw foods. Since they are more difficult for your body to process, they are then culprits in the formation of dampness. Your body needs food to be approximately body temperature before it can begin to break it down and your digestive system can begin the process of extracting energy from the food. In this way, cold food, which requires your body to heat it inside you, puts pressure on your energetic resources and, over time, can weaken your energy system. Optimally, any type of grain (such as rice) needs to be well-cooked and vegetables lightly cooked to allow the digestive system to begin extracting energy immediately. Even though the process of cooking foods does reduce some of the enzyme and nutrient content, it is considered to be less than what you would lose in the process of warming the foods internally whilst simultaneously trying to draw out the energy.

Vegetables

Vegetables are packed with life-giving nutrition and play a major role when it comes to draining dampness. A variety of colours provide a wide range of nutrients and antioxidants that promote health and vitality. The texture and taste of vegetables play a significant role in appetite regulation. Colours and textures create a combination that pleases both the palate and the eye. Ideally, you begin filling your plate with a large quantity of lightly cooked vegetables. As a guideline, this would be around half your plate. A wide variety of vegetables ensures satiety and you will want to include lots of nutrient dense and balancing leafy greens.

Rice

In TCM, rice is considered to be an easily digested and balanced food that gently drains dampness from the body. Depending on which one digests most easily for you, white or brown rice are interchangeable. In a TCM way of eating, rice would fill one quarter of your plate.

Protein

The TCM way of eating includes a small amount of animal protein or beans. Animal proteins, which are considered 'building' foods, require more energy to digest — thus the importance of a 'small' portion. A serving size of animal protein is typically 60–120g, three to four times a week. Beans absorb dampness, provide fibre and protein and so can be eaten more regularly. Your protein choice would fill the other quarter of the plate.

Sugar

According to TCM, dampness is quickly created by consuming concentrated sweets, such as soft drinks, lollies, biscuits and ice cream. TCM therapy considered the flavour of 'sweet' as nourishing and the majority of foods on the Chinese diet are thought to be primarily sweet. 'Sweet' to the Chinese means rice and most vegetables. You can imagine the overwhelming sweetness of a handful of lollies if vegetables are considered sweet! Concentrated sweets weaken the body's processes for transforming food into energy and wastes for elimination, whereas the sweet flavour of rice and vegetables are of benefit to the digestive organs. This partially transformed food becomes dampness and can accumulate over time. That's how TCM views these foods that in the West we also typically classify as being choices that don't nourish us.

In TCM, all foods are considered to be made of five different flavours: sweet, sour, pungent, bitter and salty. Balancing these flavours in accordance with someone's individual body type, disease pattern and season are all part of TCM therapy.

No dairy

There is no cheese, butter or milk used in TCM eating as they believe these foods have a tendency to create dampness. Dairy's energetic nature is cold regardless of whether it's heated or served cold. This hinders digestion, according to TCM principles. Dairy is considered to be suitable only for undernourished people as it is a building food. When consumed by already well-fed people, it becomes very stagnating.

Eating seasonally

TCM principles follow eating and cooking modifications according to the seasons. In winter, people are naturally drawn to eating more warming foods, such as stews and soups. Equally, we tend to be drawn to cooler, lighter types of foods like steamed vegetables in summer. Adjusting your food choices to align with seasons can help to keep your body in sync with the natural environment. Aligning your choices with the weather — warmer foods in the cold, cooler foods when it is warm — promotes health across all seasons.

In the same way, choosing foods that grow locally in the region you live in will also help to keep your body balanced. This simply means that if you live in a colder climate, you're probably not likely to find tropical fruits in your area, so if applying TCM principles, you would do better to avoid them, even if your local supermarket flies them in from other parts of the world. In other words, if you live near the equator where the weather is more consistently warm, you would choose to eat differently to those people who live in more extreme,

cold climates.

Although this only covers one area of TCM dietary principles — dampness — you can see the similarities between this and a common-sense way of eating: plenty of vegetables, small amounts of protein and complex carbohydrates, little to no processed foods, such as refined sugars and flours. Also, the simple messages of eating seasonally and considering your climate when making food choices. In other words, a nutritious choice in the middle of a New Zealand winter is unlikely to be a salad.

> Reflect on the simple messages of eating seasonally and consider your climate when making food choices.

Think about it. You can imagine how hungry you'd be if that is all you ate for lunch in winter. Some leftover casserole from the night before is far more likely to sustain you through a winter's afternoon. When I think of winter food, the words that spring to mind include 'warm', 'slow' and 'cooked'.

Of course, TCM has highly specific ways of treating symptoms and illnesses and again, if this appeals to your own sensibilities, it can be useful to consult an expert in this field, obtain guidance, trial it and then tune into yourself about how you feel eating in this way.

Your body knows best.

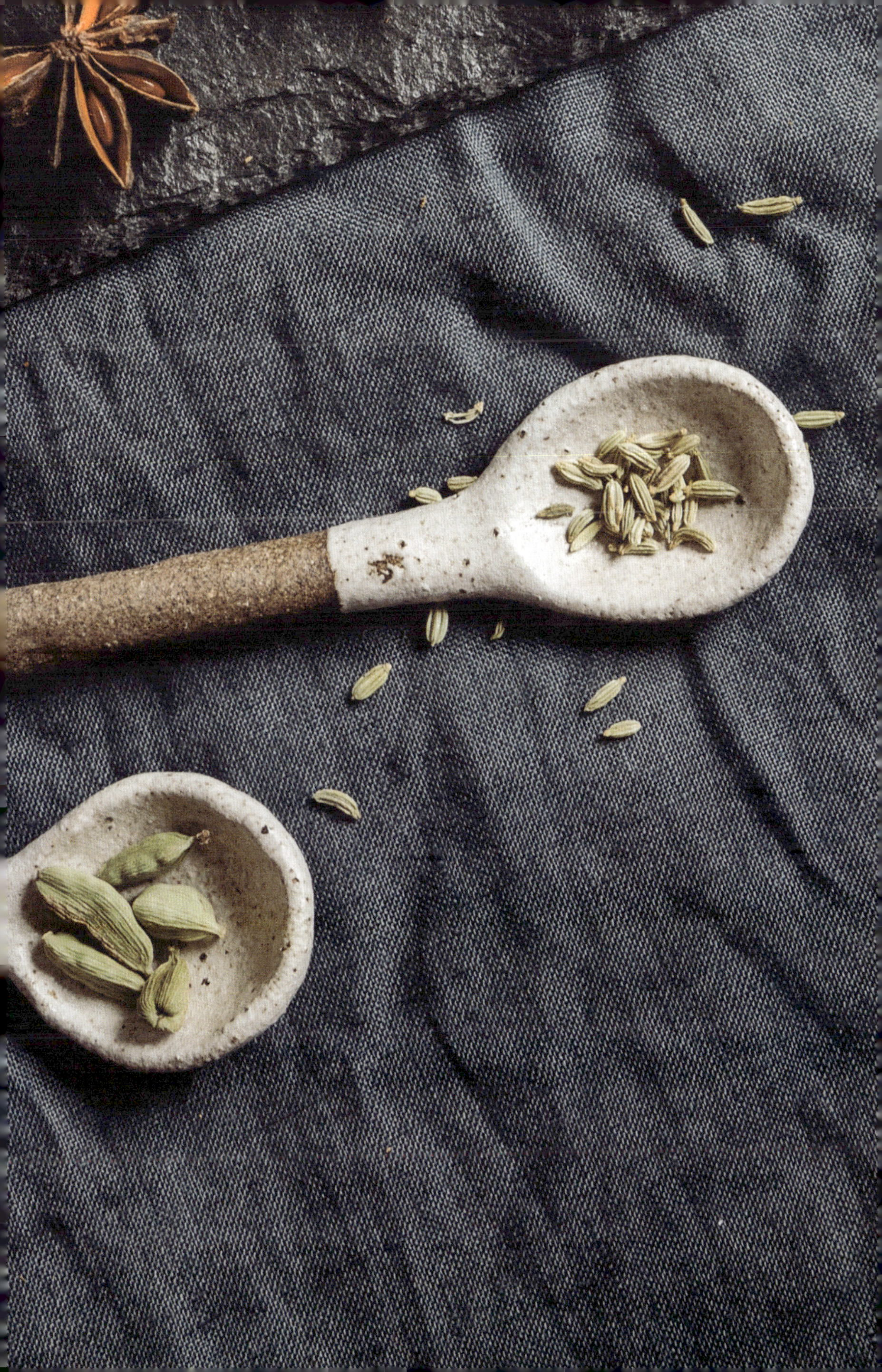

Consuming stress

WHAT ARE YOU MISSING OUT ON?

Many people suffer with digestive problems such as IBS, indigestion and heartburn, some of which is due to foods and some of which is related to stress. These conditions are a by-product of the body's biochemical response to being in a constant "fight or flight" state.

My other books go into detail about this but in a nutshell, adrenalin diverts blood flow away from the digestive system, meaning digestion and the absorption of macro- and micronutrients can become compromised.

When you make adrenalin, your body thinks it is because your life is in danger and it makes interior adjustments to allow you to fight or escape. So this is one reason why it is important to change what you can when it comes to stressful situations in your life and accept what you can't alter right now. Adjusting our attitude and the responses and meanings created in situations can be highly beneficial. As can decreasing the consumption of caffeine and examining our perceptions of pressure and urgency, as all of these factors lead to the production of stress hormones.

> "Do your best to eat in a calm state to maximise nutrient uptake."

Diaphragmatically breathing also lowers stress hormone levels rapidly and is a wonderful practice to incorporate for maximum nutrient absorption, as well as a host of other significant health benefits.

WORKSHEET

Write down all the things in your life that are causing you stress. Keep going until you've written everything down.

Pick your top five stressors from the previous page, circle them and rank them in order from one to five (with one being the most stressful to you).

1 ______________________ 4 ______________________

2 ______________________ 5 ______________________

3 ______________________

Take the stressor you have labelled number five and write it into the following sentence.

I acknowledge that _ is causing me significant stress right now.

Look up from your workbook.

Notice something out the window or a thought that brings a smile to your face.

Write that here: I notice _ is making me smile.

Now complete this sentence.

I acknowledge that _ is causing me significant stress right now and I can also see that the (thought/thing outside) _ is bringing me a smile.

While it's important to acknowledge the things in our life that are causing us stress, it is also helpful to see that there is often space outside of this stress as well. It can be very easy to envelop ourselves in our stressors and this creates a constant cascade of harmful biochemical reactions in our bodies. Adjusting your perception won't necessarily dissolve a stressful situation but it will help you to feel better equipped to deal with it.

Repeat this exercise on a separate piece of paper with the rest of your stressors and try to notice something else that makes you smile each time.

Sustenance for great sleep

- Protein foods, as they contain substances that your body converts into sleep hormones.
- Nothing containing caffeine such as chocolate, coffee, colas, tea or energy drinks.
- Eat a small meal before bed.
- Avoid spicy food at night.
- If chickpeas don't give you excessive gas, include them or eat hummus as chickpeas are rich in a substance that the body converts into tryptophan (a sleep hormone).
- Eat regular meals as, if blood glucose goes too low, you will make adrenalin which will lead to the release of glucose, while also bringing its sleep disrupting stress effects.

Eat magnesium-rich foods consistently, such as plenty of leafy green vegetables and nuts.

Eggs and/or almonds can help as they are rich in vitamin B_6, a nutrient essential for the body being able to make sleep hormones.

Eat calcium-rich foods as these help the relaxation response, such as green leafy vegetables, tahini, nuts, seeds, particularly sesame seeds, figs, salmon with edible bones.

Try to eat before 6:30pm. It can be hard to fall asleep and stay asleep if you have only just finished dinner.

Chamomile tea contains substances that help us to relax.

Note: this is general information, as if, for example, you need to be low FODMAP, then you will need to be mindful about how much of some of these foods you consume; there is no one size fits all.

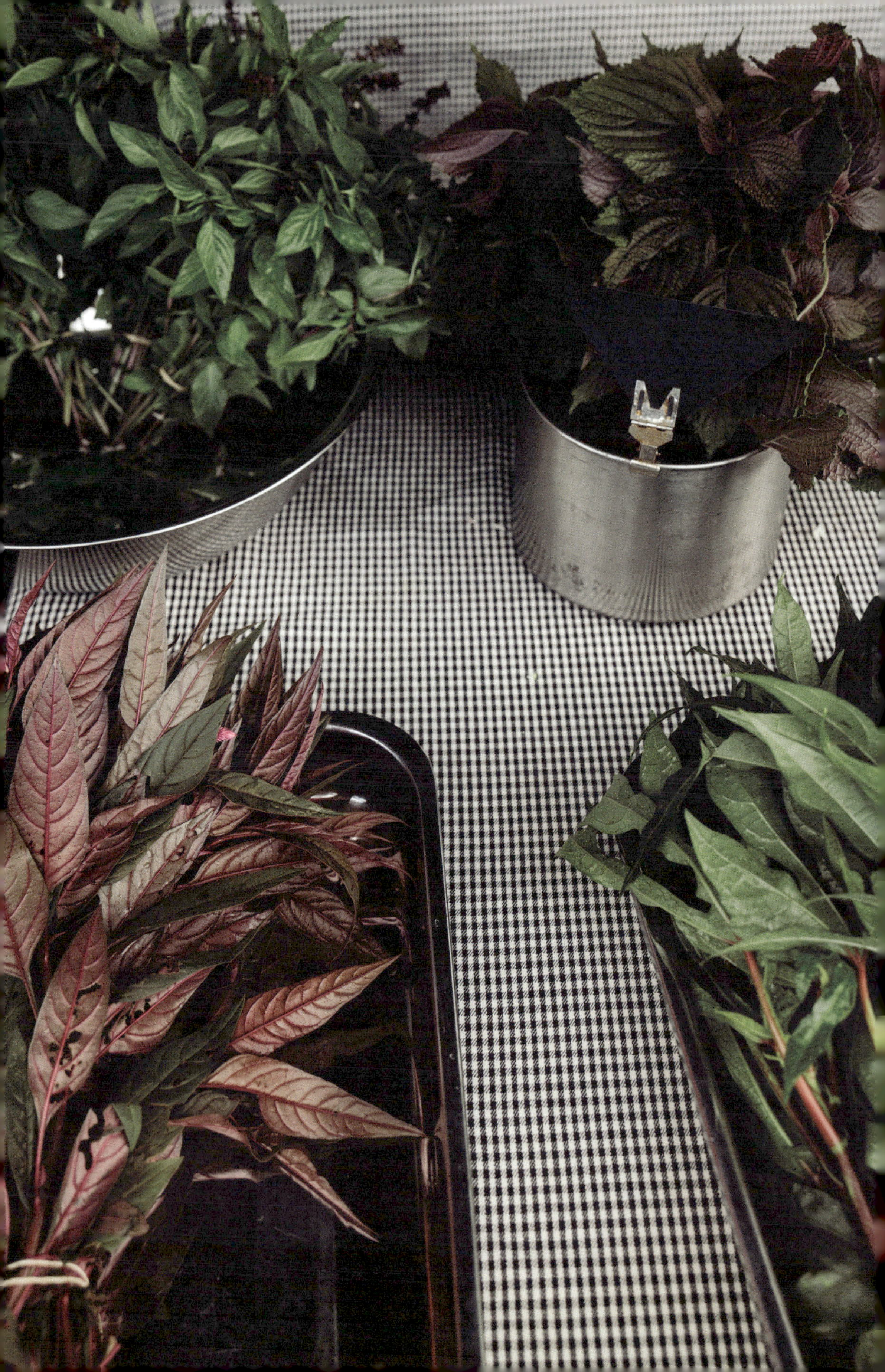

Food fads

THE CYCLE OF NUTRITION TRENDS

When I was at university, it was during the period when the public health message of the day was that a low-fat, high-carbohydrate diet was the way to eat for good health. The food industry responded and started to provide consumers with the "low-fat" versions of their conventional packaged foods.

For example, where once there was just an ordinary frozen apple pie in the freezer in the supermarket, there was now a low-fat version. And if you were a health conscious citizen at this time wanting to take care of yourself and potentially a family, then you bought the low-fat apple pie. However, when a food company removes the fat from a processed food, they leave a great big gaping hole. So guess what they filled that hole with? Refined sugars. But if you had been eating the ordinary apple pie and then you started to eat the low-fat version and it tasted sickly sweet — much sweeter than the original apple pie — you would realise what had happened. And so to mask the addition of the refined sugars, the food companies added salt, as salt masks sweetness. So if you followed a low-fat diet back then and you ate processed foods, you more than likely ate more sugar and more salt than ever before in human history.

> "If you followed a low-fat diet, and you ate processed foods, you more than likely ate more sugar and more salt than ever before in human history."

It was during this period, too, when the waistlines of the Western world grew bigger than ever before.

There were now fast-food outlets on every second corner and family situations had begun to change. Often both parents were working for myriad reasons and so had less time to prepare food from scratch. These and many other factors, paired with the increased amount of refined sugars and starches that were now available and easy to access via processed foods, can help explain why the waistlines of the Western world were expanding.

The powers that be then decided that carbohydrates must have been the enemy, as people had been told to eat them during the low-fat era. So around rolled the low-carb, high-protein era, which was nothing new. A number of the more well-known high-protein diets of today were first released in the 1970s and, for those who have been around long enough to recall, you will recount that nutrition information tends to move in about 30-year cycles. Yet when you are in it, it feels real and as if it will always be this way. But the information will shift again.

The way not to get caught up in nutritional fads is to remember that when it comes to food, Nature gets it right and it is potentially human intervention that can get it so wrong.

Of course, within the whole, real food category there can still be foods that you as an individual don't digest well. For example, some people with arthritis suffer worse joint pain when they consume vegetables from the nightshade family, which includes potato, eggplant, tomato, capsicum and chilli. However, this is best guided by a health professional.

Your living is determined not so much by what life brings to you, as by the attitude you bring to life; not so much by what happens to you, as by the way your mind looks at what happens.

KAHLIL GIBRAN

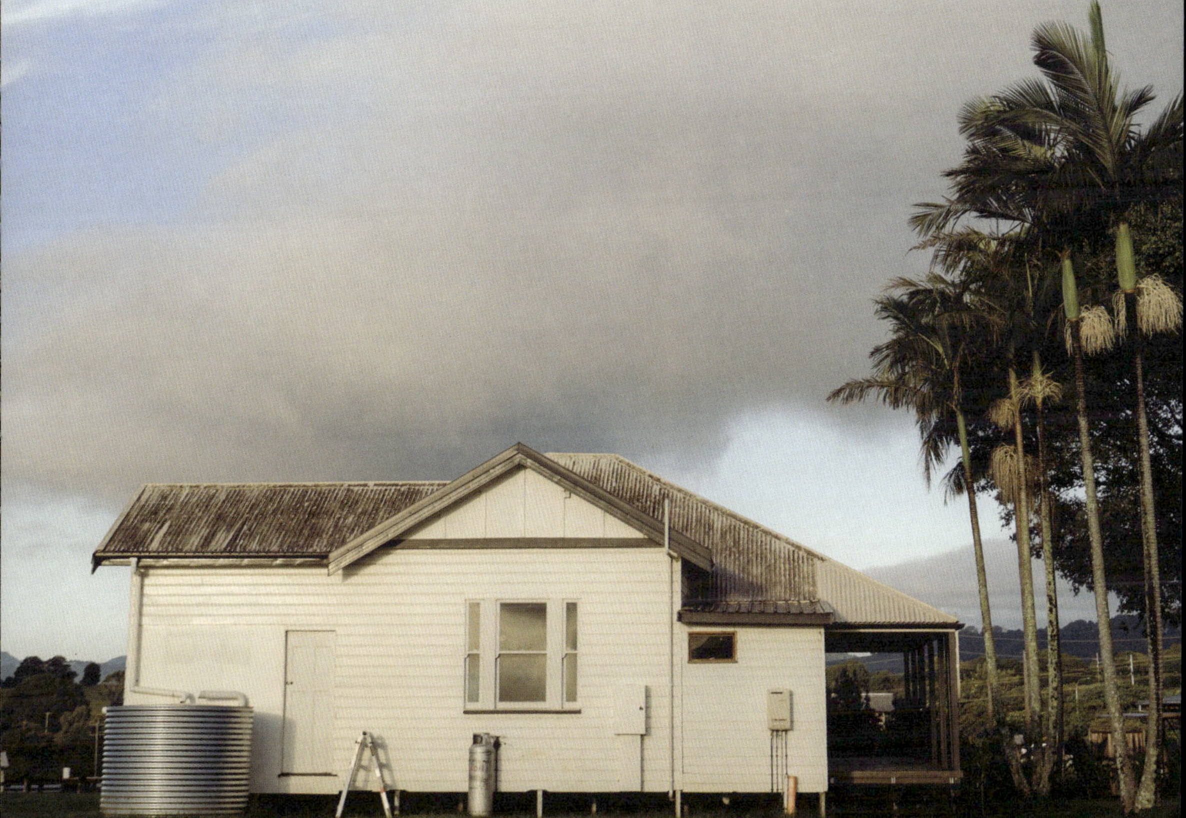

I don't eat that badly

THE PERVASIVENESS OF SUGARS

It's a phrase I have frequently heard over the past two decades. "I don't eat that badly", which is usually followed up with a question along the lines of "so why I am experiencing... [insert health or body challenge]?"

People want to be healthy and they want to make nutritious food choices for themselves and their families, yet unfortunately this does not unfold for too many people. Please know that I don't say this as a judgement. I say it because 'not eating that badly' has become the new norm in a world where we have an abundance of packaged food products masquerading as 'healthy' (not nutritious) at our fingertips. And the pervasiveness of sugars — even in foods that don't necessarily taste sweet — in our food supply is a big part of this.

A typical day of eating for someone who is likely to make the aforementioned comment may look something like the outline on the opposite page. It demonstrates just how much sugar you eat each day (perhaps without realising!), while also pointing out how few sugars whole, real food contains. It is a generalisation, but you'll get the gist.

It equates to about 65 teaspoons of sugar for the day, and that's with a real food dinner! It's also without any soft drink, most of which have about 10–15 teaspoons of sugar per can. I included the real food dinner so you could see how few sugars real food has — yes, even a dinner with potato. So many people are amazed that I don't recommend avoiding potato: ditch the processed foods instead.

I also included nutritious foods that are naturally high in sugar, such as fruit. Fruit seems to polarise people these days — some are afraid to eat it at all because of the sugar content, while others eat as much as they can because it is a 'healthy' food. Yes, fruit is nutritious, but our biochemistry is not designed for us to eat like a fruit bat. Two pieces per day is great (if you digest it well).

ON WAKING
Coffee with milk 1 cup
15g SUGAR
4 TSP

BREAKFAST
Acai bowl topped with fresh fruit and granola
55g SUGAR
13.5 TSP

ARRIVE AT WORK
Coffee with milk 1 cup
15g SUGAR
4 TSP

MORNING TEA
Fruit yoghurt 200g
25g SUGAR
6 TSP

SNACK
pack of sultanas 40g
26g SUGAR
6.5 TSP

LUNCH
Sandwich with egg, lettuce and mayonnaise
7g SUGAR
Banana smoothie
40g SUGAR
12 TSP

DESSERT
3 scoops of ice cream
33g SUGAR
8 TSP

DINNER
Chicken and vegetables with 1 small potato
2.5g SUGAR
0.5 TSP

DRINK
2 glasses of white wine 200mL each,
42g SUGAR
10.5 TSP

DAILY TOTAL
65 TEASPOONS OF SUGAR
260.5 GRAMS

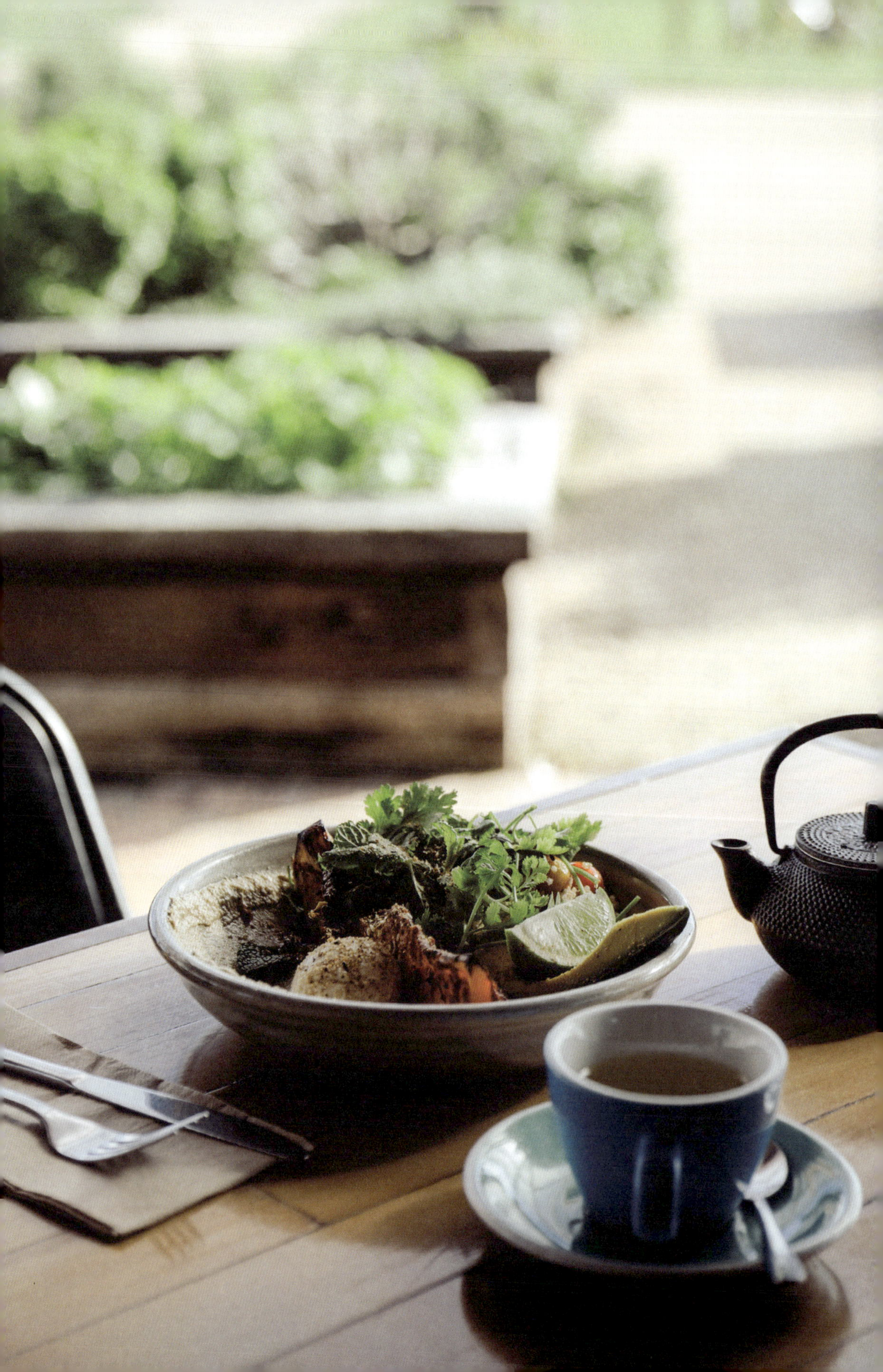

Eating out

NO NEED TO DITCH YOUR STANDARDS

Who doesn't love eating out? Having someone else cook for you, enjoying the company of loved ones, or simply having a convenient option on those big days are great draw cards. However, an irritable tummy, puffy eyes, or even breakouts can quickly replace the novelty. So how can you eat out without experiencing a "food hangover"?

One of the most important solutions to maintaining your ability to choose nourishing options when dining out is to seek out and support restaurants that offer real food options. Vote with your wallet and restaurateurs will have to listen. As consumers, we have greater power than you might think, especially in the hospitality industry. I am so encouraged by the number of people in this space who are making conscious decisions — offering organic, fair-trade, free-range and locally-sourced options; who are openly discussing what oils or sweeteners they use, the farms they buy their meat from and involving us, the customers, in these decisions.

I also encourage you to read the restaurant menu before you go. It not only helps you to determine whether it is somewhere you'd actually like to eat, it also means you don't end up selecting something at random because you feel like you're holding everyone up.

Don't be afraid to ask questions, about how the food is prepared, where it is sourced, what the sauces or dressings contain and if you can have them on the side, that way you can add them as you go. We are often too nervous to ask questions about how things are prepared, because we don't want to be a bother — but chances are the wait staff already know the answer to your question and have been asked it before. Plus, they are there to meet your needs, to help you have an enjoyable evening.

Customers are certainly more discerning when it comes to food choices than they used to be. And remember that asking more questions prompts greater awareness in the community and guides restaurateurs towards offering the options that people are enquiring about.

A sure-fire way to increase your chances of making poor food choices while dining out is to arrive at the restaurant ready to demolish anything and everything in your path. Watch out — the bread basket, fries, appetisers, you name it! If you are ravenous before you head out, have a nourishing snack before you go; for example, a handful of nuts, some vegetable sticks with dip or good quality crackers and hummus. This also prevents you from ordering whatever seems the most "filling", as opposed to the most nourishing, and ensures you don't end up overfull. If you love flavour and variety, opt for two entrées as opposed to a main and you will likely end up very satisfied.

To ensure you are able to get enough vegetables, it can be helpful to order a soup or a salad to start, or order a side of vegies. It astounds me how often meals don't come with vegetables nowadays. Take your time and eat slowly, particularly if you are a food "inhaler". Put your fork down and pause between bites if it helps.

I know it sounds old-fashioned, but potluck dinners are a wonderful alternative to eating out. Not only do you get to catch up with your friends, you can generally do so in the comfort of your own home. Combine this with the ability to prepare more nourishing options and you may enjoy this more than eating out in the first place!

Of course, if you eat out infrequently, it can be a soul-nourishing evening, where your focus is on the company you are in, rather than the nourishment the food may or may not provide. Refer to the information on page 136 for more about this.

EATING WELL WHEN TRAVELLING

“I cannot encourage you enough to simply eat when you are hungry and turn down any other meals you are offered.”

When it comes to health and wellness, many of us have formed habits that we can effortlessly do on a daily basis, particularly in the comfort of our own homes and lives. However, how do you stay healthy when routine goes out the window or when you are unable to cook your own meals? Travelling is often an exciting time, but that excitement can quickly wear off after a few days of not eating well or moving. I regularly hear people exclaim that they can't wait to cook their own meal again after travelling for weeks at a time, because they're tired of not having fresh, nourishing options available. Travelling may present some challenges, but here are a few ways you can prioritise your health and wellbeing while away from home.

Avoid the alcohol/mindless eating on the plane

Eat lightly, stay hydrated and avoid coffee or alcohol if you're on long-haul flights; these will only dehydrate you further and disrupt any sleep that may be forthcoming. It's particularly easy to fall into a mindless eating trap on a plane, as food can become an occupier activity. As many of us have been raised to "eat what we're given", it can be challenging for people to turn down meals. I cannot encourage you enough to simply eat when you are hungry and turn down any other meals you are offered.

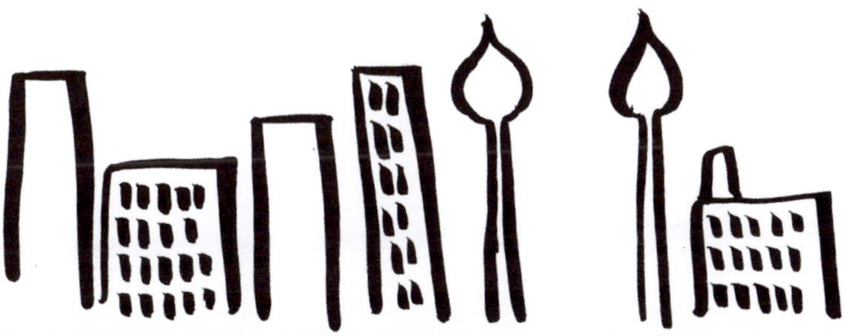

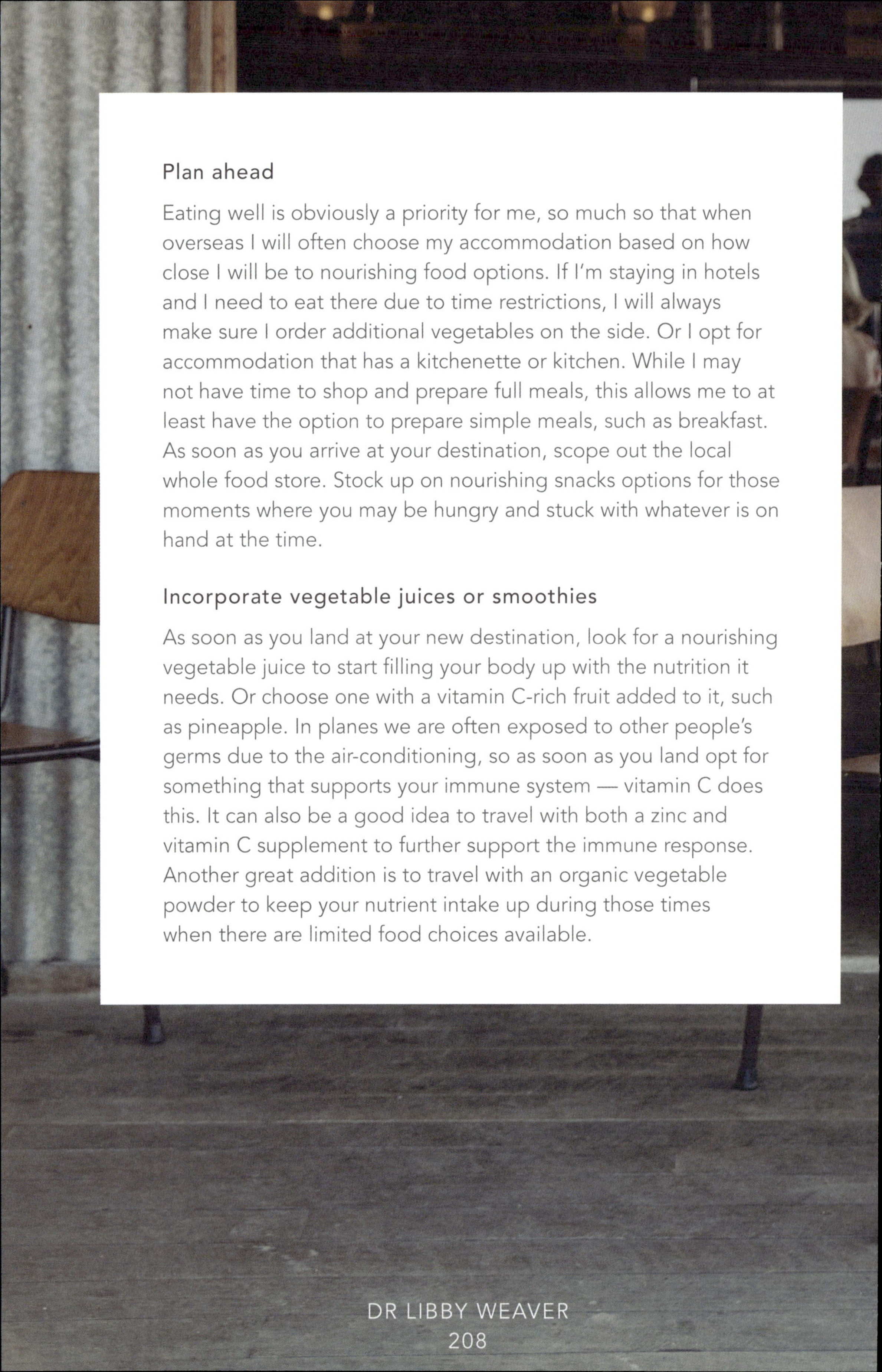

Plan ahead

Eating well is obviously a priority for me, so much so that when overseas I will often choose my accommodation based on how close I will be to nourishing food options. If I'm staying in hotels and I need to eat there due to time restrictions, I will always make sure I order additional vegetables on the side. Or I opt for accommodation that has a kitchenette or kitchen. While I may not have time to shop and prepare full meals, this allows me to at least have the option to prepare simple meals, such as breakfast. As soon as you arrive at your destination, scope out the local whole food store. Stock up on nourishing snacks options for those moments where you may be hungry and stuck with whatever is on hand at the time.

Incorporate vegetable juices or smoothies

As soon as you land at your new destination, look for a nourishing vegetable juice to start filling your body up with the nutrition it needs. Or choose one with a vitamin C-rich fruit added to it, such as pineapple. In planes we are often exposed to other people's germs due to the air-conditioning, so as soon as you land opt for something that supports your immune system — vitamin C does this. It can also be a good idea to travel with both a zinc and vitamin C supplement to further support the immune response. Another great addition is to travel with an organic vegetable powder to keep your nutrient intake up during those times when there are limited food choices available.

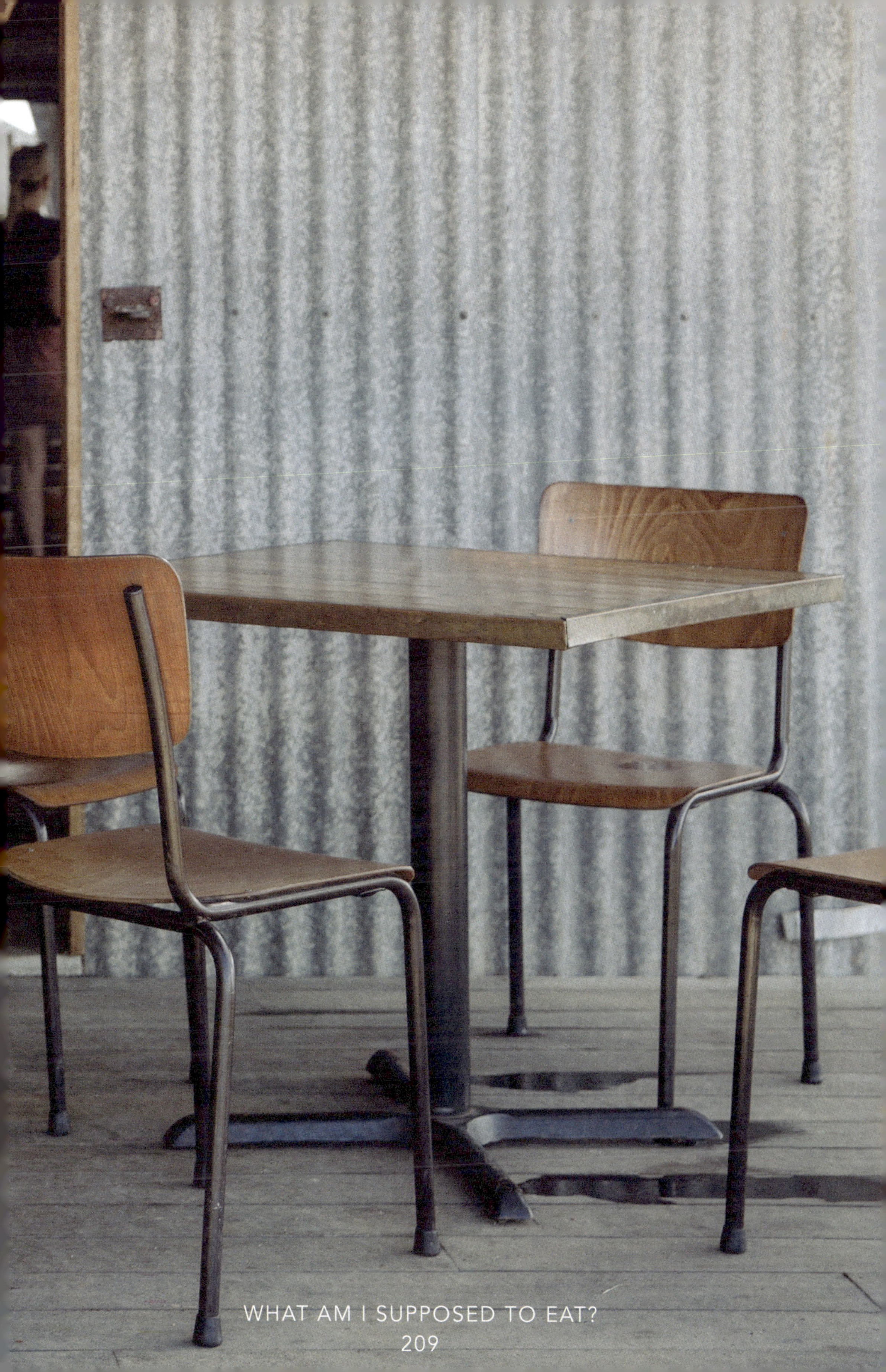

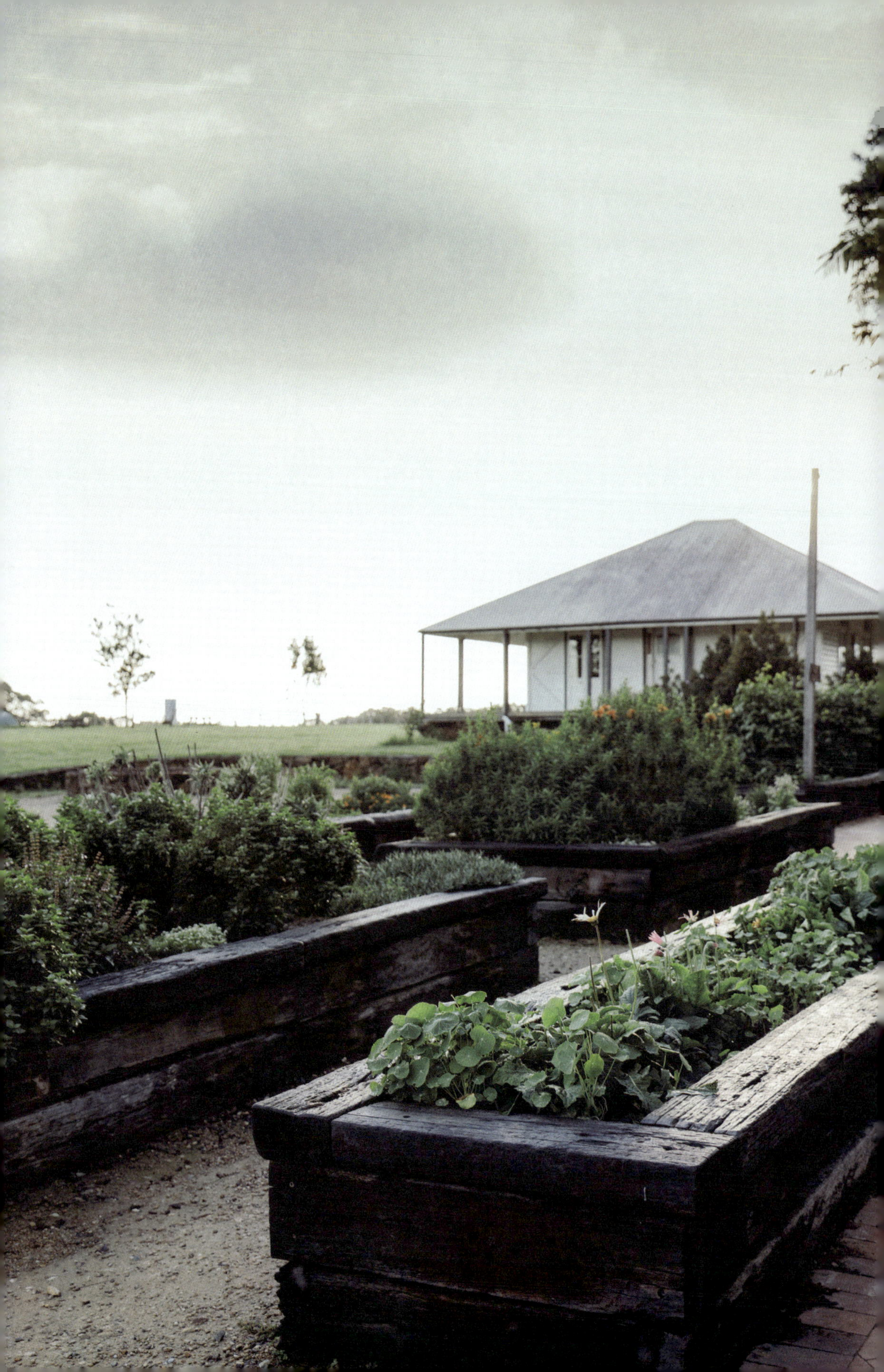

Could you grow it?

REDUCE THE TIME FROM PICKING TO CONSUMPTION

Imagine basing your meals on what is ripe and ready in your garden and being able to add oodles of parsley and basil to your meals, because it is quite literally growing at your back door. Growing your own food is not only a wonderful skill to have, it also provides a sense of accomplishment and connection to the earth like nothing else.

As the human population becomes more urbanised, many believe they have literally lost the space to be able to grow their own food. Or those who have the space may simply have lost touch with the importance, the pleasure and satisfaction that comes from producing our own food.

The reality is, you don't actually need a lot of space. Many have adapted to space restrictions by growing crops in hanging baskets or window boxes, in raised beds or containers, and having pots on balconies providing lemons and herbs. Where you live is no longer an excuse for not giving something a 'grow'!

Growing your own food is not only beneficial for the environment, it's also more nourishing for you. Home-grown produce is generally more nutritious, because the time from picking to consumption is significantly reduced, meaning there is minimal nutrient degradation. It also tastes better. How good does a cherry tomato taste picked straight from the vine, compared to one that has been sitting in cold storage for three months?

Unless you regularly buy your produce from a farmers' market or directly from a farmer, chances are your produce has spent some of its life in cold storage. Those apples you buy from the supermarket have likely been in storage for months before they're put on display in the 'fresh produce' aisle.

Not to mention the nutrient degradation the produce has suffered if it has been shipped from halfway across the world. Opting for local produce really does make all the difference. And you can't get more local than your own home!

You don't have to have a garden that is the envy of everyone — start small. Start by growing some leafy greens and a variety of herbs, and then, once you've found your green fingers, extend a bit further. Get your children or grandchildren involved. They can help weed, water and tend to the garden. Or, better still, give them a section they can keep themselves, and help them learn from a young age the value of growing their own food. Not so long ago I witnessed a group of children aged between five and 12 helping their parents to dig for potatoes. They thought it was great fun finding them! Then there was a dinner I was invited to recently, where initially the young boy refused to eat the green things on his plate, but, after learning that they came from his garden, his face lit up and he ate them. Growing some food can make a difference for many reasons.

Ask your parents, grandparents, friends, colleagues or neighbours for tips. Don't let years of gardening knowledge be left unheard. Ask the farmer selling seedlings at the farmers' market for tips, or the attendant at the garden centre — you may be surprised how easy it actually is.

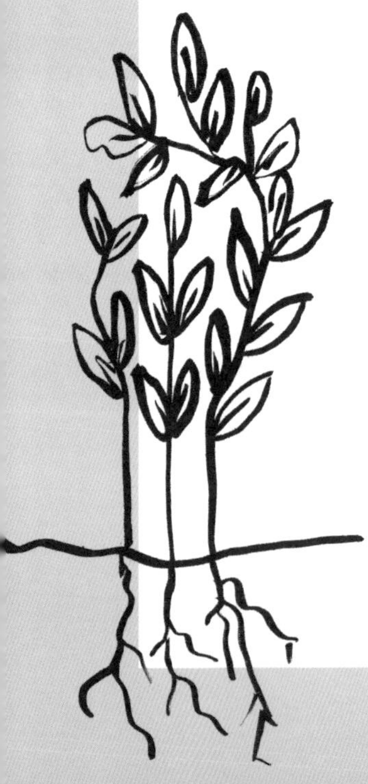

As if you needed another reason for growing your own, but another one close to my heart is how it offers much greater input from you over what goes into your food. It allows you to keep your produce spray-free, using fertiliser and pest control methods that you are comfortable with and that are better for the environment. Knowing what is (or is not used) in the growing process and being able to control how they're grown is enough of a reason to grow your own vegetables. It will certainly give you great insight into the true cost of food and may help you to value spending a bit more to purchase produce that has been grown organically and ethically.

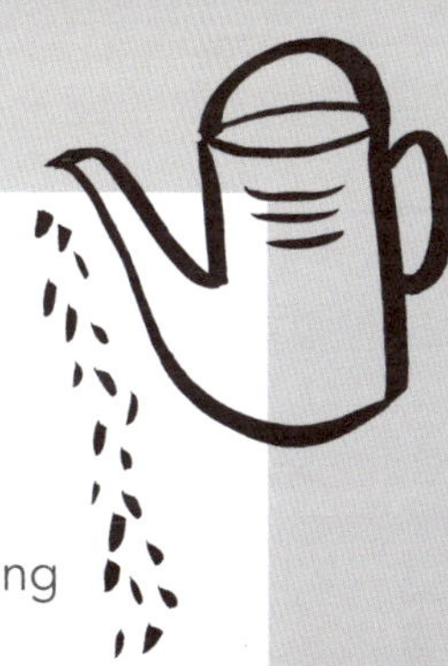

You will be amazed at the community of people who are passionate about growing their own food; it is somewhat contagious. Who knows, maybe you might even inspire your friends, family or neighbours to start putting in a plot or adding some planters to their apartment balcony.

COMMUNITY GARDENS

The concept of community gardens is something that's springing up all over the world. They provide a shared space for communities to work together to grow their own produce and, of course, obtain new skills. They benefit individuals by providing them with access to fresh, often organic or at least spray-free produce and promote physical activity. Community gardens also have many social benefits — they promote interaction, build a sense of community and provide a place to meet new people. They also offer fresh food to people who may be struggling financially.

There are also community gardens where you can have your own allotment, which is perfect for an apartment dweller or if you don't have a spacious backyard. The social benefits of community gardens are also a joy to be part of, not to mention that they offer a cost-effective way to grow your own (spray-free or organic) vegetables.

In the past few years, the New Zealand health sector has begun to identify gardening as a possible way to help reduce the high prevalence of avoidable chronic conditions among communities with poor health. More and more organisations are becoming aware of planting edible gardens — from which everyone benefits! I have noticed in my travels that gardens that would have probably originally have been planted with flowers now also contain herbs and sometimes even leafy greens. It is so wonderful to see.

I encourage you to explore and find out more about the community gardens close to you and how you might contribute to and benefit from their establishment and growth.

WAYS TO AMP UP YOUR VEGIES

By now you will understand the importance of increasing the amount of vegetables you eat each day. Often we can *know* something, but it's when we take the time to think about *how* we're going to change that things really begin to transform.

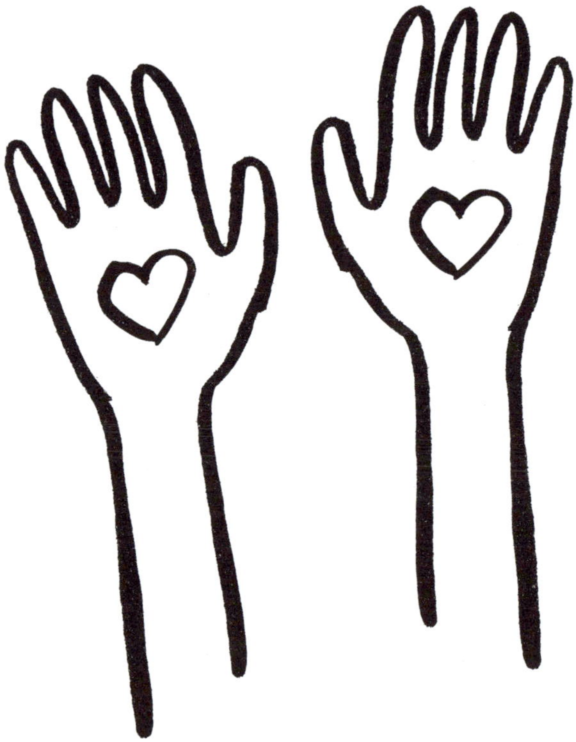

ONE SERVE OF VEGETABLES

One serve is considered to be about ½ cup of cooked vegetables or about 1 cup of salad. So you don't have to measure food (as I find this prompts a poor-quality long-term relationship with food), this is about one palm cupped of cooked vegetables and two palms cupped of raw salad vegetables, just to guide you.

Always order a side of steamed vegies when you eat out

Swap crackers for vegie crudités

Drink an organic greens powder mixed in water each day

Introduce a "breakfast salad" to your mornings

Add sprouts to salads and stir-fries to amp up their nutrient density

Add sauerkraut to your meals

Swap your snack for a green smoothie (be mindful of the amount of fruit you add)

When planning your meals, start with what vegetables you'll eat and then add fats, protein and carbs from there. Make sure vegetables take up half the room on your plate

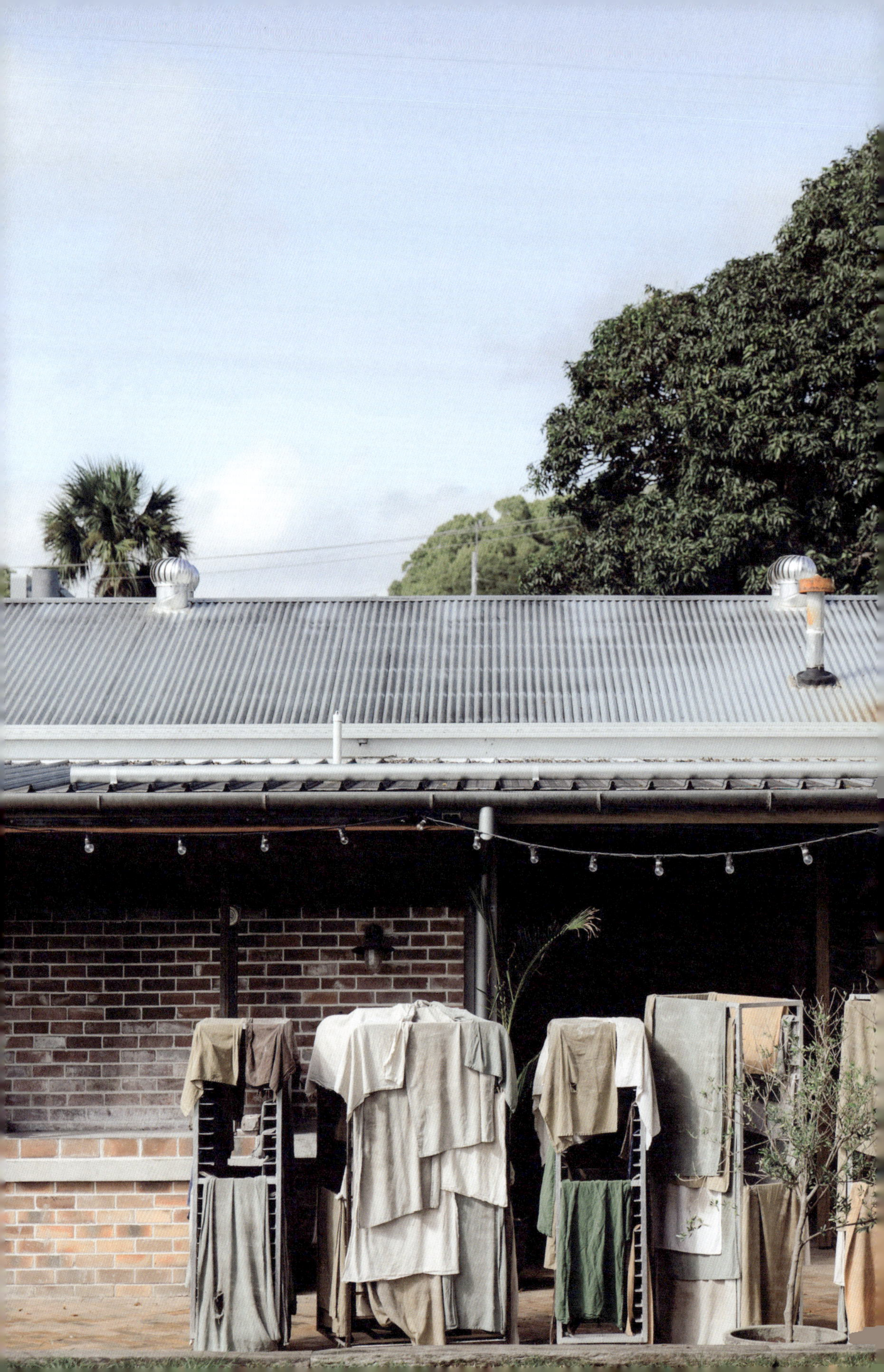

Nutrition conundrums

THE IRONY OF IRON

There are scenarios where, even for nutrition experts, there is confusion. Here is one that is top of mind. The recommended dietary intake (RDI) of iron for women through the menstruation years is 18 milligrams (mg) per day (post-menopausal women and men require 8mg per day). However, it is a common nutritional deficiency among this population.

Iron is an essential mineral that is required for the transport of oxygen around the body. It is also critical in a healthy immune response, for energy production, as well as storing oxygen in muscles (this is why muscles are red in colour).

Symptoms of iron deficiency:

- fatigue
- lack of concentration
- increased risk of infection
- headache
- pale skin
- weakness/dizziness.

Who is most at risk?

- women in reproductive years
- young children
- pregnant women
- vegetarians
- vegans.

WHERE DO I FIND IRON IN FOODS?

There are two types of iron that we obtain from foods. Iron from animal sources is called haem iron and iron from plant-based sources is known as non-haem iron.

Due to its structure, the body absorbs haem iron more efficiently than non-haem iron.

Animal food sources of iron include (per 100 grams):

- liver 11mg
- beef 3.5mg
- lamb 2.5mg
- salmon 1.3mg
- pork 0.8mg
- chicken 0.4mg
- snapper 0.3mg

Plant-based iron (*non-haem iron*) sources include:*

• kidney beans	1 cup	3.1mg
• green lentils	1 cup	3mg
• tofu	100g	2.9mg
• chickpeas	1 cup	2.7mg
• cashews	30g (20 nuts)	1.5mg
• spinach	1 cup	1.2mg
• rolled oats	30g	1.1mg
• almonds	30g	1.1mg
• broccoli	1 cup	0.86mg
• cooked brown rice	1 cup (140g)	0.7mg

** Note that these serving sizes vary, so you can't compare them directly to the haem sources, above. Nutritional values sourced from Nutrition Australia*

Eggs are also a source of non-haem iron and contain 0.7mg iron per egg.

To meet your iron needs, you need just over half a kilogram of beef or six cups of lentils per day — who can eat that much?

> To meet your iron needs, you need just over half a kilogram of beef or six cups of lentils per day. Who can eat that much?

Yet, as I've mentioned, the World Cancer Research Fund and numerous other cancer authorities suggest that to minimise your risk of numerous cancers, including bowel cancer, it is important to eat less than 500 grams of red meat per week.

If that isn't enough conundrums already, here is the next question.

Is the risk that science has found between red meat consumption and numerous cancers due to what animals are now fed? Up until relatively recently, cows ate pasture.

Now they are fed grains — usually corn, soy, canola (rapeseed) — instead of grass. We know that this changes the fatty acid profile of the meat dramatically; meat from a cow that eats pasture its whole life contains the anti-inflammatory omega-3 fat. Grain-fed animals have a fat profile that is very poor for human health. So is the cancer risk in humans the result of what the animal we eat, eats?

And as a nutrition professional, how can I ensure through food that a woman obtains her daily iron needs? It's almost impossible. Yet when we are deficient we suffer, as do children born to iron deficient mothers. It is a serious problem.

This is a massive reason why I believe in supporting a nourishing diet with food-based supplements, because I can't see how we can meet our iron needs through our diet these days. While I wish we didn't need supplements, in this day and age, it is my opinion that we do.

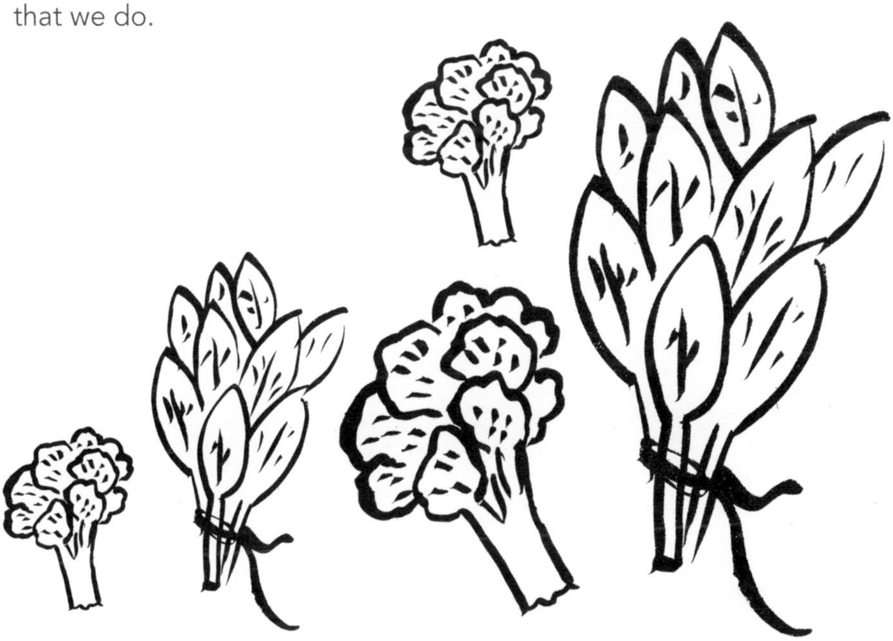

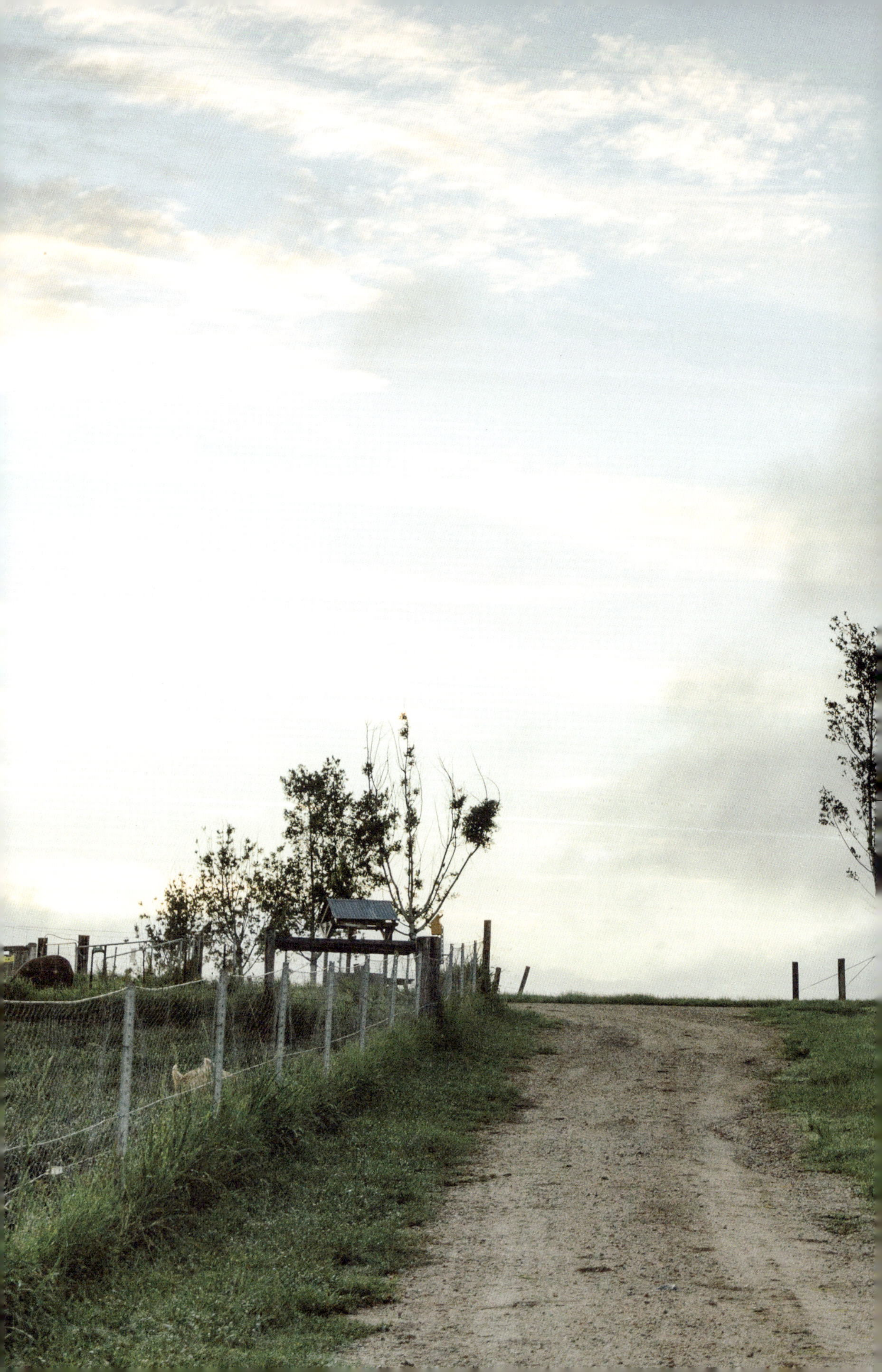

Nutritional blind spots

ESSENTIAL SUBSTANCES YOU MAY NOT BE GETTING ENOUGH OF

I am not suggesting that you eat or don't eat in a certain way. That is your choice. However, if you do eat in a certain way, there are nutrients that you need to be particularly aware of, as they are easily at inadequate levels in some diets.

You can do it, of course you can. I'm simply bringing your awareness to essential substances that you may not be getting enough of if you eat a certain way.

Following are some common ways of eating and their subsequent potential for nutrient deficiencies.

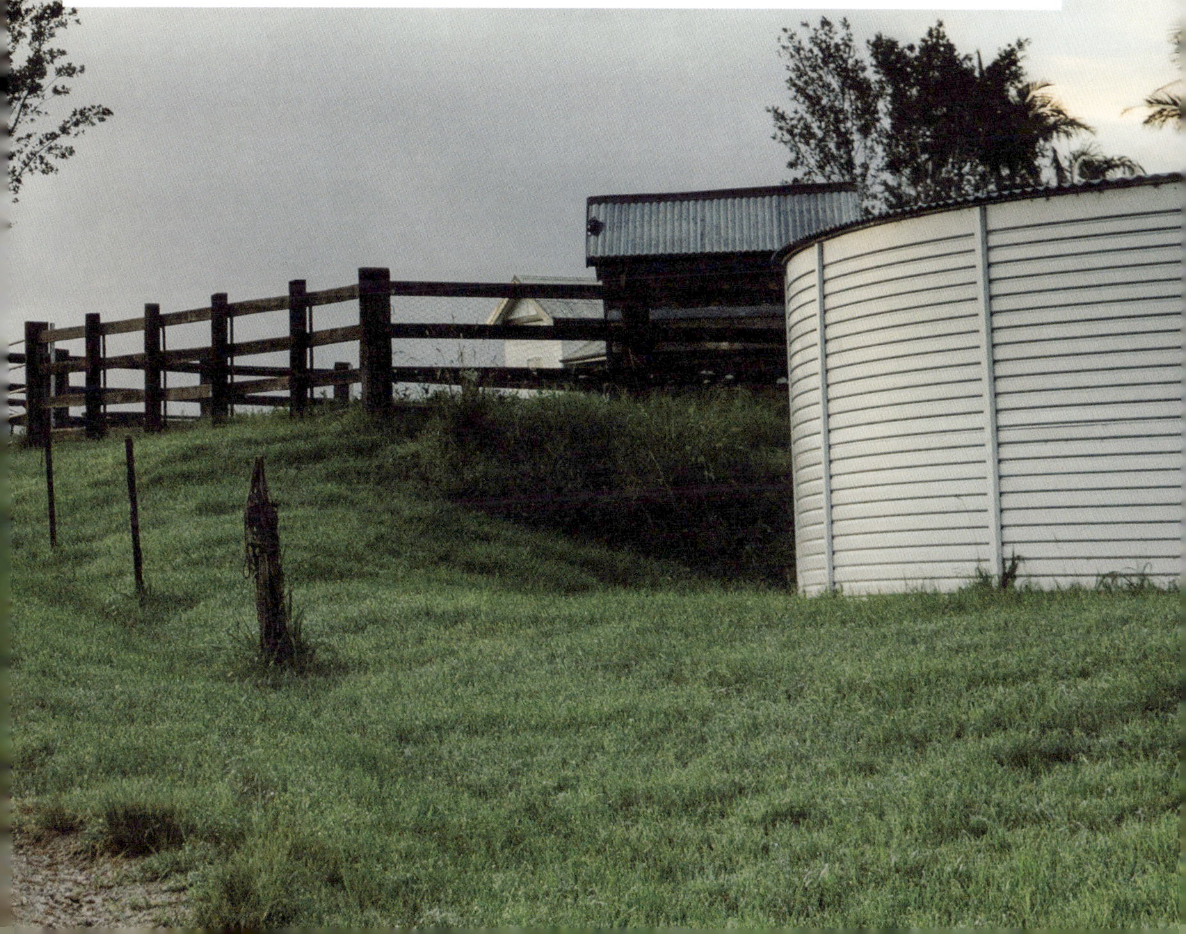

VEGETARIAN

If you eat a vegetarian diet, the nutrients for you to particularly focus on include:

Iron (even more so if you are a menstruating female): Food sources of iron for you include eggs, green leafy vegetables, and dates. However, although iron is present in these foods, it is not at high levels, nor is it in a form that the body easily absorbs without vitamin C. If you are a menstruating female, you need 18 milligrams (mg) per day. If this is you, you may need to supplement your iron intake. Eggs are the richest vegetarian source of iron at 0.7mg of iron per egg. You can see how easily a deficiency can occur when you need 18mg per day.

Zinc: Food sources of zinc for you include eggs, sunflower seeds and pumpkin seeds. You require 8–14mg per day, and these seeds contain 0.9mg per 100 grams (remembering how little seeds weigh). Eggs contain 1.2mg of zinc per 100 grams which equates to about 0.5mg zinc per egg. So you will usually need to supplement this nutrient.

VEGAN

If you eat a vegan diet, you need to ensure you obtain optimal levels of specific nutrients that can be too low when you eat this way. In addition to those that are underconsumed in a vegetarian diet (keeping in mind that eggs aren't eaten on a vegan diet), these include:

Vitamin B_{12}: From the time you become vegan, your B_{12} stores will last between two and five years. After that you will need a supplement. Or don't let yourself get depleted; supplement from the get-go.

Calcium: If you drink caffeinated drinks or soft drinks, your requirements for calcium will be higher than if you don't. Green leafy vegetables, figs, sesame seeds and tahini are some examples of vegan foods that contain calcium for you to focus on.

Omega 3 fats, particularly DHA: The body can convert ALA from plants into EPA and DHA (found in algae and fish) yet in many people this is inefficiently done. Sources of ALA include flaxseeds, chia seeds and walnuts.

GLUTEN-FREE

If you eat a gluten-free diet, make sure you obtain enough:

B-group vitamins: These are more likely to be deficient if you don't eat offal meats. Refer to more detailed information about B vitamins on page 76.

LOW-CARB

If you eat a very low-carb diet in any form, you also need to ensure you obtain enough B-group vitamins.

LOW-FAT

If you eat a low-fat diet, make sure you obtain optimal levels of:

Essential fats: The omega-3 essential fats are found in oily fish, flaxseeds, chia seeds, walnuts and pecans, while the omega-6 essential fats are found in evening primrose oil, borage oil and whole blackcurrants.

Fat-soluble vitamins: Vitamins A, D, E and K are widely spread throughout foods that contain fat, and were discussed in a previous section on page 70.

If you eat in one of the above ways, be mindful to ensure you are obtaining all of the nutrients your body needs for optimal health and function.

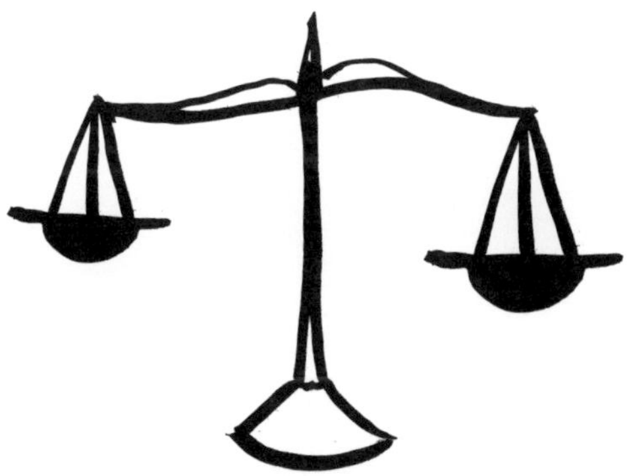

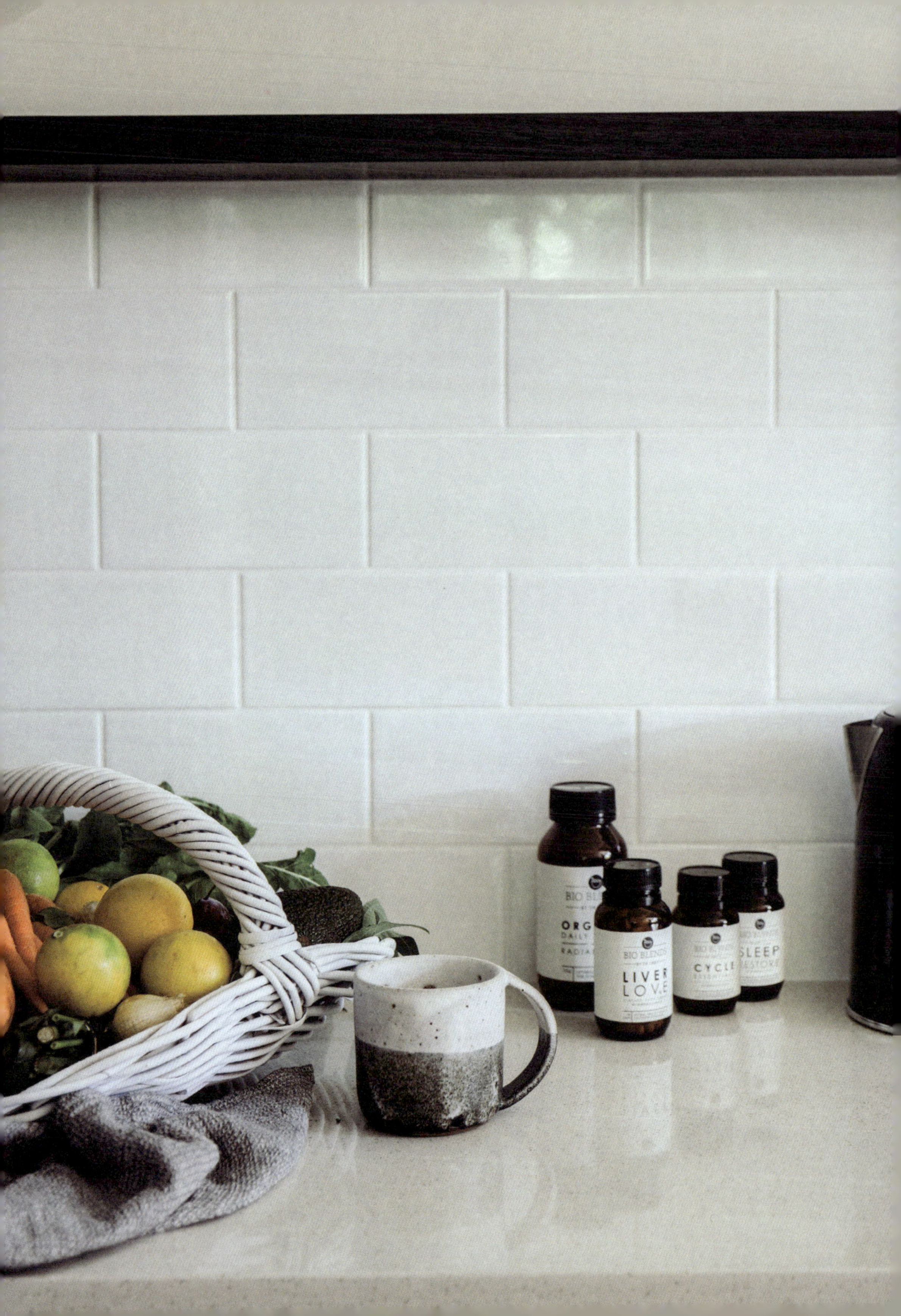
BIO BLENDS
LIVER
LOVE
CYCLE
SLEEP

Supplement your food?

OR USE FOOD AS YOUR SUPPLEMENT?

Supplementation is an area of confusion for many people. There are those who say it's unnecessary as we get complete nutrition from our food. While eating a varied and abundant diet of mostly plants to ensure you are eating in a nourishing way is vitally important to your health, I have found that nutritional supplementation is also commonly required. However, the quality and source of the nutrients in the supplements, as well as what other nutrients they are packaged with, all play a role in the bioavailability (usability) of the supplements in your body, so it's important to choose carefully.

Practitioner-only supplements, for example, will provide much higher doses of targeted nutrients than those you can buy off the shelf from a chemist or supermarket. And as the name suggests, these will need to be prescribed to you by a practitioner. However, food-based supplements are always the best choice since what's included in the supplement is not made synthetically in a lab and the supplements simply contain concentrated levels of food-sourced nutrients. There is so much power inherent in our food, yet remember that the nutrient density in the food is completely reliant on soil health.

Most nutritional supplements are synthetic, which means the nutrients included in them are made in a laboratory. Now some will argue that vitamin C is vitamin C no matter what. And on the one hand that is correct. Vitamin C is ascorbic acid and ascorbic acid can be created in a lab or by Nature, where it is found in an orange or a lemon, for example. Ascorbic acid from both sources does behave as vitamin C in the body; however, studies examining the effectiveness of nutrients, based on their source — synthetic versions or nutrients from food — reveal that the food-sourced nutrients win almost every time when it comes to absorption, and sometimes by an extensive margin.

It appears that compounds that are unique to food make nutrients from food sources highly bioavailable. So, in a world where soil is depleted and our nutritional needs are greater than ever before, I have seen great health be obtained and maintained through eating well and supplementing with additional nutrients and herbs from whole, real food sources.

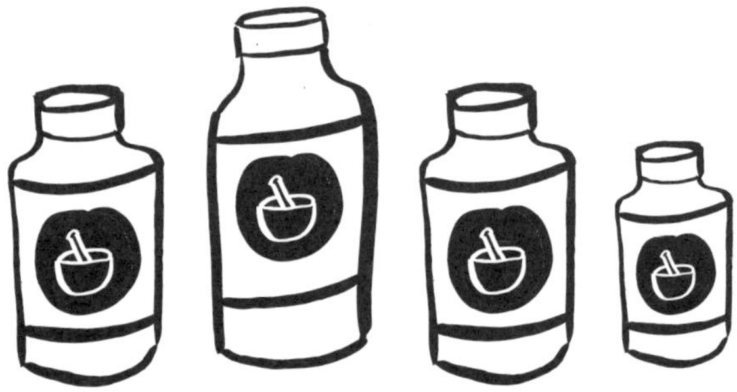

Here are a few reasons why I believe in good quality nutritional supplementation and find it essential for most people:

- The nutrient density of our soil is significantly lower than it was even 50 years ago and if a nutrient isn't in the soil, it can't be in our food.
- When we make stress hormones, especially at the level that many people do today, it changes how we breathe to more shallow and rapid. This turns over more oxygen and as a result, more free radicals are generated. These free radicals have the potential to damage our tissues in a process called oxidative damage, which is one of the ways we age and degenerate from the inside out. To combat the effects of more free radicals we must consume more antioxidants. We also make free radicals during detoxification, so the more toxins and pollutants we are exposed to, the more free radicals we will generate as well. We primarily get our antioxidants from coloured plant food, yet here's another big change that has occurred in the recent past: the effect of artificial sprays. As I've already shared with you, plants

big change that has occurred in the recent past: the effect of artificial sprays. As I've already shared with you, plants have the ability to protect themselves from pests by making substances within themselves to fulfil the need that act as antioxidants to humans. But when we spray the plant with pesticides or herbicides, the plant no longer needs to make that substance itself so the antioxidant levels in our foods have dropped dramatically in the relatively recent past.

- Modern living sees us exposed to an increasing number of pollutants, from what we eat, drink and breathe to what we put on our skin. These pollutants require detoxification via biochemical pathways that change problematic substances into less harmful versions of themselves. So, if we are asking more of our detoxification and elimination pathways, it makes sense that we would require more nutrients today, not fewer. Yet, when you couple less nutrient rich food, and the change in food and lifestyle choices, with the increase in stress hormone production, we have a situation that sets us up for under-nourishment. When so much of our health, energy and disease prevention is related to detoxification and elimination, and nutrients are required for these processes to work effectively, it's so important we amp up our nutrient intake.

PLANT SOURCES

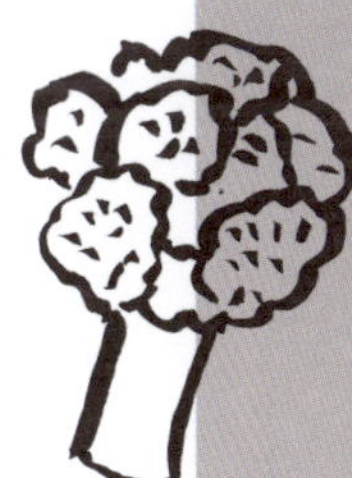

I'm also a fan of getting as much nutrition as we can from our food, particularly plants. Plants are little superstars when it comes to what they are able to do for you. Here are some of the standouts.

Brassicas

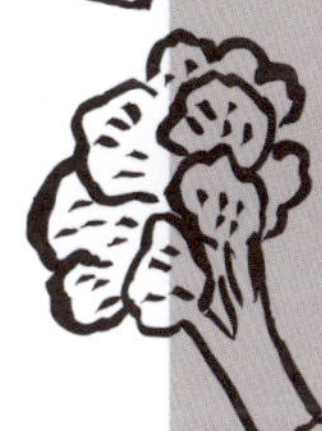

Not only do they contain vitamins, minerals and fibre, but also substances unique to this botanical family. These substances (some of which we've already talked about) are known as indoles and glucoraphanin. Glucoraphanin gets converted into the ultra-superstar sulforaphane. These substances support the optimal functioning of some of your most important biochemical pathways

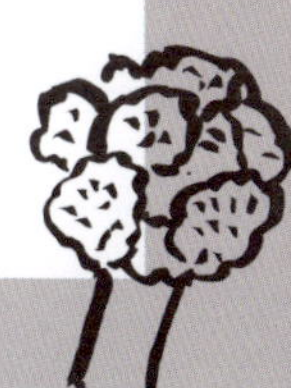

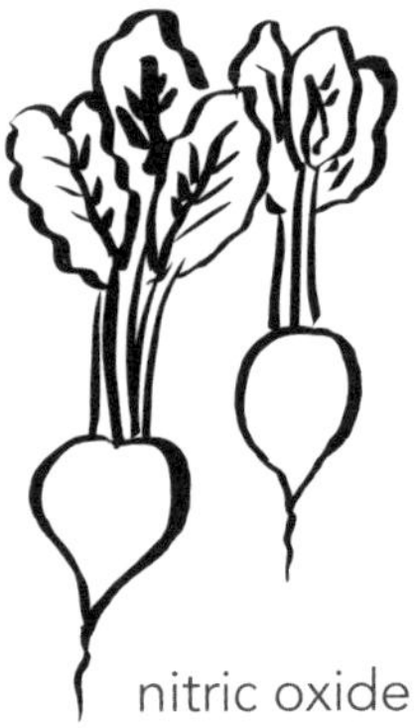

— those of the liver, particularly those needed for estrogen and pesticide detoxification. Both really matter, obviously.

Beetroot

This richly coloured plant contains many nutritious substances, including nitrates which convert to nitric oxide. This can help regulate blood pressure and provide better oxygen delivery to the tissues — again essential for great energy, anti-ageing and disease prevention.

Blackcurrants, grapes and berries

With their seeds kept in, these superstar fruits are high in oligomeric proanthocyanidins (OPCs), which are a set of bioflavonoid complexes that act as free radical scavengers in the human body. Think of OPCs like a nutrient with super power, it supports virtually every metabolic system in the body. Research has shown that decent intakes of OPCs help protect against cardiovascular and other degenerative diseases and have numerous other benefits, including lowering LDL cholesterol levels, reducing platelet aggregation (you don't want your blood to be too sticky for so many reasons), increasing the strength and elasticity of blood vessels, helping collagen repair itself, reducing fluid retention and inflammation, relieving functional problems associated with varicose veins, lessening the tendency toward diabetic retinopathy and improving skin health. All of that from Nature.

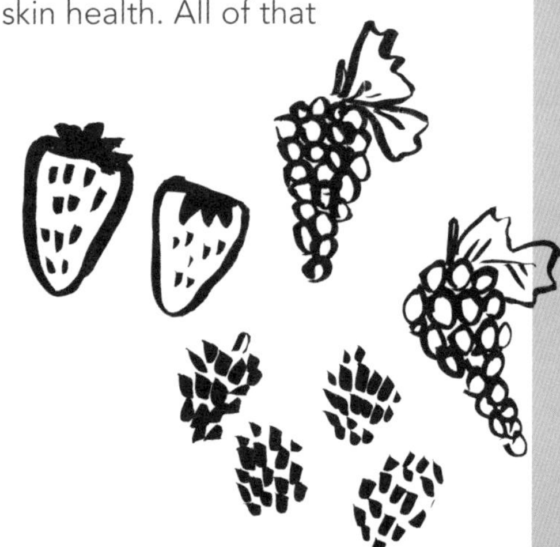

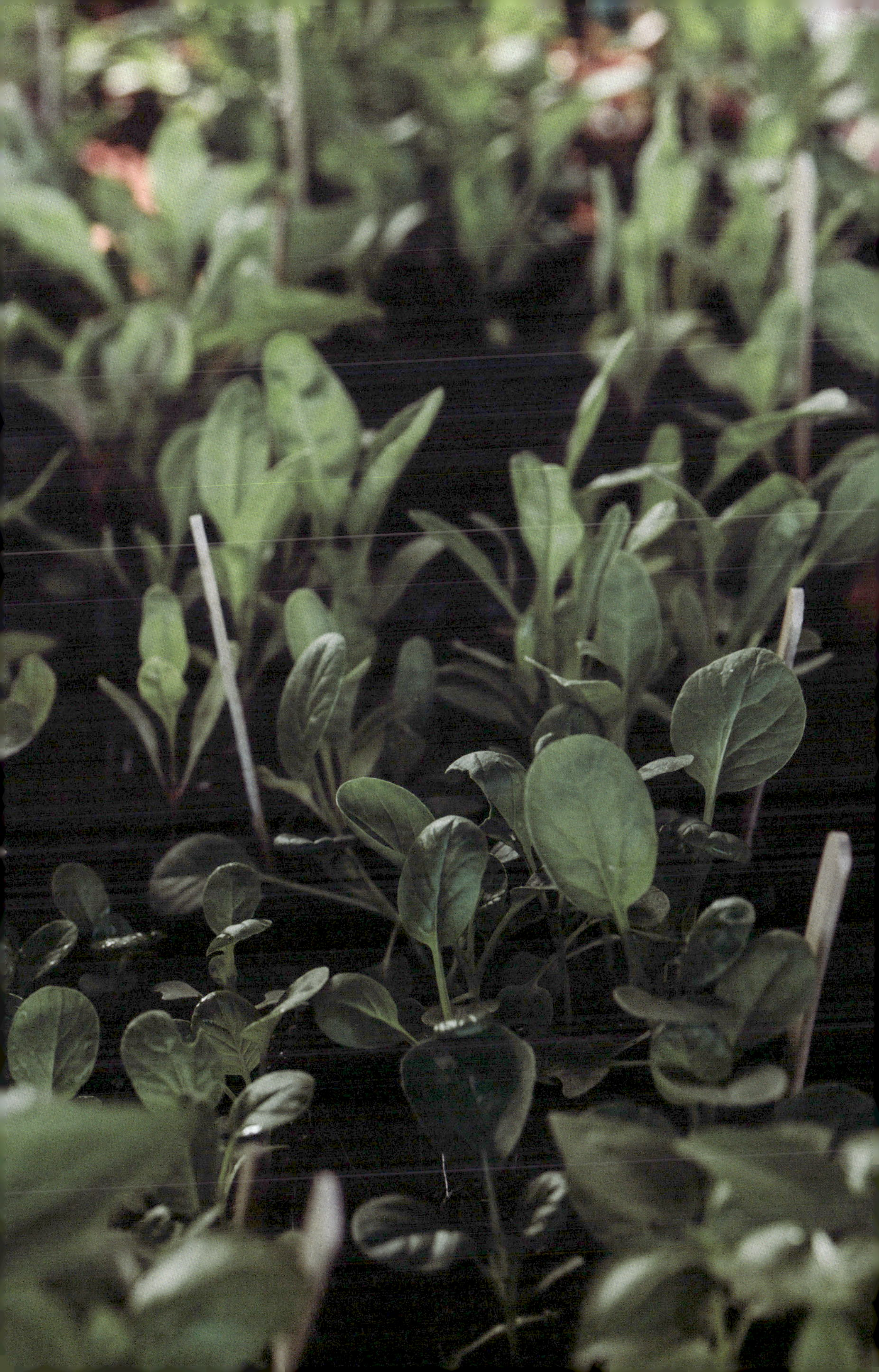

Food frequency

DO YOU NEED TO SNACK?

Another area of food confusion for many people is how often they are supposed to eat. They will ask whether it is better to eat three meals a day, or five or six smaller meals. The answer is within you.

Let's first explore, however, how this even came to be a question. When did the concept of 'snacking' first come to be a named thing that was at first considered extravagant or excessive, to then be considered the norm? Or even necessary. The low-fat era.

When you reduce how much fat you eat, you get hungrier. You also give your body the message that, because fat is restricted in your world, it is not safe for you to use it for energy. So, you had better utilise more glucose (colloquially and not quite accurately referred to as 'sugar'). When you predominantly use glucose as your fuel, your blood levels of glucose (BGLs) go up and down constantly and when they are low your body gets the message that it needs to replace what has been used. So you want/crave sweet food to top up your levels. Your hunger won't stay at bay for more than about four hours when you live like this, and you can end up in a vicious cycle of eating too much sugar, despite knowing better.

Factors other than carbohydrate intake that influence whether your body is getting the message that it needs to burn more glucose relative to body fat include anything that leads you to make adrenalin, as this requires glucose to be supplied to power you for the fight-or-flight response that adrenalin elicits. What leads us to make adrenalin? Caffeine. And fear, both real and perceived. A real fear might be the stability of a riverbank after a flood. A perceived fear might be the "pressure" of your email inbox. They are both the same to your nervous system and it all

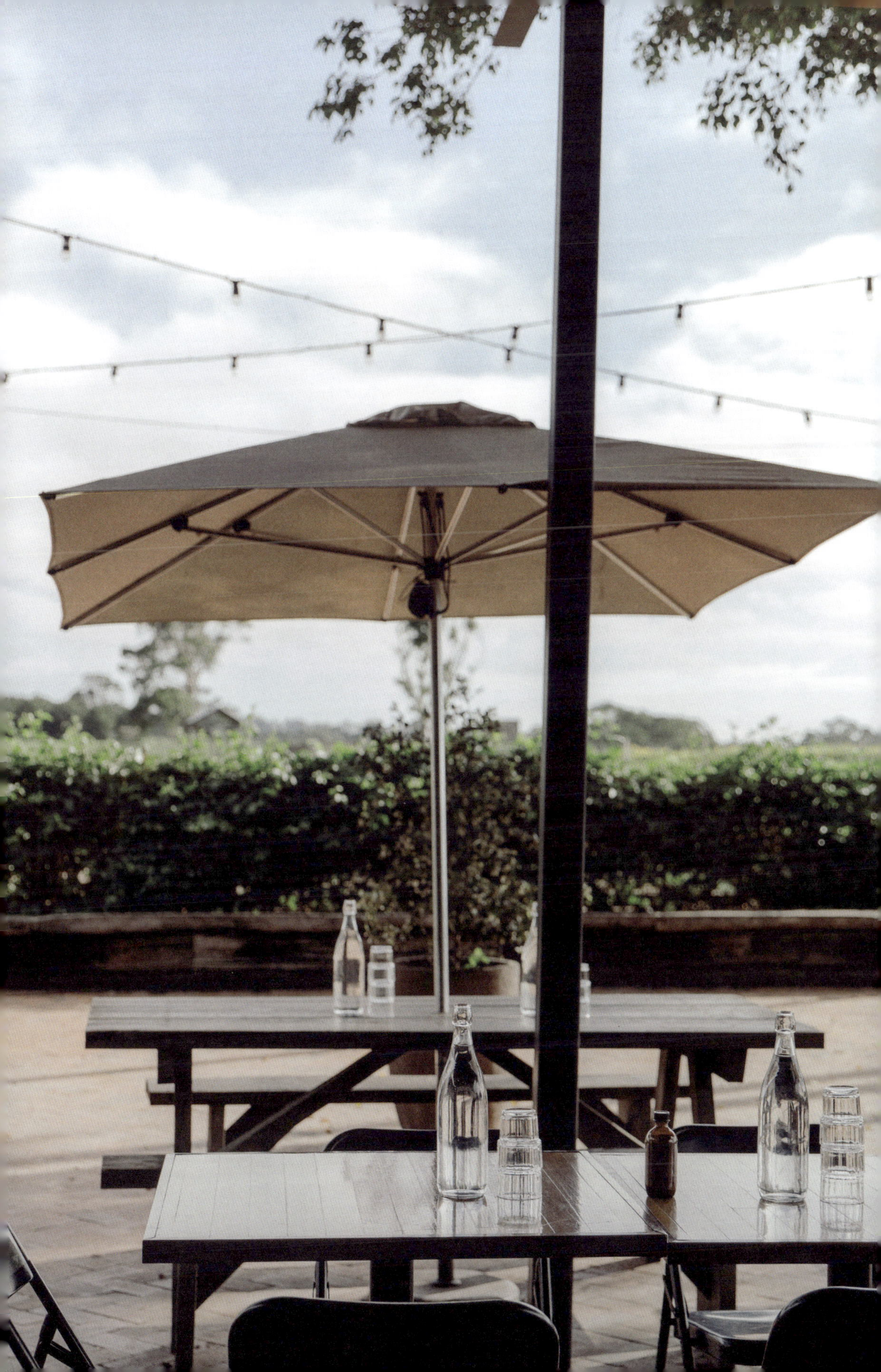

drives your body to believe that it predominantly needs to use sugar as its fuel. This will make you want to snack.

Yet when you eat fat, you are more satisfied. You also communicate to your body that it is safe to use body fat as a fuel as there is more available. You use less blood glucose and stored glucose (glycogen) this way, so BGLs don't fluctuate so much. This means you will usually be satisfied with three (or even two) meals per day.

> "When you are an efficient fat-burner, not only is your energy consistent across the day, but your clothes fit you better and you don't have all of the lousy consequences that burning mostly sugar gives you."

When you are an efficient fat-burner — meaning your body feels safe to use your body fat and the fat you eat, as fuel — not only is your energy consistent across the day (with no slumps), but your clothes fit you better and you don't have all of the lousy consequences that burning mostly sugar gives you.

When we burn mostly glucose (sugar) as an energy source, we are likely to experience sugar cravings, regular and sometimes excessive insulin production (which signals fat storage and increases risk of insulin resistance, impaired glucose tolerance and type 2 diabetes), inflammation, and excessive free radical production — which is how we age and degenerate from the inside out.

So start to notice:

- How often do you feel hungry? If it is an hour after eating, what you ate did not serve you.
- What do you crave? If it is sweet food, you are either trying to meet physical needs by topping up blood and/or stored glucose, or emotional needs and looking for food to give you sweetness or joy in your life.
- Is there a time of day you are more likely to crave sweet food? If there is a pattern to this, increase your whole food fat intake at the meal before your craving kicks in. For example, if you are desperate for sweet food mid-afternoon, increase the fat content of lunch (perhaps from oily fish, avocado, nuts, seeds or organic butter) and notice if this changes your sweet food desires after a week of doing this consistently.
- If you choose nutritious, real food snacks, do you find you eat less across the day because you aren't ravenous for main meals? Or does even real food snacking lead you to eat too much across your day?

There is no right or wrong; there is simply what best serves your body. And this will likely change over time or even from day to day.

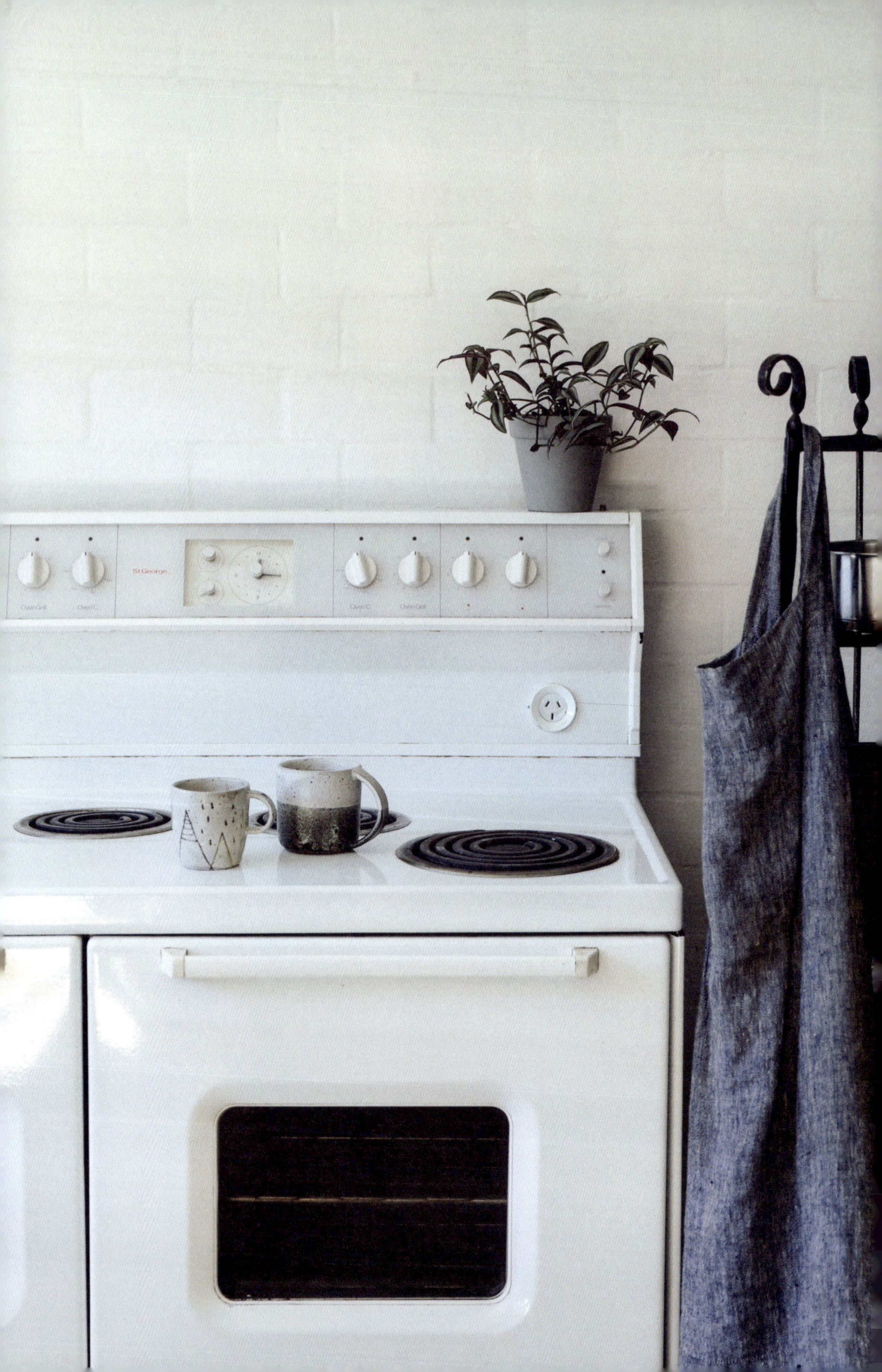
St George

What fuels your hunger?

IT'S NOT JUST WHAT YOU EAT IT'S WHY

Over the years, I have observed not just what people eat, but also why they eat. Hunger is one obvious reason but there are others. And having read widely on this topic (the work of Louise Hay, Lise Bourbeau, and Geneen Roth in particular) in an attempt to better support my clients and those attending my women's health weekends, here is a list of six other reasons people eat. There may be more — we are always learning — but explore these six to see if any of them resonate for you.

- theory/principle/ethics (fear)
- habit
- emotion
- sensory pleasure
- reward
- lethargy/laziness/convenience.

Please know there is no right or wrong, good or bad here. My goal is to simply help you see why you make some of the choices you do, if this is something you need assistance with, on your road to getting back in touch with what will truly nourish your own individual body.

If you are motivated by ethics when you eat, you are influenced by the notion of good and bad, or fear.

In this category, you would find any of the situations of the following pages.

FEAR

Fear of wasting:

- Eating or drinking any substance before it goes bad, or before the best by date.
- Finishing what is on your plate rather than discarding, sharing or donating leftovers.
- Finishing other people's plates.
- Ordering and eating the full meal at an all-inclusive restaurant e.g. bread, entrée, main, dessert, just because they are all part of the deal.
- Choosing the cheapest food, even though it is not what you want (and your financial situation doesn't necessitate this).
- Depriving yourself because you deem the price too high, even though you can afford it.

Fear of letting someone down, displeasing them, offending them, upsetting them:

- You find it impossible to say no when you are offered something to eat or drink, even though you weren't planning to have anything and you don't really feel like it.
- Fear of sharing your dislike of something after you have tasted it (so you keep eating).

Fear of judgement:

- You do what others do out of a fear of what they will think or say about you if you don't — think office morning tea or a function where alcohol is offered — you don't want to partake but you do anyway.

Fear of consequences:

- Eating because you feel like you have to, despite a lack of enjoyment, only because you perceive (or have been instructed) that your body needs nourishment in this particular form — think a salad for lunch when your instinct tells you that a warm, cooked meal would nourish you better and get you further into your afternoon.

HABIT

You are motivated by habit if:

- You often or always eat the same thing e.g. porridge with three prunes for breakfast.
- You often or always eat at the same time.
- You do what you learned in childhood and have done ever since, like eating three meals a day, never skipping breakfast etc.
- You hesitate or refuse to try a new food because you have never tasted it before.

EMOTION

You are motivated by emotion if:

- You know you aren't really hungry but something inside you prompts you to eat anyway or perhaps you're constantly thinking about what you might eat next.
- You are angry, frustrated, hurting or lonely and you eat or drink for lack of being able to let out your feelings in some other way.

SENSORY PLEASURE

You are motivated by sensory pleasure if you are motivated by one or more of your senses:

- You eat or drink because it smells good.
- You cannot help yourself (amount-wise) because it is 'just so good'.
- You are attracted to a certain type of food once you have seen it, while a few minutes earlier you had not even thought about it.

- You cannot refrain from sampling a dish once you have set eyes on it.
- You want to eat the same thing as the person next to you.
- You are attracted to a certain food once you have smelled it or touched it — you like its aroma or texture — think popcorn at the movies.
- You let yourself be influenced by what you hear, for example, when a waiter gives a glowing description of an item on the menu.

REWARD

You are motivated by the need for a reward if:

- You have just completed a task you are proud of and now feel you need to eat or drink something, knowing very well it is not necessary at that particular moment.
- You have exceeded your limits — you might have worked non-stop without taking a break — and you think that eating or drinking something will now make you relax.
- You feel frustrated or unhappy because no one complimented or thanked you so you eat whatever you feel like (this also can be motivated by emotions).

LETHARGY/ CONVENIENCE

You are motivated by lethargy/convenience if:

- You accept what someone else cooks for you, rather than having to prepare something yourself (see note below about families).
- You are home alone so you choose a dish that doesn't require any preparation.
- You choose not to eat rather than to have to make yourself something.
- You buy takeaway or a frozen meal as you leave work.

Lethargy isn't always a motivation as such — it can be a state due to health or relationship issues you are experiencing at the time. Of course, people who are part of a family or group will accept what someone else has prepared for them as being part of the family unit/group that evening. With the statement above, I refer more to a flatmate situation or living alone.

Note that you could also choose to drink something for any of these reasons — wherever it says 'eat', you can replace it with drink as we have these same motivators for drinking, almost anything other than water. And of course there are times when we eat a food for a number of reasons. For example, you might eat some biscuits for emotional reasons and as a reward.

If you make food choices during a day or night that you know in your heart of hearts does not serve you — does not nourish you — whether that is poor quality food choices, too much food or starving yourself, then reflect on why you chose this. Bring curiosity, rather than judgement.

Start a notebook that you keep in your kitchen or bag if you like. And consider what happened in the hours or minutes preceding your poor quality choice. After a week or so you will start to see a pattern, and for some of you, this will allow you to better guide your own nourishing food choices far more often.

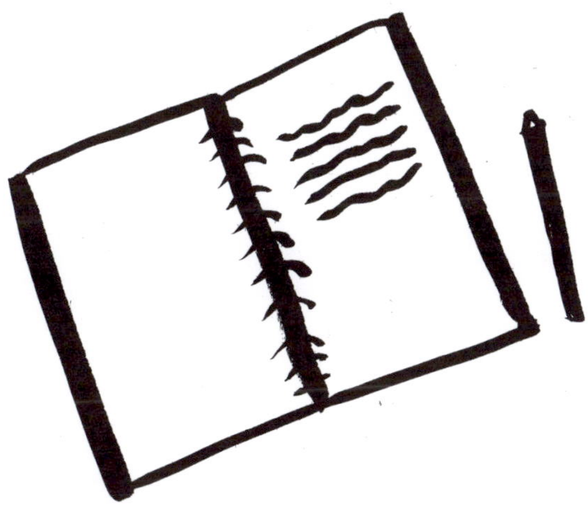

WORKSHEET

1

The first step to begin to change non-hungry eating is to see WHY you make certain choices.

Reflecting on the previous article, think of the last time you ate when you weren't really that hungry.

Tick the boxes that relate to why you might have opted to eat at this time:

- ☐ Fear of:
  - ○ wasting
  - ○ letting someone down
  - ○ judgement
  - ○ consequences
- ☐ Habit
- ☐ Emotion
- ☐ Sensory Pleasure
- ☐ Reward
- ☐ Lethargy

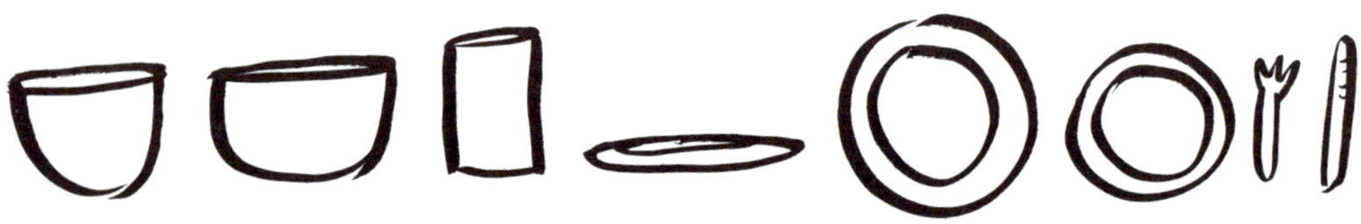

2

Now you have identified why you made that choice, what else could you do or focus on the next time this feeling or situation arises?

e.g. 'I always have something sweet after dinner'. What else can you do or focus on that would bring you that feeling of sweetness?

A good way to know if you're truly hungry is to ask yourself "Would I eat a serving of vegetables right now to curb my hunger?" If the answer is no, perhaps you're not truly hungry.

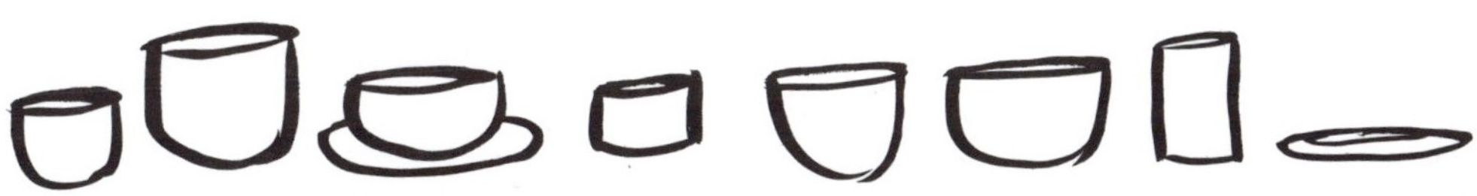

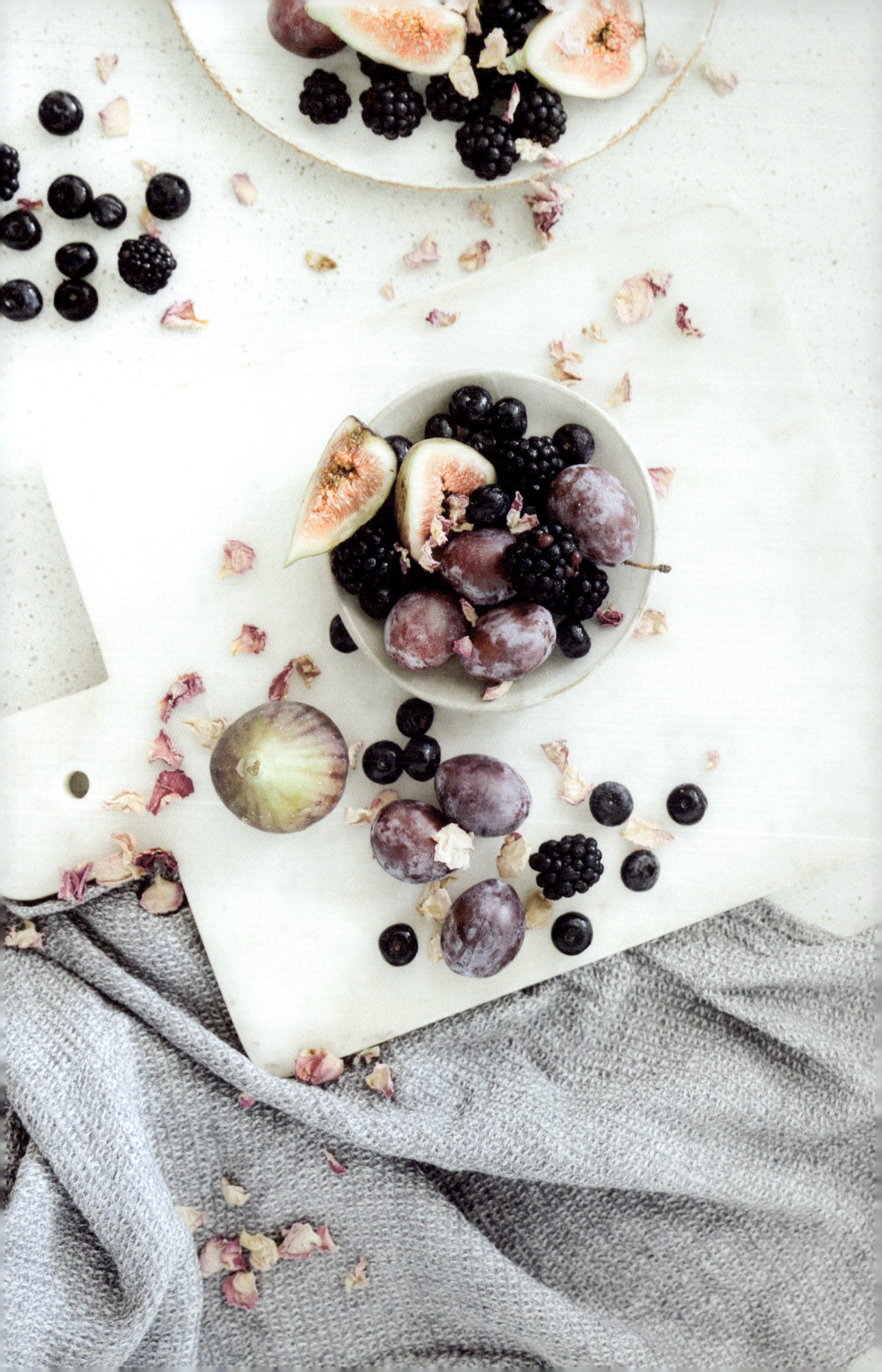

I just need something sweet...

WHEN TASTE BUDS TAKE OVER

There are countless people who make great food choices for breakfast and lunch and then at three o'clock in the afternoon they feel like someone else has taken over their body! The desire for, and subsequent consumption of, sweet food at this time of day can take hold without you really knowing why or what to do about it. Too many people reach for sweet food that doesn't serve their health; in fact, it may contain substances that actually have the potential to take away from their health, yet they feel powerless to live any differently, having 'tried' to change their sweet food habits many times.

And if it's not reaching for sweet food at three o'clock, it's reaching for sweet food after dinner or late at night. Many people grew up in households where the meal wasn't complete unless there was a dessert or at least something sweet and it can be particularly difficult to move past these habits.

There is a big difference nutritionally between a couple of squares of dark chocolate and the whole block, or a homemade fruit and nut ball versus a packet of store-bought biscuits — you get my drift. However, the often-relentless guilt that consuming something that is perceived as 'bad' or 'unhealthy' is in my opinion just as damaging to your health as the actual poor quality food. Remember from an earlier chapter, that food is not healthy. Humans are, or aren't.

Food is nutritious, or it's not. This shift in language alone can assist people to make better food choices.

TRANSITIONING TO LESS AND MORE NUTRITIOUS SWEETNESS

When it comes to reducing your reliance on sweet foods, a gradual reduction can work to change taste preferences. The taste buds on our tongue are a truly unique sensory organ. Taste buds renew every 10 to 21 days and because of this short renewal time we can train our taste buds to enjoy food with less sweetness. By changing the source of the sweet foods from highly refined sugars to sweetness from Nature, and hence decreasing the intensity of the sweet flavour, you can lower the threshold level of sweet food you prefer. For example, commercially-made products usually contain large quantities of refined sugars, but when you make real food at home you can control the level of sweetness and choose the source of that sweetness, so that each mouthful provides you with the nutrients you need for great health and vitality, and nothing that takes away from that.

Another way to shift your taste bud profile away from sweetness is, if you have smoothies made entirely of fruit, you can slowly, week by week, start replacing some of the fruit with green leafy vegetables which are naturally bitter. Eventually, once you have gotten used to vegie smoothies with only a small amount of fruit, you will find a fruit-filled smoothie too sweet for your taste buds.

When I worked in health retreats, we would serve guests essentially a refined-sugar-free diet, but to soften this transition we would serve them tahini balls (which were basically tahini, nuts, coconut and a little bit of honey to sweeten and bind them). The guests didn't receive them until the back end of their experience and they always loved and appreciated them. They loved them so much because they had just massively reduced their sugar consumption across the week, so these balls, that were subtly sweet, tasted much sweeter to them than if they had eaten one in the middle of their normal day-to-day lives.

REDUCING RELIANCE ON SWEET FOOD

Some people like to completely overhaul how they eat and feel energised and excited by doing so. For others, though, making small, committed changes over time means you can work towards consuming less processed food and enjoying more real food.

I'm certainly a big believer that it's what you do every day that impacts on your health, not what you do occasionally. Often our craving for sugar has more to do with an emotional need that isn't being met. 'Something sweet' is often perceived as a symbol of joy and we become conditioned to need something sweet to feel complete or satisfied. Here are five strategies you can use to reduce your reliance on sweet food.

Fuel yourself for longer

For far too long people have been afraid to incorporate good fats in their diets, due to the belief that 'fat makes you fat'. Try adding more fat to your meals, particularly at lunch, in the form of avocado, nuts, organic butter, coconut, tahini, or oily fish, and observe whether your desire for sweet foods mid-afternoon diminishes. Good fats slow down the release of glucose into your bloodstream, meaning you actually stay full for longer.

Slow down

If you amp yourself up on caffeine, live on adrenalin due to your perception of pressure and urgency, or push your body intensely during cardiovascular exercise, your body will predominantly burn glucose and you will crave sugar to replenish your stores. Slow down! I cannot emphasise enough the importance of activating the rest-and-repair arm of the nervous system (the parasympathetic nervous system), using breath-focused movement, which allows your body to efficiently use body fat as a fuel. Not only will you feel a greater sense of calm, you are also far less likely to experience hunger that results in you eating the entire contents of the pantry.

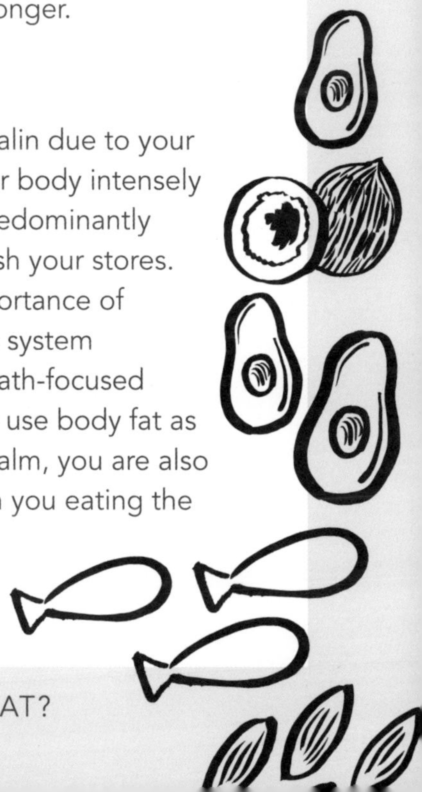

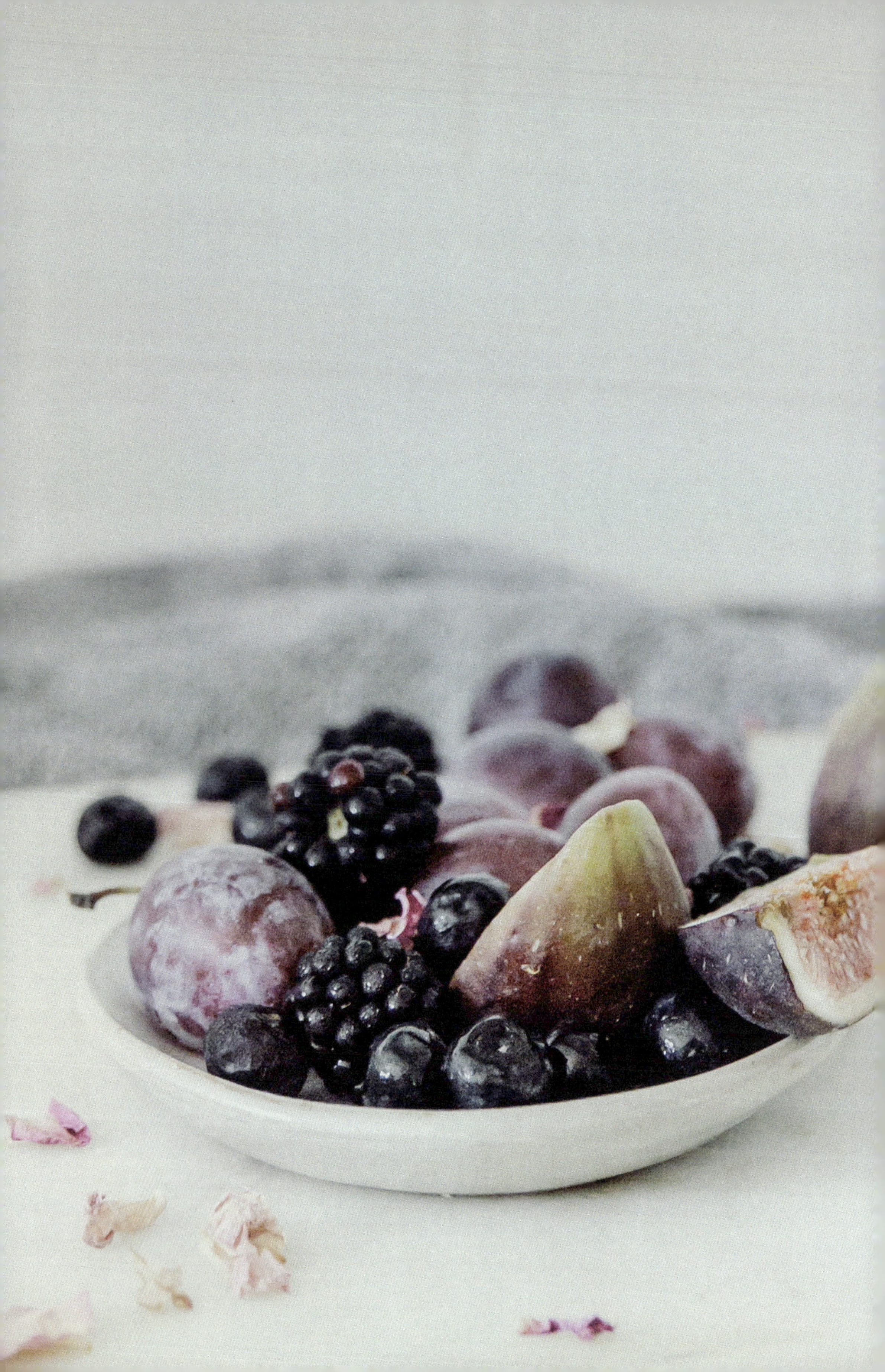

Increase your consumption of leafy green vegetables

Leafy greens tend to be bitter, which helps reduce cravings for sugar. If you eat sugar when you're feeling stressed and depressed, experiment by adding more leafy greens, like silverbeet, kale, spinach and mustard greens to your meals every day.

A couple of squares of dark chocolate

When I say dark chocolate, I'm talking about 70 per cent cocoa content and upwards! A little goes a long way, and it's a good source of antioxidants. The more bitter varieties of dark chocolate tend to mean you are satisfied with only one or two squares.

Explore the emotional connections to sweetness

Often our craving for sugar has more to do with an emotional need that isn't being met. Identify other non-food-related activities that give you a feeling of sweetness and joy and incorporate more of these into your life. Get up and watch the sunrise every morning for a week, go for a walk in Nature, write a list of all the things you are grateful for, watch your children or grandchildren sleep, or book a getaway with friends — whatever spins your tyres — and notice whether having things to look forward to diminishes your sugar cravings.

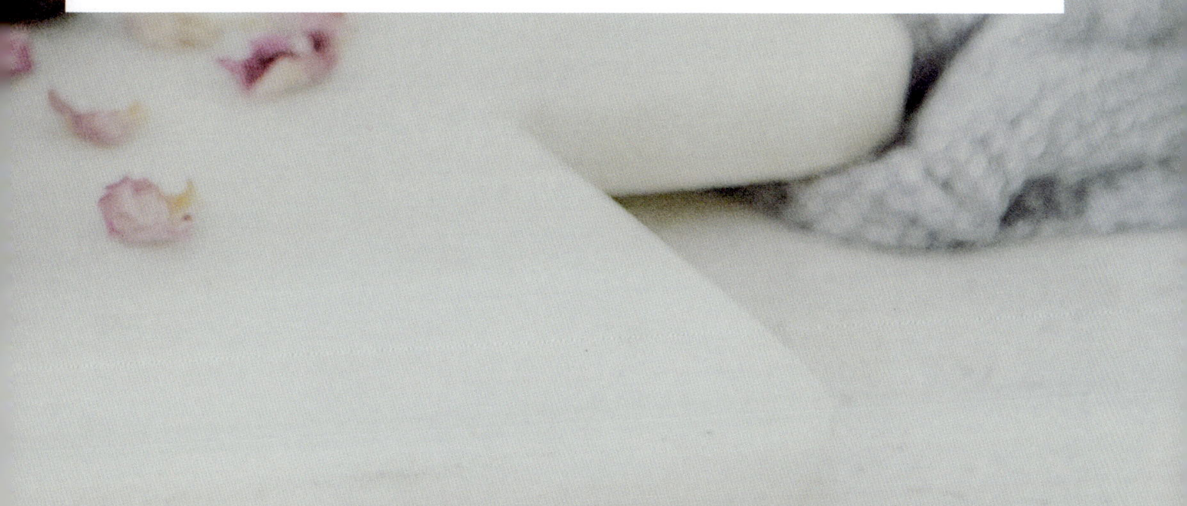

I've ruined it

BRINGING CURIOSITY TO YOUR CHOICES

Have you ever found yourself making nourishing food choices day after day until one day you don't? A common phrase I hear is "I've ruined it".

Okay, so first things first. You haven't ruined anything. All you did was eat some…umm, I don't know…let's say biscuits. Yet in your head you are telling yourself that you have ruined everything. Do you think telling yourself that you've ruined it leads you to make nourishing food choices for the rest of the day? No. It does the opposite. You decide you may as well polish off the whole packet of crackers, the whole block of cheese, the whole container of dip…You told yourself you'd have one glass of wine and, before you know it, you've had the whole bottle — so now you really feel like you've ruined it.

So you eat dinner and decide you may as well eat dessert to top it all off, because you ruined it all ages ago!

You might eat unresourcefully for another day, or week, or it might be years before you start to make nourishing choices again — all because you ate some biscuits! Remember, nothing in this world has meaning unless we give it meaning, and when you create a meaning that you've ruined everything from eating something that you know is not great for you, you run the risk of continuing the lousy eating patterns.

If you bring curiosity to your choice (of biscuits), rather than judgement, you open yourself to learn something. Instead of judging and berating yourself, ask: "I wonder what led me to eat the biscuits?"

Were you actually hungry, in which case you'd do well making some nourishing snacks each Sunday for the week ahead. Or did you have a conversation with a colleague and your feelings were

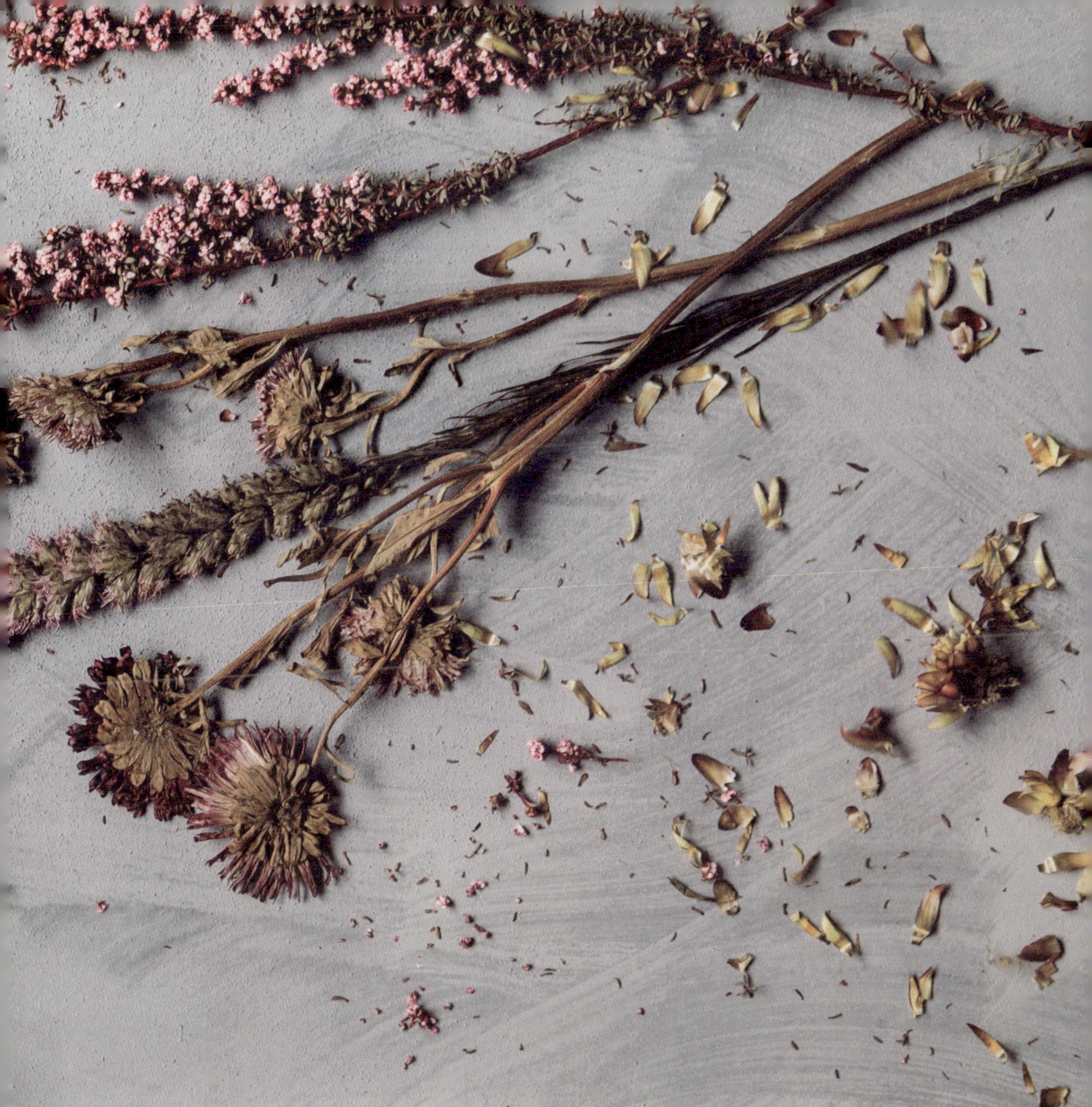

hurt, so you ate the biscuits to try to numb the pain? Utilise your poor quality choice for learning and growth, rather than allowing it to lead you to not care for yourself long term.

Another phrase that is common in these types of scenarios is "I fell off the wagon". The problem is the belief that there is a wagon to fall off! There is no wagon.

There is only your life! And it is what you do every day that impacts on your health, not what you occasionally do.

When food is frightening

WHEN HEALTH BECOMES AN OBSESSION

Disordered eating is on the rise and statistics show that even primary school aged children are more commonly becoming affected. A study in New Zealand found that out of 80 per cent of women who were polled and found to be within normal weight limits, only 18 per cent of them *thought* their weight was normal. In Australia, Canada and the United States, one in every 100 females experiences anorexia nervosa, and three in every 100 will experience bulimia nervosa. These statistics astound me and not just because it highlights the prevalence of eating disorders in the Western world. When I think about all of the women who walked through my clinic door and their relationship with food, the way that so many of them would starve themselves to lose weight, I believe that this problem is even bigger than our statistics lead us to believe.

Because it's not just an obsession with weight loss; an eating disorder that is also on the rise is *orthorexia nervosa*. The name for this relatively new eating disorder was coined by Dr Steven Bratman in 1996 to describe those of his patients who were overly obsessed with healthy eating or 'clean' eating.

I run women's health weekends for females aged 14 and up. If I ask women and girls in that room how and what they eat, countless number reply 'clean' and many have severely disordered eating. It's an obsession. And some level of health is always compromised when you are that frightened of food — when you are that frightened of yourself and your own desires.

For the vast majority of people, it is recommended to increase consumption of leafy greens, considering that research shows

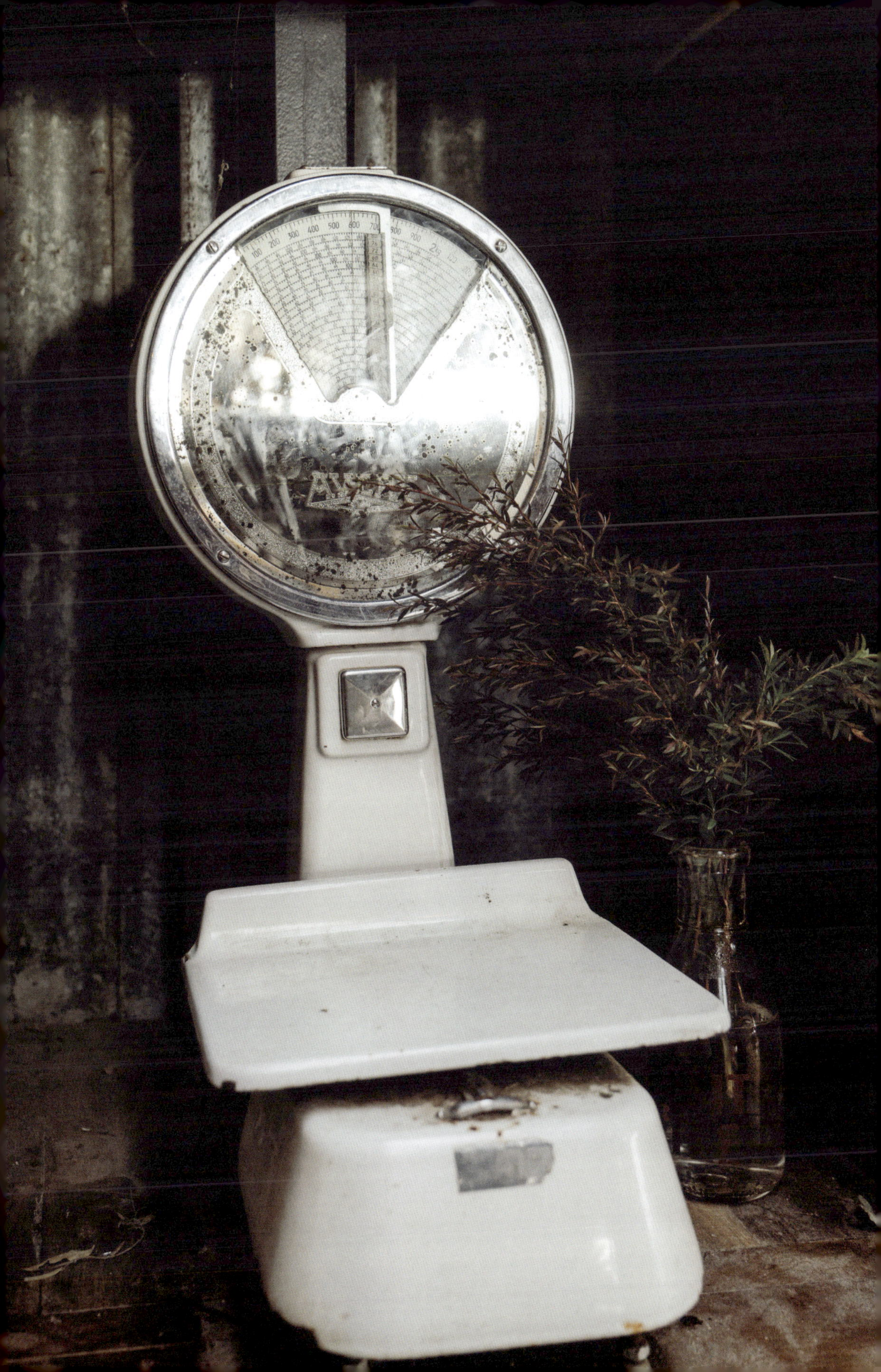

many of us do not eat enough. However, having a green smoothie, green juice, green salad and stir-fried greens in the name of health is erring towards obsessive. You all probably know someone who, after being told something is good for them, proceeds to take three times the recommended amount, because surely that means they will be three times as healthy? Well, no actually. Variety of foods is an incredibly important component of optimal health, as is chewing and when you rely too much on liquid nutrition, your stomach acid production and other digestive processes can become compromised. By all means enjoy a green smoothie! Just don't live on them.

> You all probably know someone who, after being told something is good for them, proceeds to take three times the recommended amount, because surely that means they will be three times as healthy? Well, no actually.

Orthorexia typically begins innocuously with a commitment to improve health. As the person begins to feel the benefits of eating more nutritious food, and perhaps begins to receive comments from those noticing a reduction in body size, they start to think about what else they might be able to eliminate and find themselves thinking about food with increasing regularity.

To an orthorexic, deviating in any tiny way from what they would consider to be a 'clean' diet would be met with guilt and self-loathing. They have strict food rules and plan their entire lives around food. They have difficulty allowing others to provide meals for them, because they feel the need to control everything that they put in their mouths. They can be incredibly judgemental of themselves and those around them whom they perceive are making inferior food choices.

This is the disorder at its extreme, but I actually see parallels to these tendencies within certain people who adopt a specific way of eating. When it comes to how we are supposed to eat, generally speaking as a culture we are obsessed with finding a 'plan' that works. When we find one that works for us, we become convinced that every other human on the planet would benefit from adopting it and we can become incredibly critical of those who don't eat the same way, whether we say this out loud or not. We can become so obsessed with maintaining this way of eating that it becomes incredibly difficult for others to cook for us, or to enjoy a meal out. If we deviate from that plan in the slightest, we berate ourselves for our 'bad' decision and judge ourselves harshly for 'messing up'. I think the judgment we pass on ourselves when we deviate from a set diet/nutrition or wellness plan is often more harmful than the action itself.

> *There is absolutely nothing wrong with adhering to food choices that work for your body — in fact, I encourage you to do so!*

If you know your body doesn't respond well to gluten because every time you eat it makes you gassy and bloated, then don't eat it. If you have been diagnosed with a particular intolerance, allergy or health problem that requires you to eat in a particular way, of course you need to follow that plan for the betterment of your health.

We need to be mindful that we don't become so obsessed with our food choices that they begin to rule our lives. For some people, adhering to high standards when it comes to their own nourishment is effortless and energising. For most, the pursuit of perfection is nothing more than a mask fear wears; and only you know which one is describing your relationship with food.

The way that we speak about food, the place of food in our lives and our underlying beliefs, directly affect how we eat and those beliefs can drive helpful or less helpful behaviours.

We need to try to let go of labelling food in particular ways, because in doing so we set up a whole range of beliefs that take root in our subconscious. Even something as simple as labelling food as 'clean' — seemingly the latest trend — can become problematic and set up concepts in our minds about what's okay and not okay to eat. Food isn't 'clean' or 'unclean', 'good' or 'bad', 'healthy' or 'unhealthy' — it's nutritious or less nutritious and it is far more accurate and helpful to talk about the food that we consume in this way.

Please always remember that it is what you do every day that impacts your health, not what you do occasionally. Rigidity when it stems from fear does not serve our health in any way. When we are kinder to ourselves and put less pressure on fulfilling set criteria, we are more likely to make choices in our lives that we can sustain. After all, the way you take care of yourself needs to be sustainable.

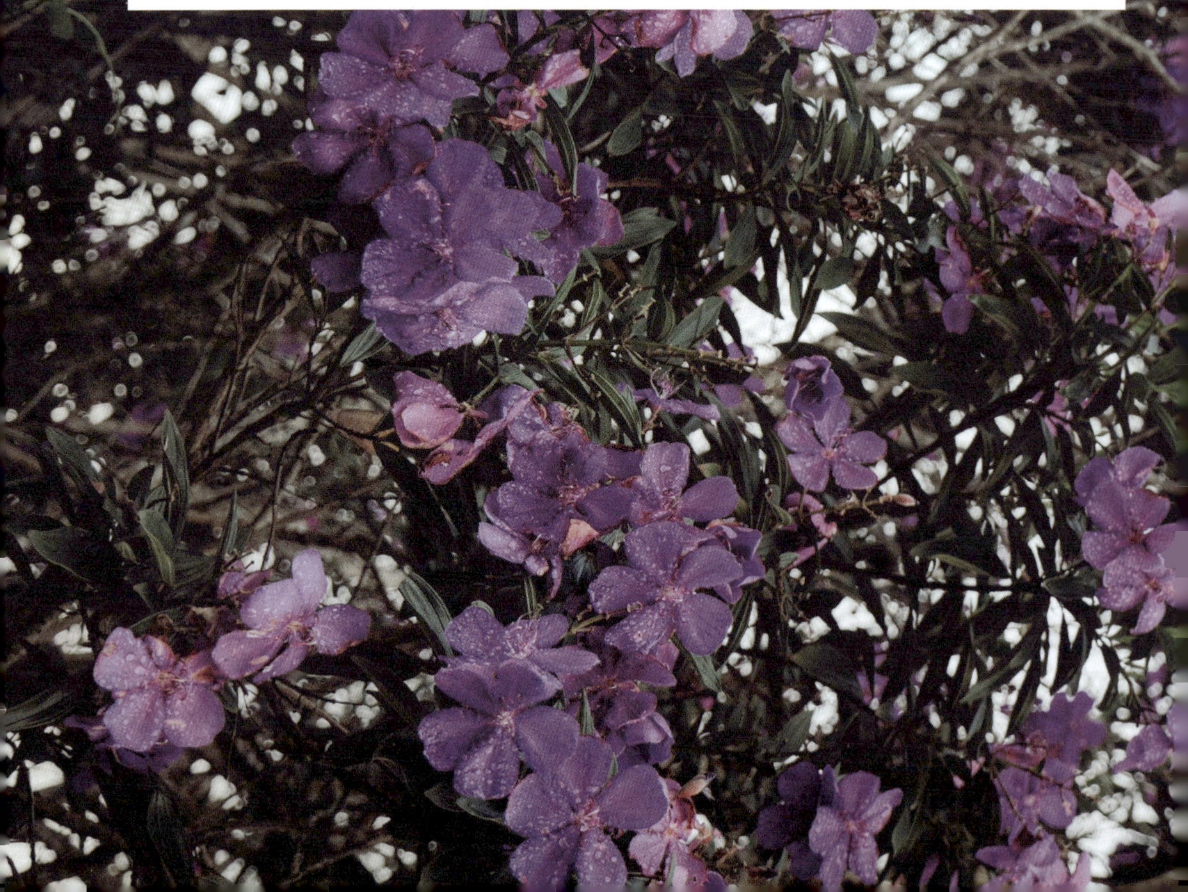

Eat from a place of love, not fear.

DR LIBBY

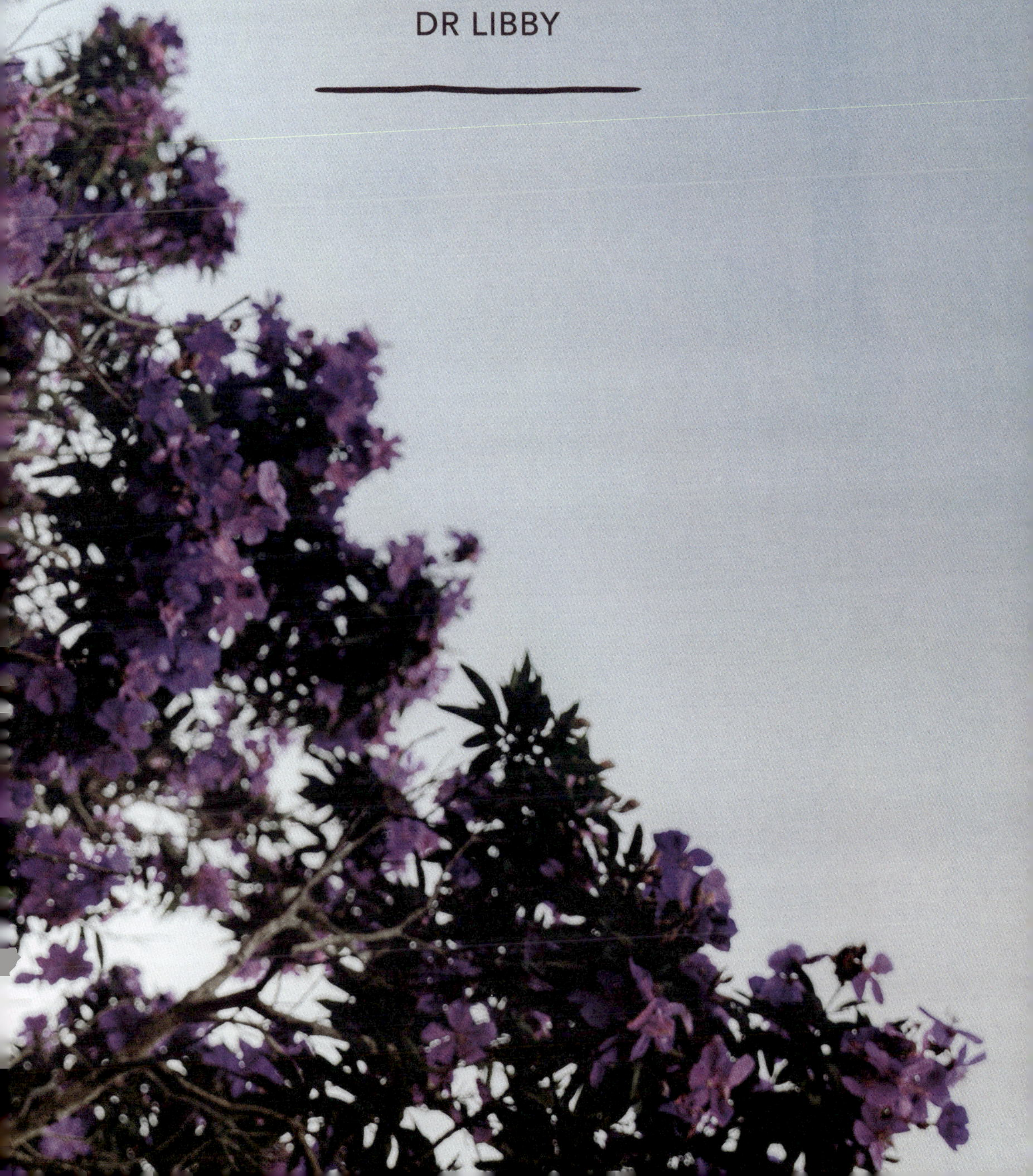

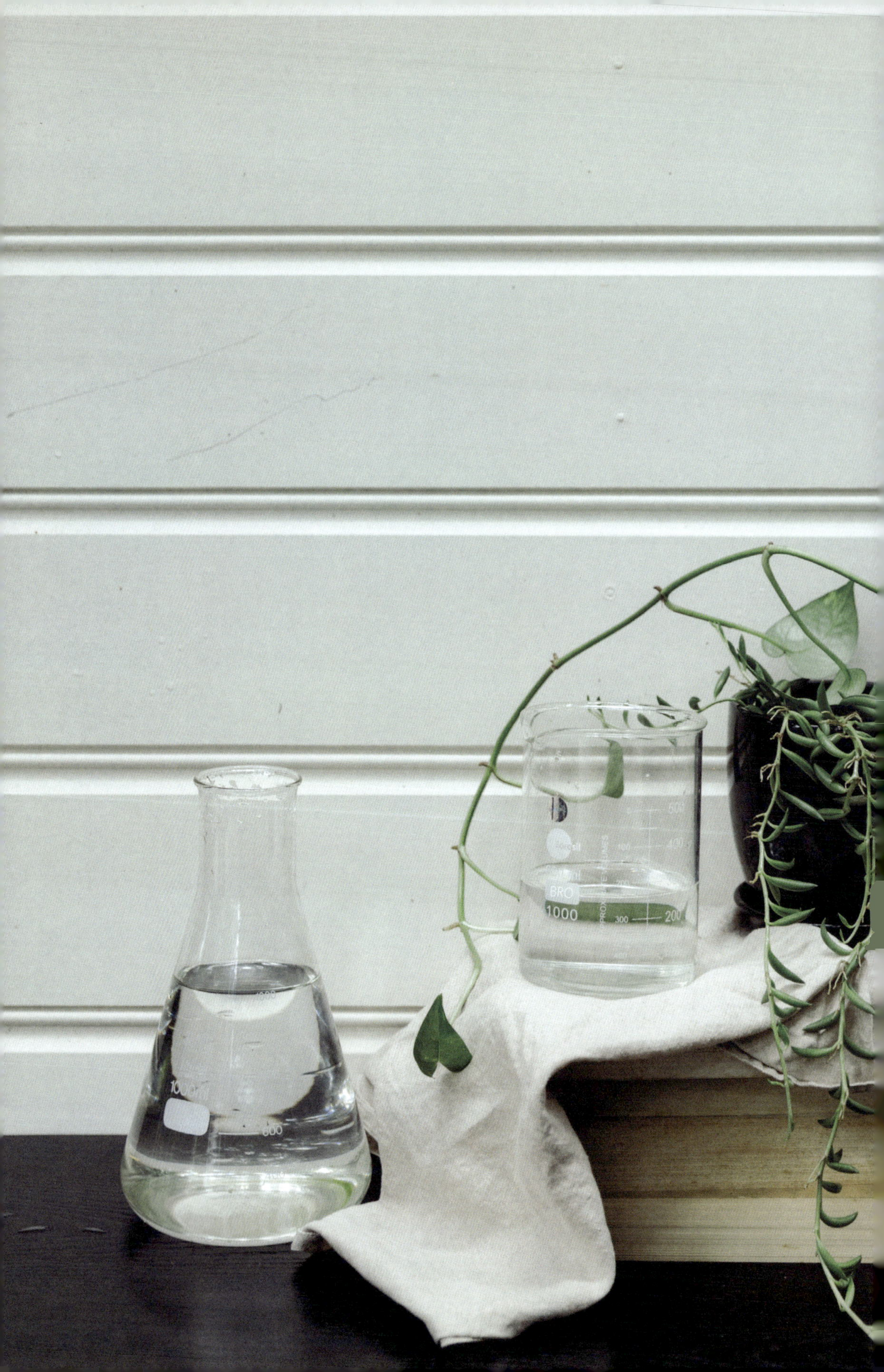
BRO
1000
300
200

Said who?

WHERE DOES YOUR ADVICE COME FROM?

My intention with this piece is to help you consider where you obtain nutrition-related information from. It is not to put anyone down or to suggest that personal experience can't play a role in supporting others. Of course, all of this can. You never know when what worked for you will assist another. There is immense beauty and kindness in that. And if you feel called to do this, then by all means share.

My concerns, however, lie in nutrition-related information being touted as the be-all-and-end-all for all people, especially when it comes from sources who have no training, beyond what they *believe*; beyond what they *do*.

> “My concerns, however, lie in nutrition-related information being touted as the be-all-and-end-all for all people.”

For example, say you go low-carb — which many people unquestionably benefit from (and, as an aside, means different things to different people; i.e. what one person defines as low-carb is another person's medium, but that is a conversation for another day). If the person guiding you doesn't know that some of what you will have cut out are some of the best nutritional sources of B vitamins for those who can digest them and that your liver requires B vitamins to fire some of your detoxification pathways, they may also not realise that unless you have replaced your grain intake with regular liver (or other offal meat) consumption — which some people do but many don't — you may not be getting enough B vitamins and this will lead to your liver not being able to do its critical work efficiently. That's what bothers me. Scenarios like this.

The advent of the internet saw people from all walks of life — both qualified and unqualified — being able to share advice. This obviously has both benefits and drawbacks. Yet part of the problem also lies in the lack of trust that has developed among the public in those who are university educated in nutrition. These people are more likely to deeply understand the inner workings of the body (the liver process, for example), but many lag behind in the food department by, for example, still promoting highly processed breakfast cereals that common sense teaches you are not highly nourishing options. You don't want to hear what is essentially nutrition marketing from a nutrition graduate. So I don't deny for a second that it's not tricky.

However, most people would benefit from simply applying common sense to food principles. For example, we all know that we need to be eating plenty of vegetables on a daily basis and we all know in our hearts whether we are eating enough of them or not. Yet, instead of simply eating more plant-based foods we might still choose to follow a diet plan set by someone else.

Too many people tend to approach food as a quick fix to get them to where they want to be and this very thinking usually sends people to seek answers outside of themselves because they don't think they know what's best for them. But if we're just approaching food as nourishing our bodies we innately know what is nourishing and what is not and our body gives us our own unique symptoms to things it doesn't feel good after consuming. Think of this as common sense paired with your own body's wisdom, again reiterating that what is supportive of one person may not be for another.

BLOGS

There are many health-related blogs out there and they tend to typically focus on improving physical and sometimes mental health. Posts often share what the blogger does themselves,

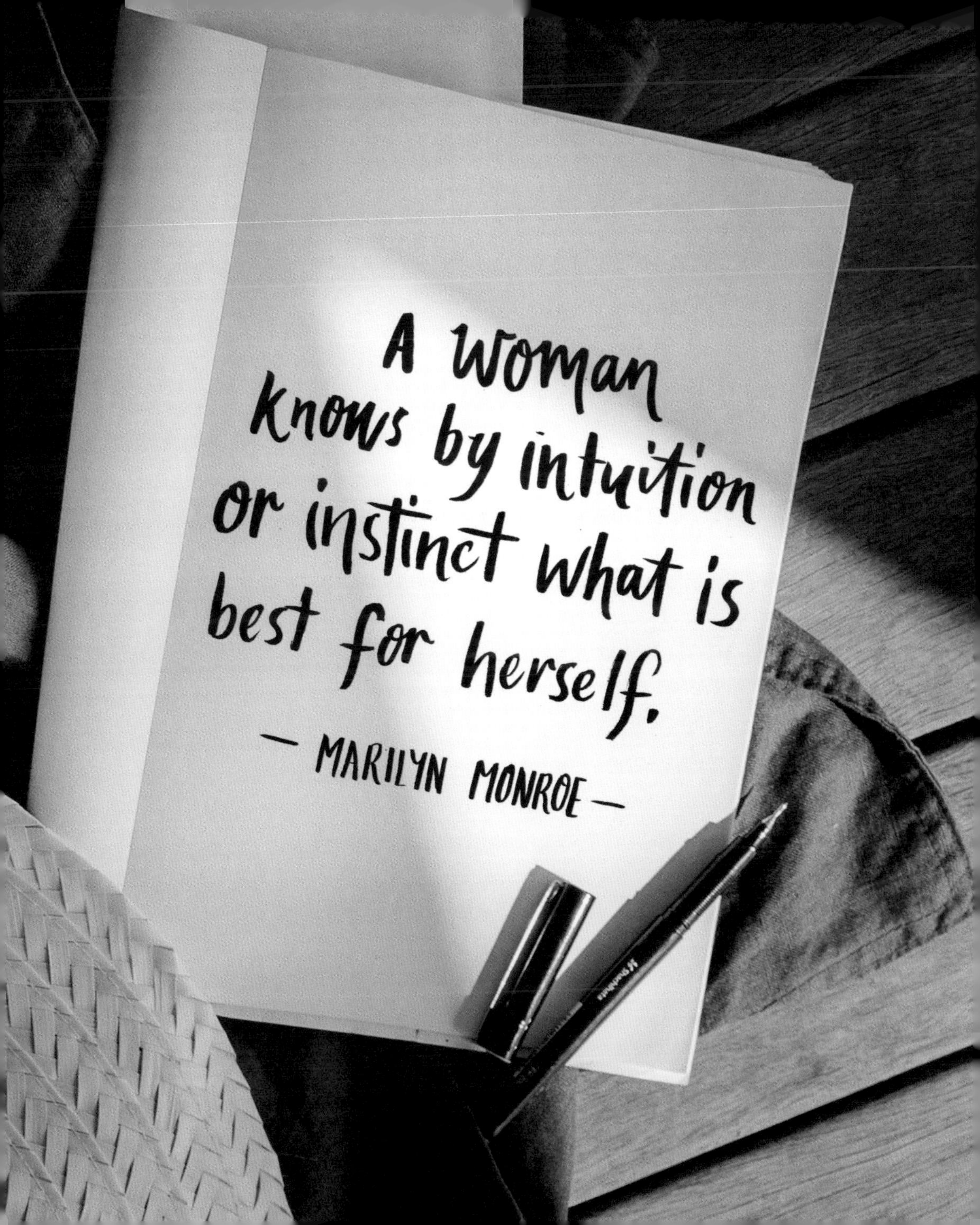
A woman knows by intuition or instinct what is best for herself.
— MARILYN MONROE —

offering insights into their lives as well as dietary and exercise routines. Many include advice about how to eat, what exercise to do and self-esteem. They are well-intentioned and often the blogger cares very much about the welfare of others.

An article in the New Zealand magazine *The Listener* prompted me to go and read some research conducted by psychologists from the University of South Florida. They investigated the types of health-related messages these laypeople were presenting.

The researchers selected 21 of the most popular messages that had received a health-related blogging award in the previous year. They then collected seven random days of posts and the 'About Me' section where the blogger described themselves.

Written content and images were analysed, with a focus on comments about disordered food/nutrition messages (such as severely energy-restricted diet recommendations or guilt messages), comments about appearance (including phrases that objectify the body), thin appearance ideals (such as praise for a thin appearance, or overweight stigmatisation) and health messages.

> "Your body has your back – let it offer you the insight into what is best for you."

The researchers identified a number of posts they labelled as 'problematic', with one such example suggesting that drinking ice-cold water to prevent food cravings would allow people to eat less.

What is concerning, both for the bloggers and for those who follow their advice, is that five of them had a history of eating disorders (and that their posts suggested may still be active), and six had menstruation or infertility issues.

While these challenges can be the result of myriad problems (some unrelated to food), having disordered eating is certainly one scenario that can create this. Many of the posts could potentially normalise disordered eating and behaviour.

Given all of this, it is no wonder the public are confused and concerned.

> *So as the availability of information continues to increase, how do you not get caught up in nutrition fads or encouragement to eat too little? The answers lie in you. Did what you just ate support your health or take away from it?*

Only you can answer that and it requires a level of honesty with yourself that might require some courage.

Use energy as your health currency. Notice your energy: what supports consistently robust energy versus what leads it to slump for you?

Your body has your back — let it offer you the insight into what is best for you, rather than an external (often well-intentioned) voice that hasn't asked you any questions about what it is like to be you, about your medical history, about your stresses or about what you feel and experience in your body. Your body is your best evidence for what works for you and what doesn't. Tune in.

Your inner wisdom

LEARNING TO TRUST YOURSELF

I meet a lot of people who are simply looking for answers. They want to know exactly what to eat, how to move and what constitutes a healthful life. They are looking for a prescription, if you like; a guarantee that if they follow the guidelines, they can get 'fixed' once and for all. In consults they are impatient to get to the bit where I tell them what I think they need to do, particularly what they need to eat. They don't believe that they have their own answers within them — that they know what's best for themselves — so they seek expert advice. And of course I understand this.

The reality is though, even if they do get the answers they seek, many of these people will not make the changes prescribed to them by the expert. Or, if they do, they won't stick to them for long. Think about your own experiences — how long has it taken you to go back to your old habits after following a plan given to you by a naturopath or a trainer or that you read in a book?

Perhaps the opposite is true for you. Perhaps you are someone who follows everything you're told to do to the letter, you're adamant that if you don't step a foot wrong, everything will come together and that plan will get you to optimal health and vitality. Even though your tummy has been upset every day since beginning a new diet that a nutritionist told you to go on, and you've been getting headaches from doing those exercises the trainer told you to do, you keep powering through anyway because they're the experts and they must know what's best for you.

Both of these examples highlight how easy it is for us to prioritise someone else's authority over our own inner wisdom. It may sound a little clichéd, but unless we dive inside of ourselves and explore our inner world — alongside getting the expert

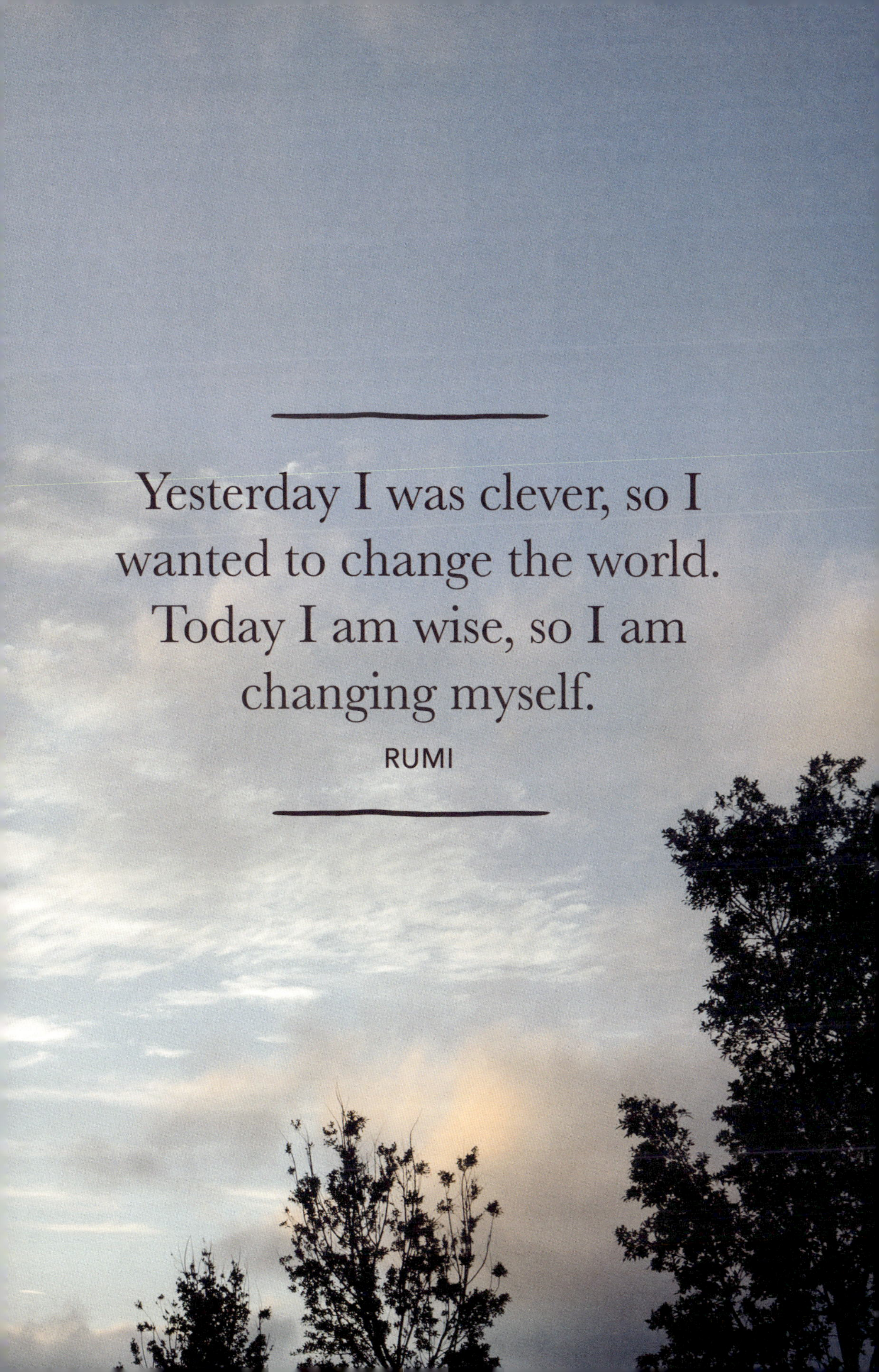

Yesterday I was clever, so I wanted to change the world. Today I am wise, so I am changing myself.

RUMI

information that will help us along the way — we are likely not to get very far. Because it's about so much more than just the food, or our lack of motivation to exercise, or whatever it is we go out there seeking answers for. We need to take into account how our unique biochemistry responds to our choices, emotional landscape and any unconscious beliefs that may be holding our behaviours, patterns and habits in place. Sometimes we need to uncover the 'why' and pay attention to what happens when we make certain changes. Unless you're curious about what might have led to you getting to wherever it is you find yourself, you're unlikely to get to the bottom of how to move forward.

We need to take ownership of our health — the choices we make and where they lead us — and learn to connect back to our body and what it's communicating, instead of automatically seeking external authority, assuming that someone else knows how to 'fix' us. We know ourselves better than anyone!

I do believe that having experts we can turn to for advice and support is helpful — don't get me wrong. I wouldn't be doing what I do, if I didn't believe in my heart that it was valuable. Education and knowledge are both part of any journey and change process. Sometimes we don't understand what's going on for us and need assistance to get to the heart of it. But when we continue to seek authority, jumping from one expert to the next, without also looking inward for our own answers, we are doing ourselves a great disservice.

There is no one set way to approach life or health that works for all of us. It might suit your friend to be vegan, but when you try it, you feel completely exhausted no matter how much or how frequently you eat. Our body gives us messages all the time, trying to help us to understand what it needs. If you bring curiosity, and look at the symptoms you experience as messages, messages that are designed to communicate to us that something isn't right, you'll likely hear a response bubble up from within you guiding you forward.

If you've had a hectic week at work and a stomach bug that has ripped through your family one by one, disrupting night after night of sleep, your body is going to ask you for rest to recuperate. If you don't give it that because you've still got a thousand things to do and, oh, there's that birthday party you're supposed to go to on the weekend and what will people think if you don't show up? What impact do you think that's going to have on your body? This is a simplified version, because of course real life throws us all kinds of different shaped and sized curve balls. But what I'm trying to communicate is quite simply that you often know in your heart what it is you need to do — you just don't trust that you know enough and you too regularly doubt your own wisdom.

Instead of getting fed up and frustrated and seeking expert advice to fix what's 'wrong', ask yourself: What is my inner wisdom trying to communicate to me? Try to connect the dots to something you've done that day (or in the preceding days, even weeks or months) and see what comes to mind. It might be that you still need to seek outside help, and that's okay, but even just the attitude shift from frustration to curiosity can make all the difference to the outcome.

GROWING YOUR INNER WISDOM

If we're sick, we are told to see a doctor. If we need money advice, we're told to see a financial planner. When you look at the way our society operates generally, it's no wonder we don't really think to seek our own wisdom on things automatically!

Here are some strategies to help you connect back to that voice within you that can offer guidance and wisdom far greater than any external authority.

Slow down.
If you're rushing around all the time without taking a moment to pause, your mind is going to be racing at a million miles an hour and you'll never hear the quiet voice of your guiding wisdom. Help to slow your mind down with a breathing practice, meditation, yoga, tai chi, qi gong or simply by stopping to enjoy the sunset.

Take a day to yourself and do whatever feels right for you on that day.
The more you allow yourself to be guided by what 'feels' right and create space in your schedule away from work, duties and chores — the more that wisdom will come through. If a whole day is beyond you, take however much time you can and do something that's just for you.

Learn to listen to your body's communication.
If you feel jittery after that second coffee, tired after eating that sandwich for lunch, or experience IBS symptoms after consuming certain foods, pay attention to these things as messages from your body that something needs to change. Avoid things that you know affect your body in this way.

Practise self-care.
We're not our best self when we're feeling tired, overwhelmed and run down. We need to prioritise looking after ourselves by nourishing ourselves with nutrient rich foods, taking time to move our body daily and making time for joy. When we practise taking better care of ourselves, we're more attuned to what it is we need.

Flex your "No" muscle more frequently.

If you're constantly running around doing everything for everyone else, always last in your own line, you're going to be completely out of touch with your own needs. Of course there are going to be things that you need to do, regardless of how you feel about it but quite often we're busy simply because we don't feel comfortable saying "No". Remember: if it's not a "Heck, yes!" then it probably needs to be a "No".

Be aware of any avoidance tendencies.

Do you reach for a glass of wine to help you wind down after work? Or veg out in front of the television because you need to switch off? While there's absolutely nothing wrong with either of these things in small amounts, we all have our ways of numbing out when we're not feeling good. We might know what we're doing isn't great for us, but we do it anyway. If we pause before rolling with a habit of avoidance, and stop to consider what might be going on for us, we can usually find a nugget of wisdom in that moment that we can then use to make different, more nourishing choices for ourselves.

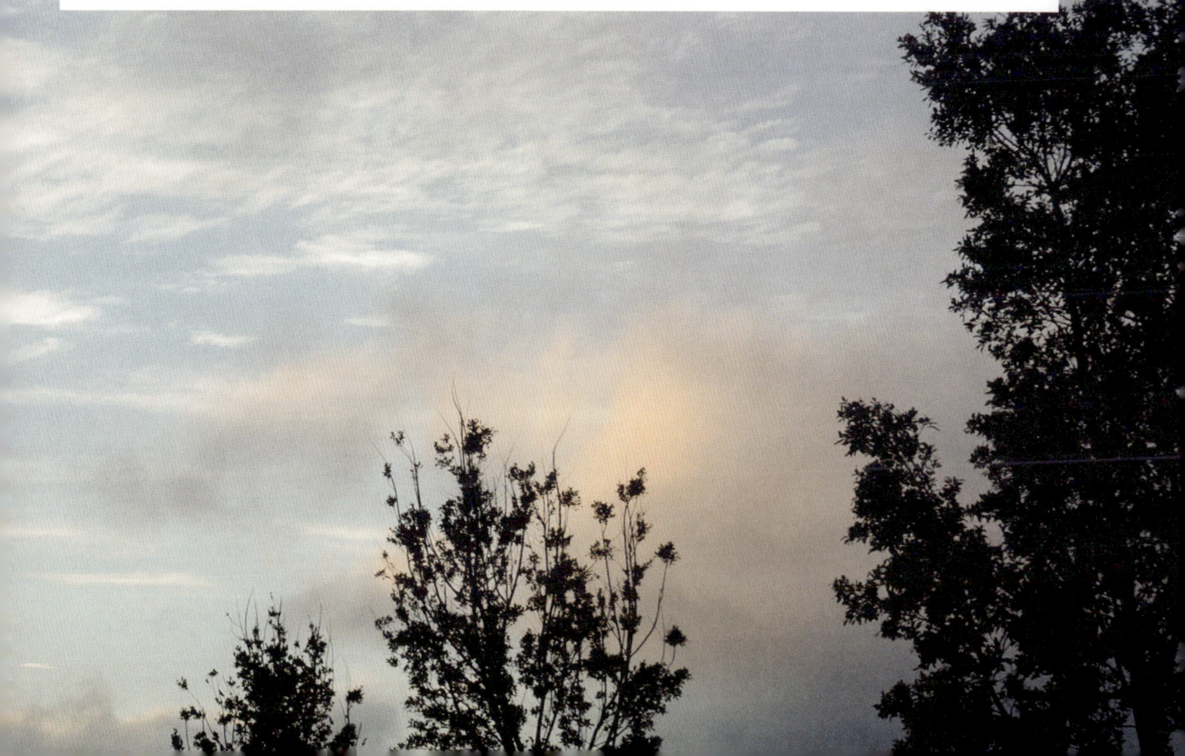

WORKSHEET

Fostering more trust in your own inner wisdom.

When it comes to your health, what area are you really focused on? It might be resolving PMS, recovering from a chronic health condition or gaining great energy, or something else.

What is the common thing that you seek expert advice on?

....

....

....

....

....

....

....

....

Could it be possible that you are seeking answers and expertise outside of yourself more often than you are listening to your own inner guidance?

☐ Yes

☐ No

☐ Maybe

IF YOU ANSWERED

YES OR MAYBE

REFLECT ON THE PREVIOUS ARTICLE AND IDENTIFY TWO OPTIONS THAT YOU COULD BEGIN TO DO MORE FREQUENTLY

SLOW DOWN

TAKE A DAY TO YOURSELF

PRACTISE SELF-CARE

LISTEN TO YOUR BODY

FLEX YOUR "NO" MUSCLE

BE AWARE OF AVOIDANCE TENDENCIES

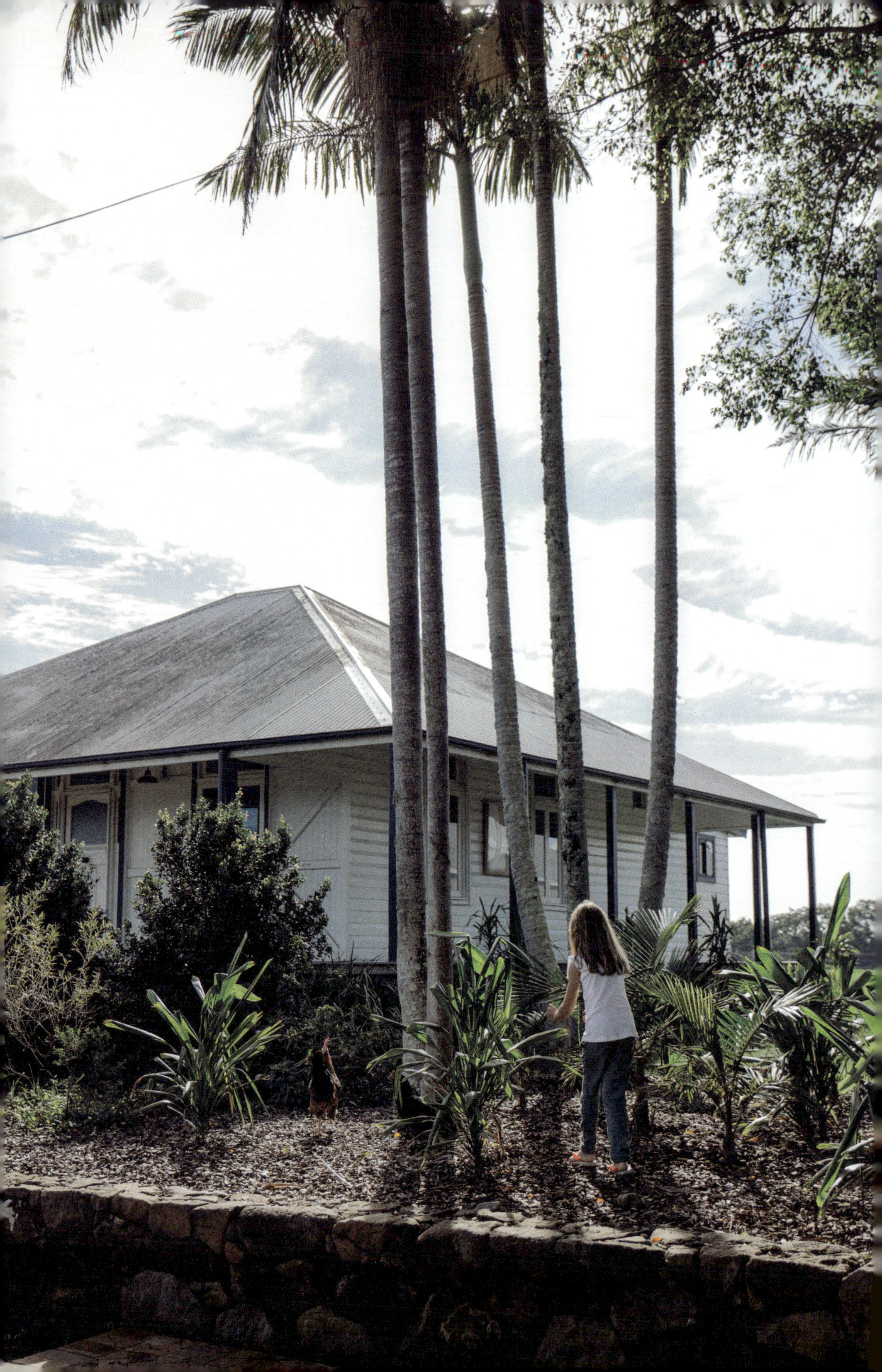

Guiding young girls

HELPING TO SHAPE THE NEXT GENERATIONS

There are many studies to support the theory that daughters are strongly influenced by their mother's relationship with food and their body. Women who have grown up in a household where the mother was regularly dieting or frequently commenting on her own or other people's weight and/or appearance are more likely to suffer body dysmorphia. Studies have shown girls as young as primary-school age are showing signs of disordered eating. Many have a negative self-image when it comes to their bodies, and the media is playing a significant role in this.

I want to preface this conversation by saying the last thing I ever want to do is create a situation where anyone experiences more guilt — goodness knows mothers especially experience enough! So please take the following information in the way that it is intended: I simply want to help you bring more awareness to how you communicate about food, nutrition and your body weight, particularly around your daughter.

By focusing on the mother–daughter relationship I'm also not saying that fathers don't have any influence. In fact, I have witnessed countless cases of disordered eating occur due to the perception that a father does not love his daughter — which is never true: it is the perception that must be addressed. And I say that all with love and with the intention to help foster the exploration of this in families where it may be relevant.

However, the focus here is on mothers and daughters, because mothers are role models for their daughters in ways that fathers are not, and because the desire or pressure to be "slim" and "pretty" is far greater on girls and women, making them more vulnerable to this influence. Additionally, it's often mothers who are unintentionally passing down their own feelings and beliefs of self-loathing, guilt and shame, to the very child they are trying to protect or shelter from external influences that do the same. If we want our daughters to have a positive relationship with their bodies, then mothers becoming aware of their own relationship with food, nutrition and weight is a critical part of this.

I have never weighed a client, as I believe a focus on weight is usually based on deprivation, and it does not promote a healthy body image. Through this process, many females are simply weighing their self-esteem. If your daughter sees that you weigh yourself regularly, it can foster a perception that this is how she is supposed to assess herself; that her weight impacts how she is and who she is and this can negatively affect her self-image.

I had a client who described how her mother used to stand naked in front of a mirror and grab her excess body fat, exclaiming, "Look how disgusting this is!" Often this would be followed by her stepping on the scales to further drive home the point that she was too heavy and was a failure, which was then followed by the solution: "That's it — I'm going on a diet."

And so her mother would prepare her own meals separately for a month or so. Now this was during the height of the low-fat era, so she would prepare steamed fish, broccoli or salad with no dressing. Later on she dabbled with the Atkins diet, tried the "protein shake" diet, and then went back to good old-fashioned calorie restriction. Basically, you name it, chances are she tried it. If it wasn't diet fads it was exercise fads — she got into running, aerobics and then zumba — but also went for large periods of time without doing any physical activity at all; not even a walk around the block.

My client also recounted how her brothers and father would eagerly chime in on this vulnerability, and, if her mother were closing a gate, they would drive off and yell out the window: "Run, run, run — run all the fat off your bum!"

We are all capable of saying and doing things like this, with no ill intent, but my client could still recall this, so it obviously had an impact on her. It is not just the mother's job to reinforce

> Help the next generation to approach food as a source of nourishment, and also understand that it's what we do most of the time that comprises our health, not what we do sometimes.

positive body image statements; it is up to the whole family. Not surprisingly, my client had also been a yo-yo dieter most of her life. She would lose 10–15 kilograms and then put it all back on as soon as she went off the "diet". She realised that a lot of her early disordered food and exercise behaviours, including calorie obsession, actually came from watching and observing her own mother's struggle and she had unknowingly mirrored this behaviour.

All of this occurred before social media existed and the impacts of what young girls now see, sometimes on a daily basis, can also take away from how she perceives herself. Do your best to become aware of the channels through which she may see images that are inaccurate — that may have air brushing and filters applied — and explain that these images are not "real", that nobody has skin without pores, and so on.

Think about your own experience of body size and shape. Are you happy with how you look, or do you often speak negatively about your body, or someone else's body for that matter, in front of your children? Do you ever discuss dieting, weight loss, being skinny or slim, bikini bodies, fitting into a pair of jeans and so on in front of your children, or leave magazines lying around that discuss these issues? How often do you weigh yourself and feel disappointed by the number that appears on the scale? Sadly, we are kidding ourselves if we don't think our children are absorbing this information, particularly girls.

I know many of you are reading this thinking "Oh gosh, now I have to think carefully about every single thing I say." Well, no, not exactly. But I certainly want to bring awareness to the fact that your children will tend to model their relationship with food, nutrition and weight around your beliefs.

Make it your mission to help them understand that food is fuel — it is neither good nor bad. Help them to focus on food as nourishment or that making more nourishing food choices can support them in their endeavours. In other words, make nutritious food related to something that they care about such as being great at their chosen sport or having clear skin. Help her to focus on health and nourishment, not on calories/energy, fats or carbohydrates. Teach her to become aware if guilt arises from food choices and to share this with you so you can assist her. Many young girls worry that what they just ate will lead to immediate weight gain yet no one will gain 10 kilos overnight by eating some French fries. Nor will anyone be nourished if they only ever eat steamed green vegetables. Help the next generation to approach food as a source of nourishment, and also understand that it's what we do most of the time that comprises our health, not what we do sometimes — so making the odd less-nourishing choice isn't the end of the world.

Sometimes dieting mentality shows up even more in the movement/exercise choices of girls if they believe that they have to "burn off" everything they eat to achieve or maintain the body they want. This thinking can be the result of exposure to the calorie equation concept being the sole determinant of body size (a concept I demystify in my book *The Calorie Fallacy*).

Stress hormones, sex hormones, insulin, gut bacteria, the fat deposition level of the liver and thyroid function all contribute to whether the body gets the message to store fat or utilise fat as a fuel and these processes in the body all work best when we are healthy — yet another reason to shift the focus from weight to health. Movement is best thought of as something that fosters great energy and vitality, a strong and functional body that allows us to enjoy and contribute to life, rather than for weight control.

Become diligent about how you offer food to your children. Do your best not to entrench in them a 'treat' mentality or that food is soothing or a reward. A more useful concept to consider is how the food being offered as a 'treat' will actually treat them. Many adults use food knowingly or unknowingly to alter their emotional states and this has usually been established in childhood when food was given to comfort them. So as appealing as it might be to connect via a tub of ice cream if you're feeling down, or happy for that matter, find other non-food-related means.

Go for a walk together, have a cup of herbal tea, and so on. Spend time together and be present: switch off your phone and allow her to feel that you are there with her, not thinking about what you need to cook for dinner, or how little of your to-do list you've ticked off today.

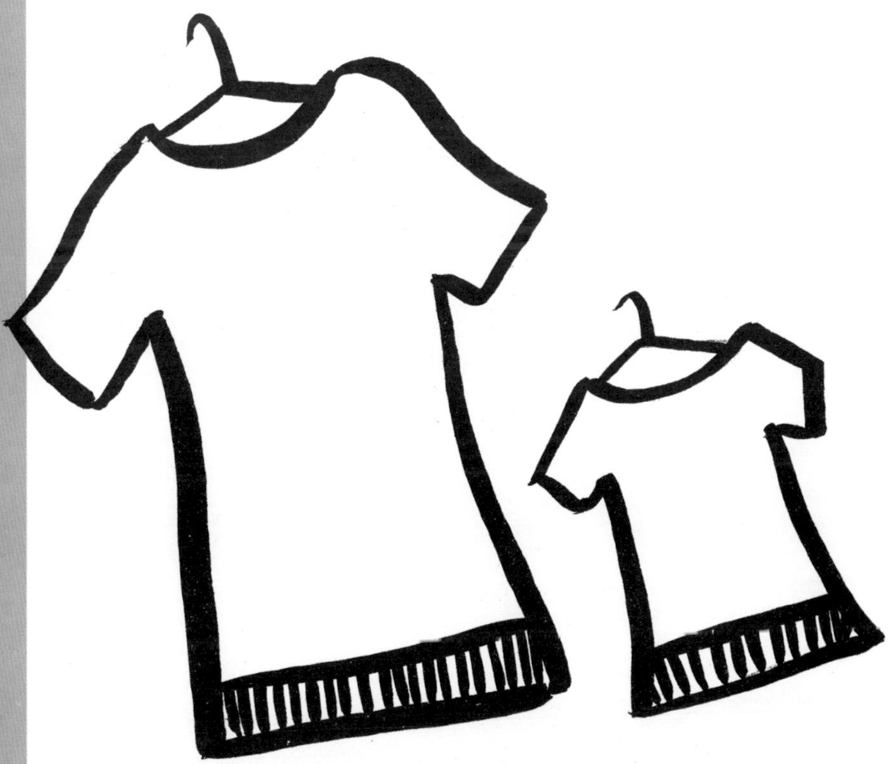

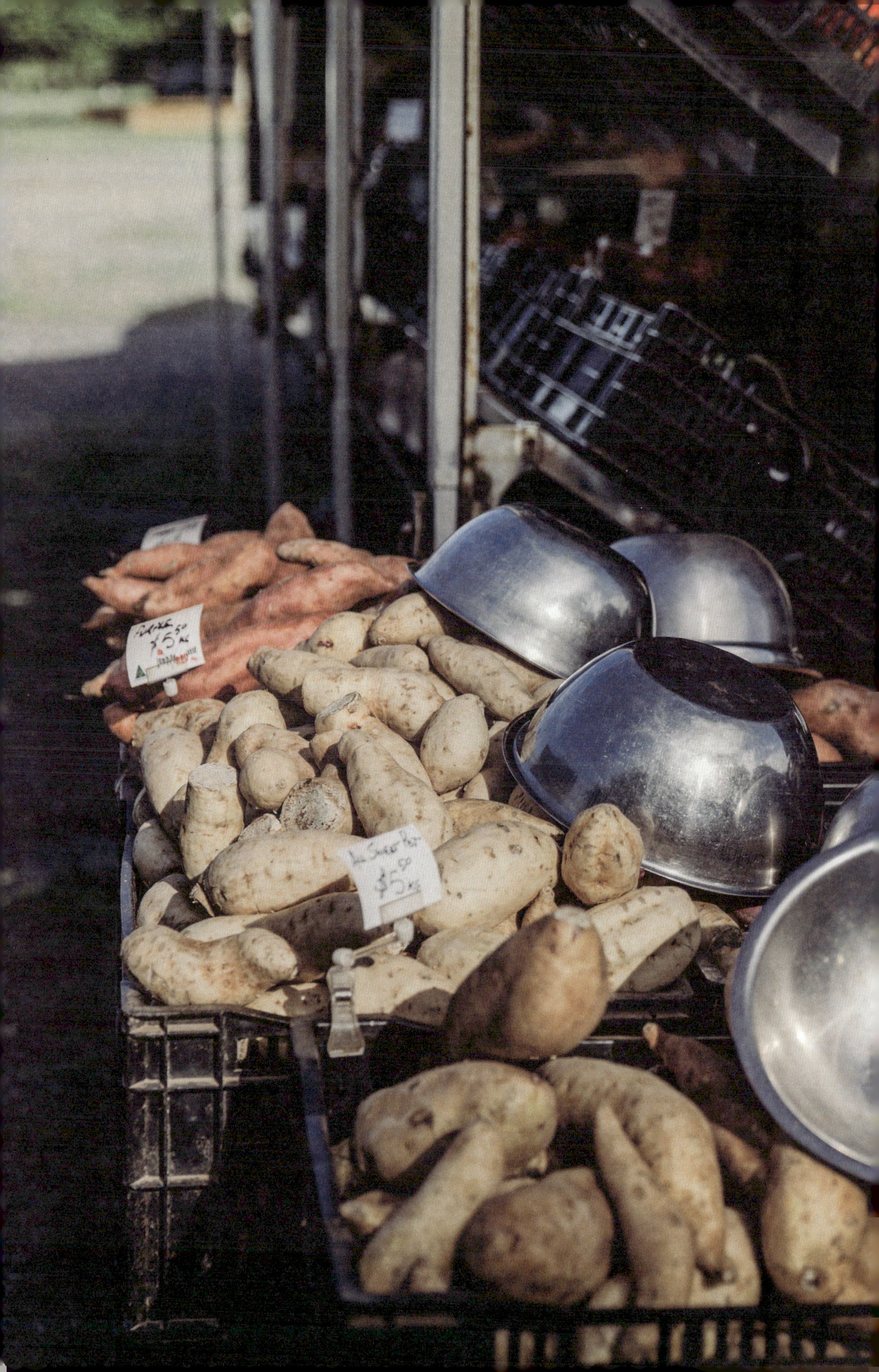

Packaging: tread lightly

HOW IS YOUR FOOD WRAPPED?

Another consideration in what you eat needs to be the packaging. How many single-use plastic things do you use? Sandwich bags, for example, can be washed and dried and reused if you need to use them in your house. Do you buy takeaway juices or coffees? It's wonderful if the cafés are using biodegradable cups, that's so much better than those that aren't. Yet can you take it a step further? Bring your own cup to grab your takeaway drinks. It only takes you to remember to do this a few times and then you will have formed a new habit.

How often do you now see organic and non-organic vegetables packaged up in a plastic tray covered in more plastic? Buy your produce loose. You don't need that packaging. Teach the shop owners through your purchases what you do and don't want.

If items must come in packaging, choose those than can be recycled. There is also a growing number of companies that, although using plastic packaging, are using plastic that has been created from sugar cane and will fully decompose.

Become aware of the additional costs to the environment if we don't move hurriedly towards a more sustainable future when it comes to packaging. Vote with your wallet.

In a figure that is almost double that of many European nations, statistics say that the average Australian consumes 90 kilograms of resources in packaging each year. We can help to minimise the amount of waste going into landfill and reduce our use of natural resources like energy and water simply by reducing the amount of packaging we purchase.

So, where possible, choose the least packaged products.

HERE ARE SOME IDEAS TO HELP YOU GET STARTED

1 **Fruit and vegetables.**
Avoid purchasing vegetables and fruit that come wrapped in plastic as these foods come in their own beautiful packaging and only require a basket or reusable bag to pop them into.

2 **Second-hand products.**
Buying pre-loved items helps the Earth in more ways than one. Reusing products protects the Earth's resources, saving resources that would otherwise be used in the production and transportation of brand-new products. As an additional benefit, buying or donating pre-loved items helps those in need. A partially-used item that still has use left in it doesn't need to go into landfill, when it can be of use to someone else, often purchased at a cheaper price than a new one.

3 **Buy in bulk.**
Why not try to buy in bulk? Not only does it reduce the amount of packaging you consume but it can also be a wonderfully cost-effective way to purchase products you use in larger quantities. Some supermarkets, markets, wholesalers and most health food stores sell nuts, beans, fruit, vegetables, cleaning products, toilet paper and many other household products in bulk. You can also buy many things direct from the farmers. Stock up on large airtight plastic and glass containers which are excellent for storing bulk items. They are commonly sold at wholesalers, supermarkets and hardware shops. If bulk-buying doesn't feel like the right option for you, it can still be helpful to avoid single serve and individually wrapped products in supermarkets. For example, it's better to buy one large, five kilogram tub of washing powder than to buy 10 smaller 500 gram containers. It saves both resources and money.

4 Minimise takeaway food.

While what you do in your home can make a significant difference, don't forget what you do when you're out and about too. Fifty per cent of all packaging is consumed by people outside the home, mostly in the form of takeaway food and drinks. Look for opportunities to bring your own reusable resources. Coffee is a great example. If you want to get your coffee to go, have a reusable coffee cup on hand and ask them to pour your coffee into that instead. Many cafés offer discounted prices for those who bring their own cups. Of course there are times when we don't feel like cooking, and takeaway tends to be more appealing. You might like to consider cooking in bulk at home and having a stock of frozen meals for those days. This is also much better for your nourishment! And if you do feel like something different, consider eating out at your favourite restaurant instead and avoid the plastic containers altogether. That said, there are many takeaway shops that are doing their bit to reduce packaging consumption so look out for those who stock biodegradable takeaway packaging (made from materials like corn starch) and when you do takeaway, make sure your packaging doesn't end up as litter or landfill by taking the packaging home to reuse or recycle.

5 Reuse packaging wherever possible.

If something comes in a sturdy plastic container, why throw it out immediately? You can reuse packaging around the home for all sorts of things. Old glass bottles make lovely vases for example. There are many places where you are encouraged to bring your own reusable containers. Places such as food co-ops, markets and health food shops are some that come to mind. Remember it's important to bring the right type of containers. Food and drink containers aren't suitable for bathroom and laundry products so bring along an old detergent or shampoo bottle.

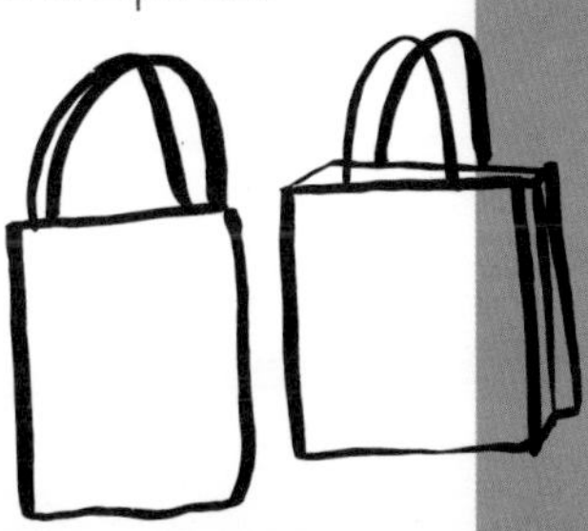

Every year Australians still continue to use four billion plastic bags so wherever you choose to shop, bringing your own basket, box or bag can play an integral role in reducing our reliance on disposable packaging.

6 **Carry a reusable drink bottle.**
Rather than buying bottled water, refill from the tap or buy a water filter station if you prefer filtered water.

7 **Recycle all your packaging.**
The good news is, most packaging can be recycled. Look for recycling symbols and make it a priority to recycle anything you don't reuse. Your local council will be able to provide more details on their kerbside recycling programme; each council has differences between the products that can be recycled. You can also find that information at your nearest recycling depot.

8 **Compost or worm-farm.**
Recycle Nature's packaging by composting, or feeding it to the worms.

WHY DOES THIS MATTER?

Unless we do something to change it, this is a problem that is only going to keep growing. Nearly everything we buy comes in some kind of packaging. Less than half of our post-consumer packaging is recycled yet each year packaging waste grows along with the growth in consumption. This excessive use of packaging has disastrous consequences for the Earth and it's up to us to change our daily habits. This is another area where voting with your wallet can make a wonderful difference. Together, we can reduce water and energy consumption, minimise the loss of precious resources, and stop landfill encroaching on our wilderness areas which endangers wildlife, increases soil, air and water pollution and reduces diversity.

Litter is also pervasive. It's not only an eyesore, it is also a direct threat to the life of many creatures and our health.

Reports of whales and dolphins choking on plastic and turtles being strangled by bags show us that packaging litter that enters our waterways has significant effects on marine species. Platypus in certain regions have been found with lacerations to the body as a direct result of packaging litter. In its Key Threatening Process in the Environment Protection and Biodiversity Conservation Act 1999, the Australian Government has classified packaging waste as a direct threat to over 20 marine species. Reduce your waste. It truly will make an incredible difference.

With thanks to Hawkesbury City Council's sustainability education for assistance with some of this information.

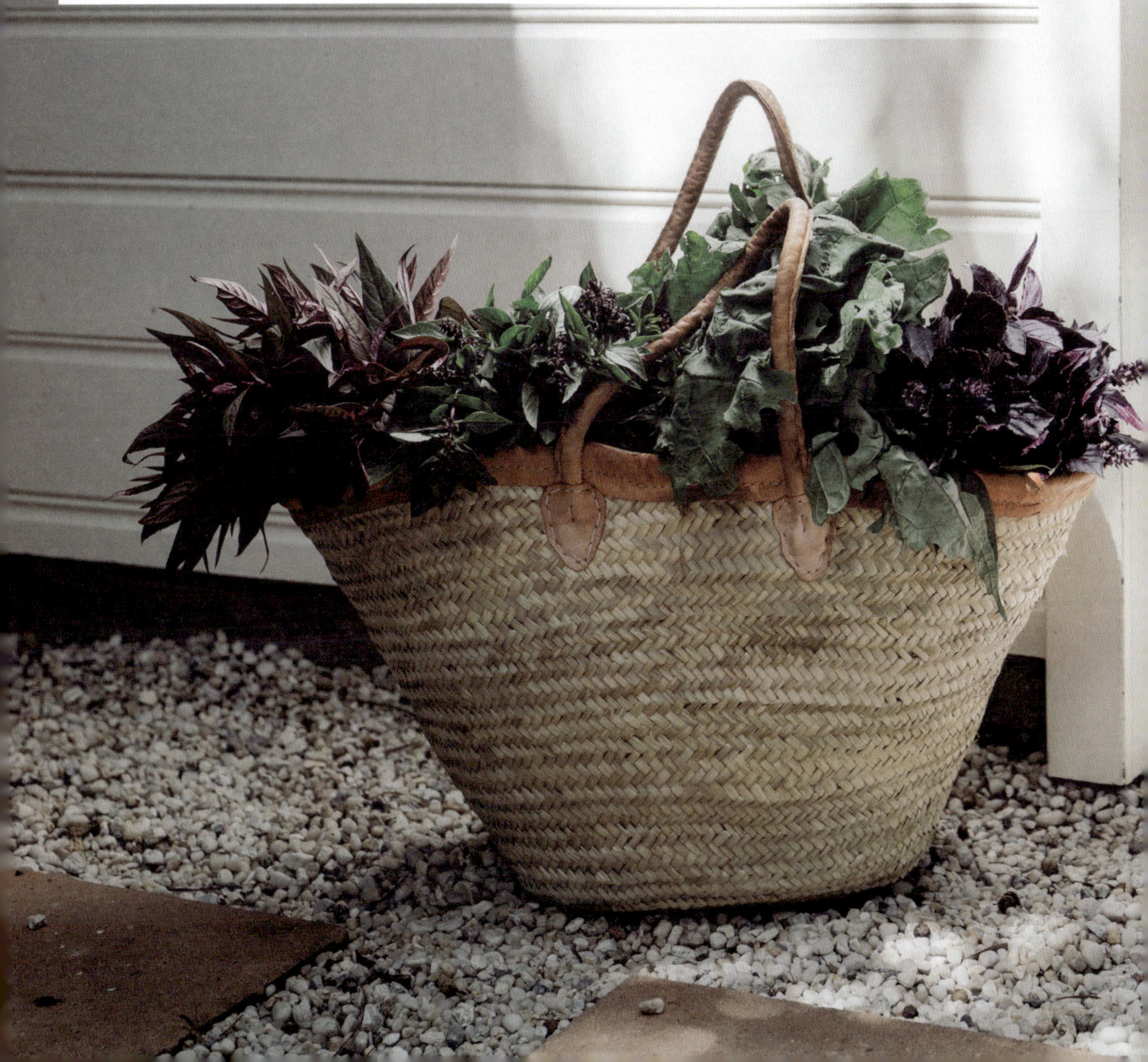

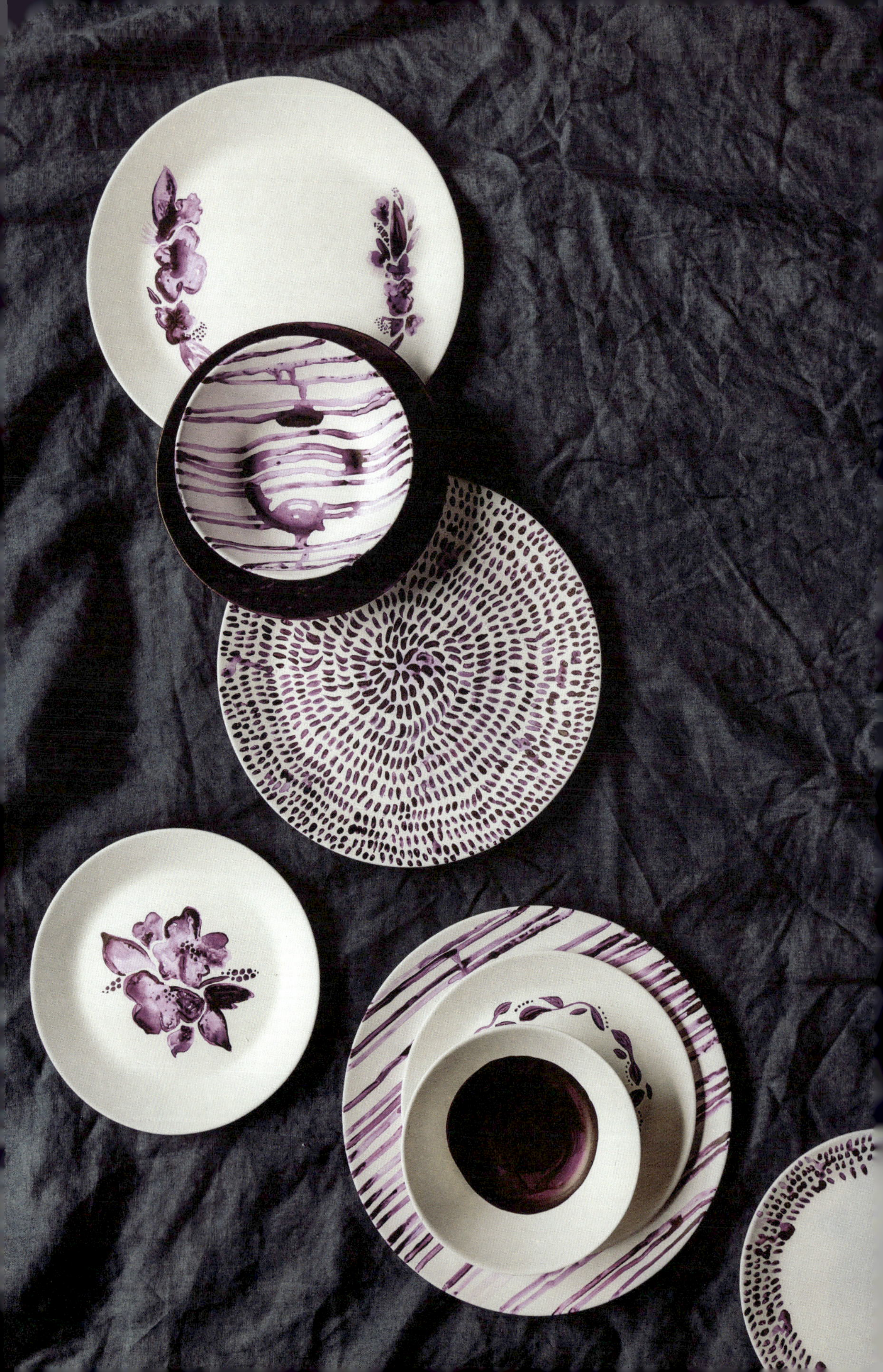

But, how much to eat?

A GUIDE TO QUANTITY

When people ask me this they're usually looking for a one-size-fits-all solution… and there isn't one. How much you need to eat is dependent on many factors, including your height, age, sex, health, job, physical activity level, genetics, body size, body composition such as muscle mass, stress hormone levels, sex hormone balance, thyroid function, gut bacteria profile and the medications you may take, just to name a few! My goal is to get you back in touch with what your body needs, rather than what your taste buds or emotional state drive you to eat and not be governed by a prescriptive way of eating that requires precise measurements.

However, I am also aware that getting you back in touch with your body's innate signals can take some time, so as a guideline use your fist size. Your fist is roughly the size of your empty stomach.

> *Generally, for main meals it can be good to eat about two fist sizes of concentrated foods (low-water foods, such as proteins and starchy carbohydrates) with as many greens as possible added to that. Snacks are ideally approximately one fist size.*

However, the higher your muscle mass, the more frequently you will need to eat these amounts. For example, someone who is sedentary may eat two to four times over a day, whereas someone who trains may need to eat these amounts seven to eight times a day to fuel their metabolism while also supporting digestion by not overeating.

Remember to include fat from whole food sources. Such foods add to the satiety factor of each meal, as well as to the nutritional content.

For the body to be able to extract fat-soluble vitamins from food, for example, they must be in the presence of fat. So often I am asked: "How much avocado can I eat?" When you start to eat more real food meals, you will be able to answer that question yourself.

Your body is your best guide and I want you to be in touch with its signals rather than having them masked by a diet full of processed fats and refined sugars and flours. There will be days when half an avocado will serve you at lunchtime, while on other days only a whole one will do.

You might begin to notice that when avocado is in the presence of lemon juice and herbs it tastes even better and taste may be one of the aspects you need in your food for it to be satisfying. Yet there will be days when you don't want the avocado or much fat from other foods at all. Begin to notice.

Eat in amounts that meet your own individual needs, remembering that these can change. Apply the principles above related to fist size guides and fat consumption, to get you started if you struggle with this and begin to notice how you feel.

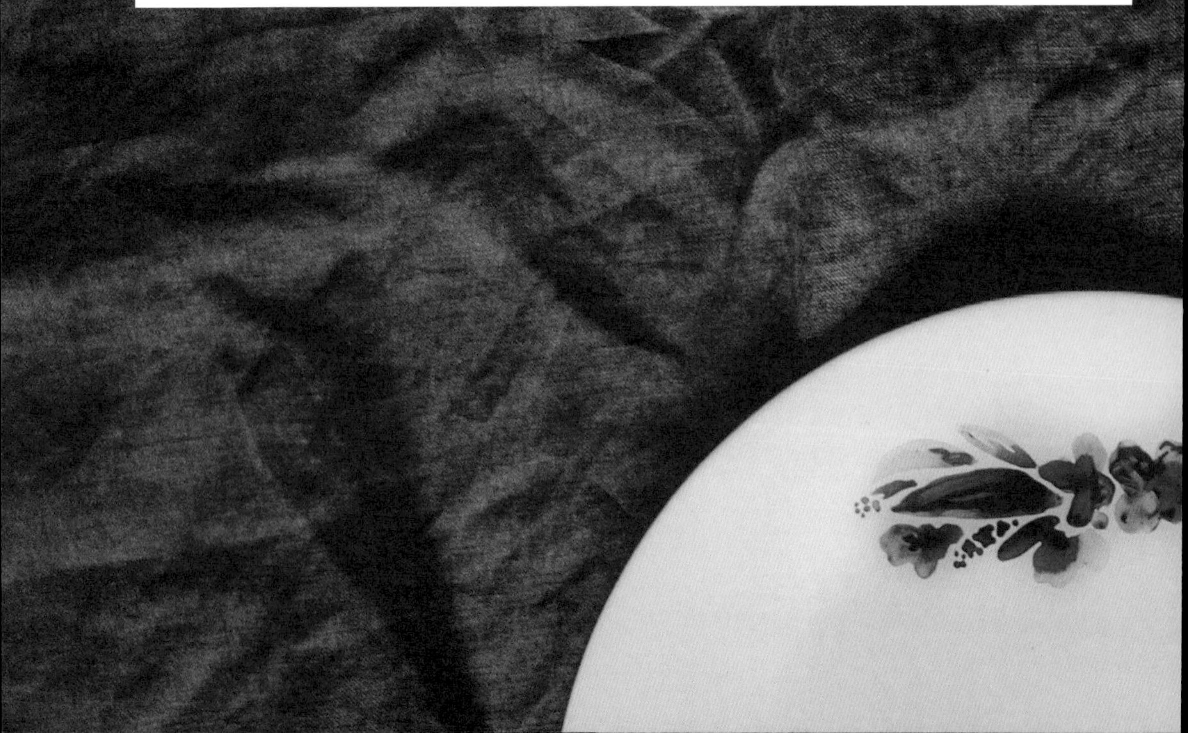

Self-compassion is a series of choices. Little, moment by moment decisions that guide you toward the things that will nourish you.

DR LIBBY

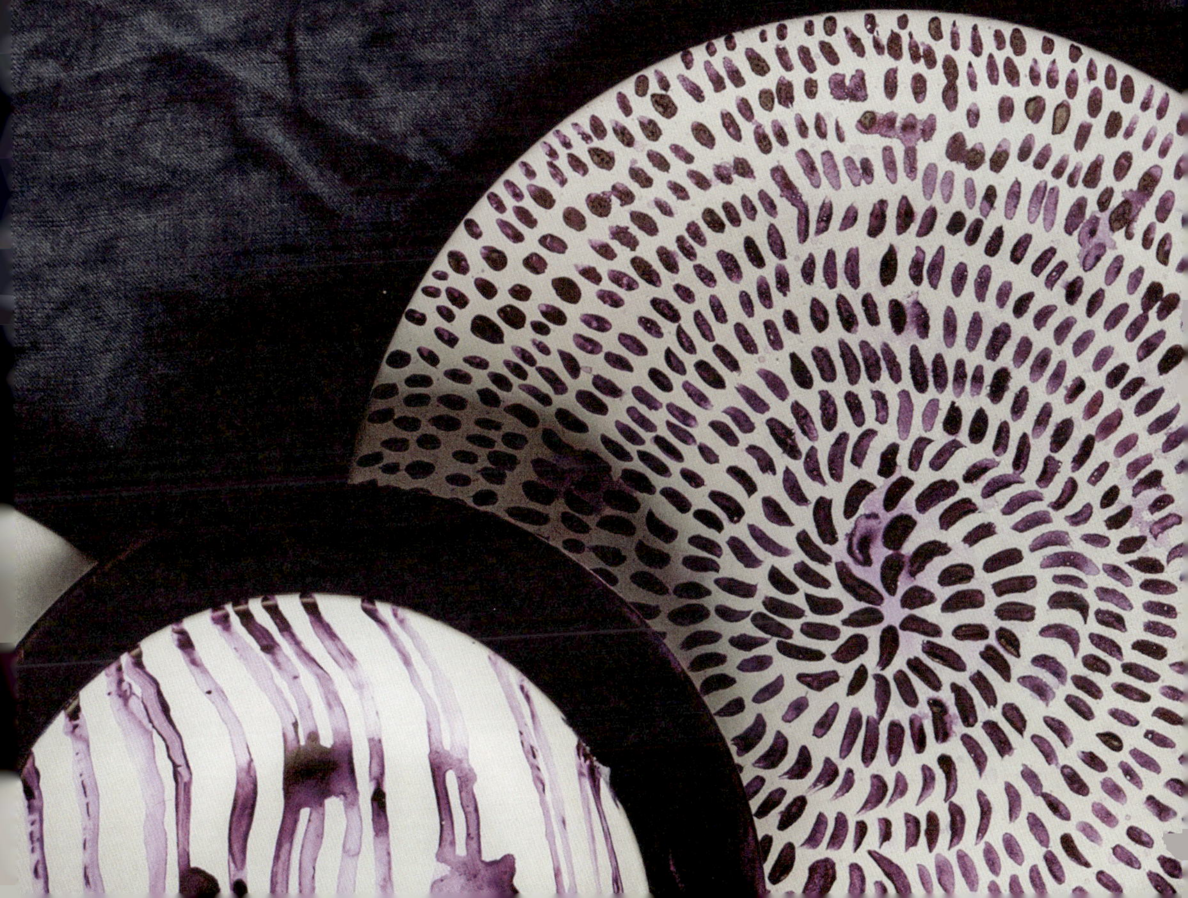

Food matrix

A GENERAL GUIDE

You will all be beginning your nutritious food journey from a different place. For some, you already only eat whole, real food. For others, you are well on your way towards this, but it's time to take it up a notch in the self-care stakes by perhaps getting organised on a Sunday and preparing a few meals or snacks for the week ahead. While for others, they are beginning a new food journey and a new relationship with themselves.

As you have read over the previous pages, one of my goals for this book is to help you get in touch with a way of eating that serves *you*. And, as a result of my experience that there is no one-size-fits-all when it comes to how to eat, I resist writing anything that looks remotely like a prescription. Because if I do, what makes it any different to any other diet? So I don't do that type of thing... However, I want to meet people where they are at on their health journey, and for some of them, particularly those at the beginning, they may have absolutely no idea where or how to begin.

So if that is you, if you are stuck with where to start, I have created a food matrix to help you make nourishing food selections. Of course you can buy a real food cookbook or borrow one from a friend or the library — go for it if that appeals. However, I am also aware that many people like simple meals.

So the food matrix is designed for you to almost throw food together for lunch and/or dinner.

Please remember this is just a guide as to the types of food you may like to eat and is not an exhaustive list.

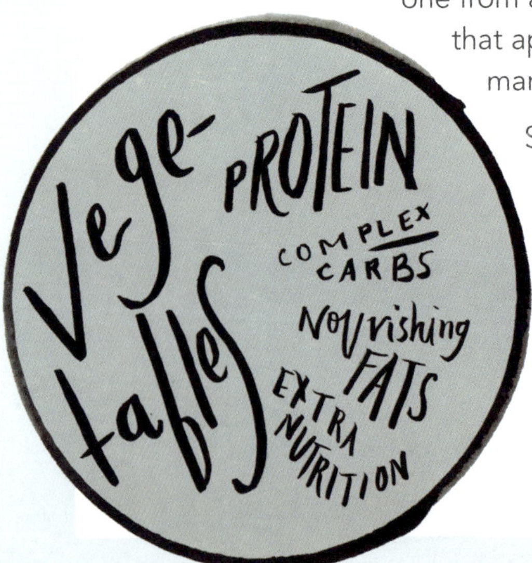

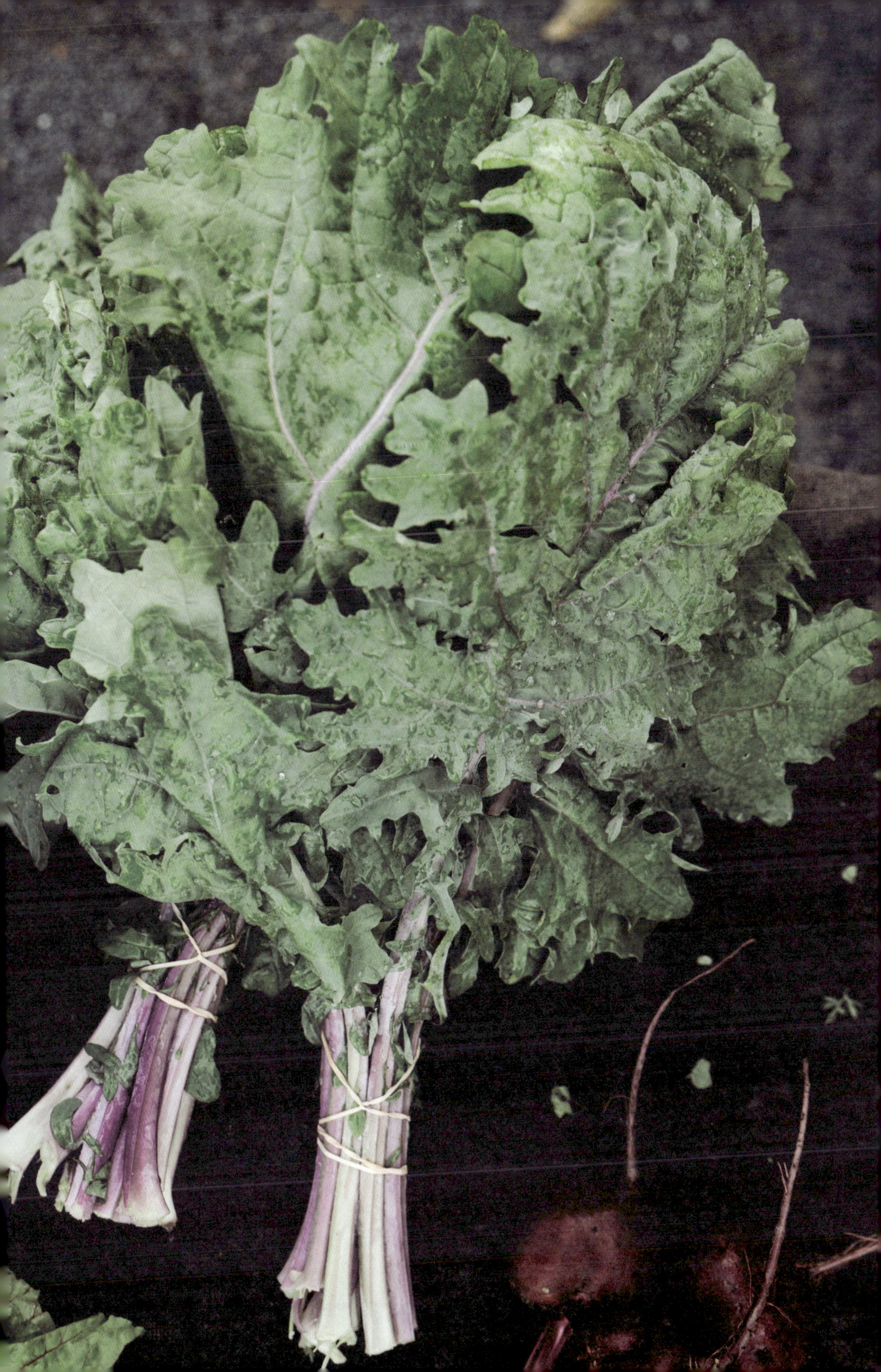

A GUIDE

1 **Vegetables (non-starchy)**	**CHOOSE 2 HANDFULS** Leafy greens. The darker, the better. *(e.g. spinach, kale, rocket, lettuce)**	**PLUS** At least 1 handful of mixed vegetables. The more colours the better.
2 **Protein**	**CHOOSE 1 OPTION**	**E.G.** 1 small fillet or, less often, small tin of wild, line-caught, sustainable white or oily fish *(e.g. salmon, sardines, mackerel)*
3 **Complex carbohydrates**	**CHOOSE 1 OPTION**	**E.G.** 1–2 handfuls of baked or steamed potato, sweet potato*
4 **Nourishing fats**	**CHOOSE 1-2 OPTIONS**	**E.G.** 1 handful of nuts and seeds *(e.g. almonds, walnuts, sunflower seeds, sesame seeds, pepitas)**
5 **Flavour/ extra nutrition**	**ADD TO TASTE**	Herbs *(e.g. parsley, coriander, basil, lemongrass)** Chilli* Aromatics, such as garlic, ginger and onion*

*Vegetarian option

E.G. Salad vegetables *(e.g. cucumber, tomato, celery, capsicum, shredded beetroot, cabbage and carrot)**	**E.G.** Roasted vegetables *(e.g. beetroot, pumpkin, carrot, cauliflower, Brussels sprouts)**	**E.G.** Steamed or stir-fried vegetables *(e.g. broccoli, carrot, capsicum, snowpeas)**
E.G. 1 handful of cooked chicken, beef, or lamb or other non-processed meat	**E.G.** 1–2 handfuls of cooked lentils, chickpeas or beans*	**E.G.** 1–2 organic free-range eggs*
E.G. A cob of fresh corn*	**E.G.** 1–2 handfuls of brown rice, quinoa, millet, amaranth or buckwheat noodles*	
E.G. ½ avocado*	**E.G.** Generous drizzle of extra virgin, cold-pressed olive oil, avocado oil*	**E.G.** Tahini*
Lemon juice Apple cider vinegar* Homemade vinaigrette*	Hummus* Sprouts*	Sea vegetables *(e.g. dulse, nori, kelp)**

Please note: this is a guide, not a definitive list. I encourage you to apply what you've learnt in the book.

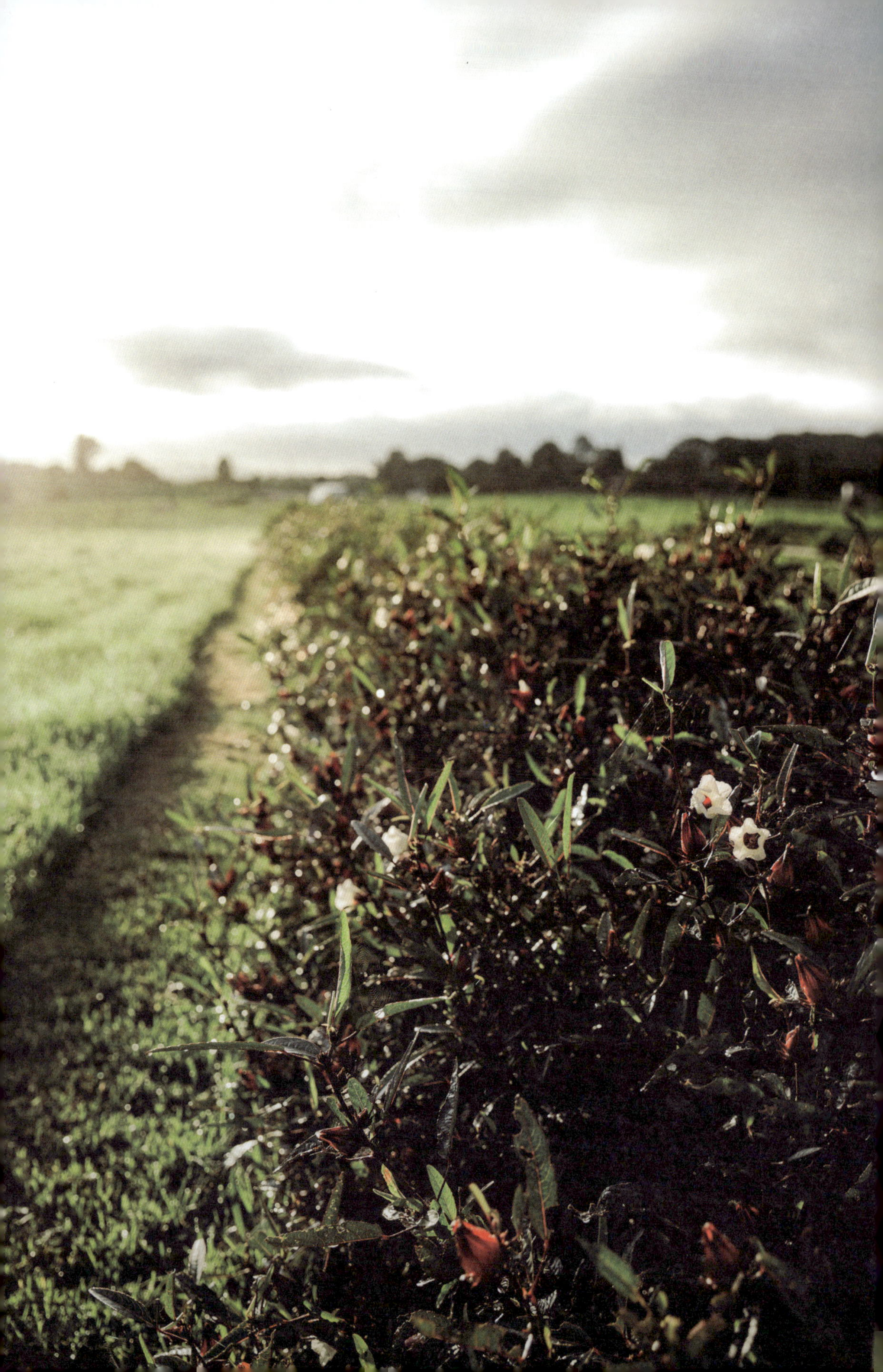

Food and false beliefs

WHAT'S DRIVING YOUR BEHAVIOUR?

Your behaviour is the expression of your beliefs. Please read that again. It is that important. What you believe about yourself, other people and the world will show in your behaviour. The emotional exploration I have done with patients never ceases to amaze me as people connect with what they believe and how this has been driving their life and their choices.

Our beliefs are usually based on stories we made up as youngsters in an attempt to make sense of a situation we were part of.

In the opening chapter of a book I read about Steve Jobs, the author recounts how on learning from a neighbour he was adopted, a young Steve zoomed home on his bike to ask his mother about it. As part of her reply she said "I chose you", which you can see would likely lead to the recipient of that statement creating a belief that he was special. And from that secure foundation blossomed one of the most creative geniuses the modern world has known (regardless of what you may think about him personally). Beliefs drive behaviour.

There are many forms of disordered eating, whether that involves eating far too much, you start eating and you can't stop, you know better but you continue to eat too much poor quality food, or the opposite ends of this spectrum — you starve yourself or you starve, binge and purge. Please hear this. In all of these situations, it is never about the food. It is merely the way you distance yourself from the way things are, when they are not how you want them to be.

The challenge is that there are no subjects at school teaching us how to go within and see what we believe, particularly about ourselves. We are usually much better at knowing what we believe about things and situations outside of us — such as what we think of the state of the environment, or what we believe about a political party — than about things relating to us, such as who you believe you have to be to be loved. Or who you can never be to ensure you fit in, are appreciated, or never rejected, or, in some people's cases, who they can never be if they want peace at home while they are growing up.

So when you eat in a way that you know does not help your health, or takes away from it, bring curiosity to what you believe about yourself that allows or drives you to continue to make these choices. For example, a woman who was sent away from her family at the age of 14 to be raised by other people believed it was because her dad loved her brothers enough to keep them, but he didn't love her enough to keep her — when the truth was that he sent her away because he loved her so much. He sent her away to give her a better quality of life. But until she experiences the truth — a new belief in seeing that he sent her away because he loved her — she eats far too much sugary food every night after dinner, despite knowing better, and despite knowing that this habit is killing her. Until she's able to see (and change) the false belief she created, she will feel powerless to stop her overconsumption. It will always feel like an uphill battle until such beliefs are addressed.

> "Bring curiosity to what you believe about yourself that allows or drives you to continue to make these choices."

Or the teenager who starves herself in the belief that, if she has a small body, she can remain a child, which was a time when her parents were still together and she felt loved and safe rather than responsible for their split (her perception, not the reality).

Or the young woman who finally realised that her patterns of starvation began with a comment she overheard as a teenager, spoken by two very young boys — "Look! There goes a big girl" — and her unconscious internal response was "even the little kids think I'm fat". (She wasn't aware she'd done this until a decade later.) As an outsider, you can clearly see that when young children make such a comment it is usually in reference to the passer-by being taller or older than them, not related to the size of her body.

What you believe about yourself — particularly when it comes to your worthiness of receiving both self-love and love from others — offers you immense insight into why you make certain choices.

If you make food choices that you don't understand, despite knowing better, then know that you have a belief behind them that needs to be explored with gentleness, kindness and curiosity. When you change the belief, the behaviour effortlessly changes and I don't say that lightly.

Why do you do what you do, even though you know what you know? You do it to avoid ever having to feel the ultimate emotional pain — the false belief that you think you aren't worthy of love.

If you have moments or stints in which you eat unresourcefully, remember this is not about the food.

> *I invite you to grab a journal and bring curiosity to your choices and wonder what might have led you to eat what you ate. Or if you start eating unresourcefully, catch yourself in the act, muster up that curiosity not judgement, pause and ask yourself,*
>
> *"I wonder what led me to do this?"*
>
> *Capture your insights.*

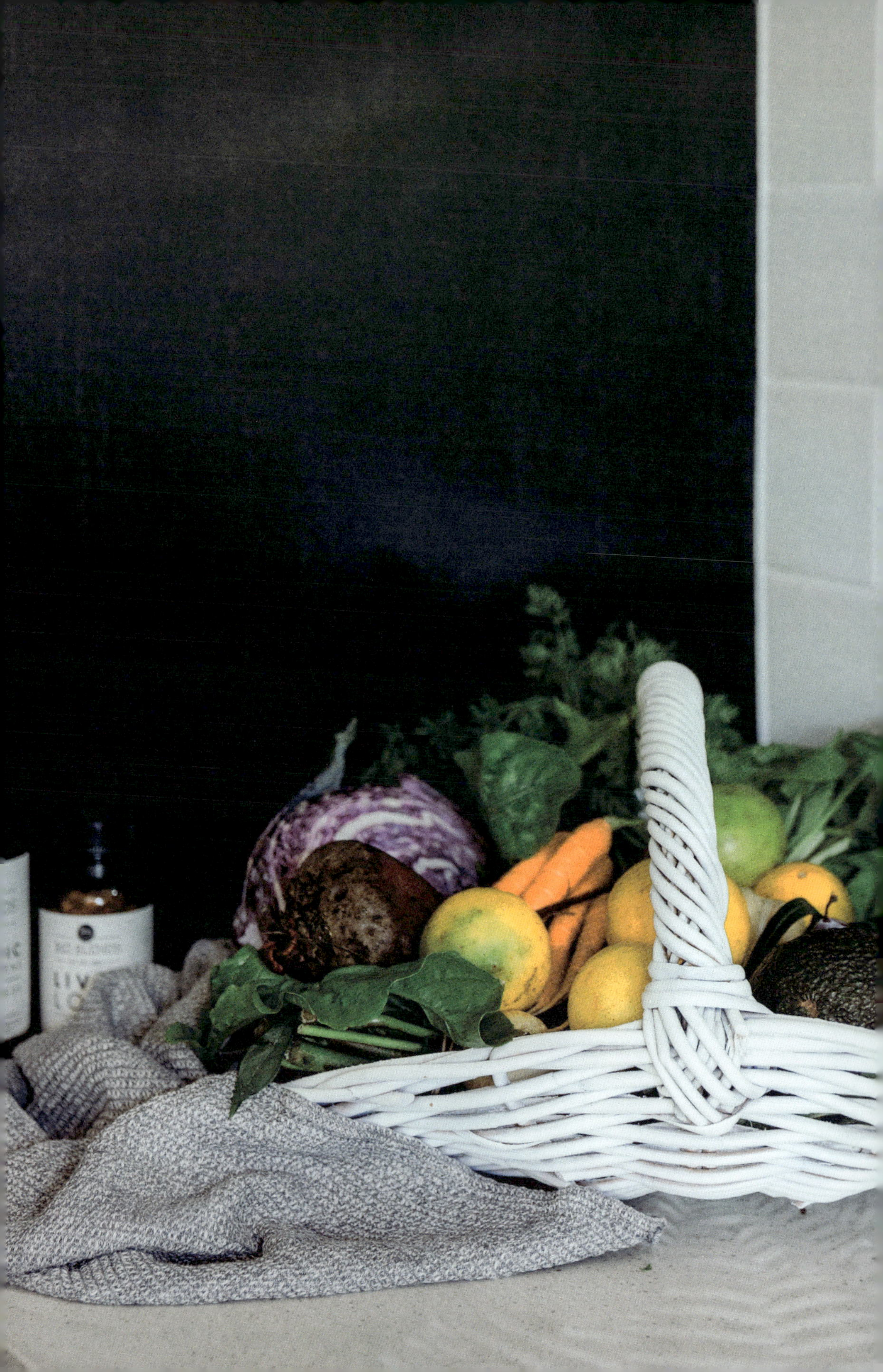

So what am I supposed to eat?

THE WRAP-UP

Thank you for taking this journey. I hope your brain and heart have been nourished with insight and information into the way you have been eating and approaching food and how this has either been serving, or not serving, your health.

I invite you to review the book again and this time, at the end of each article, answer the question, "Based on this information, what am I now considering, or what has this prompted me to change?" Journal your insights. You will be amazed at the number of small changes you can make around food and the profound impact these changes can have on your health and the way you feel each day.

As I've already mentioned, I don't believe there is one set way for everyone to eat that suits all bodies. But I also don't want you to come away from reading this book feeling as though you don't have answers to your questions.

SO TO ANSWER THE QUESTION, "WHAT AM I SUPPOSED TO EAT?":

Eat mostly whole, real foods that provide high levels of nourishment rather than processed foods (many of which are not really food at all), that might be low in calories or contain relatively little goodness or problematic substances that can interfere with the body's inner processes working optimally.

Choose nutrient dense foods for maximum nourishment. Eat plenty of plants and select a wide variety of colourful vegetables so that your body receives the powerful benefits they offer, not just their micronutrient content but also those substances that are unique to plants and are also vital for the body's biochemical processes. If you're someone who knows in their heart of hearts that you don't eat enough vegetables — amp up your intake. Try adding a daily green smoothie to your routine if the thought of consuming a plate of vegies sounds impossible. Aim to broaden the range of foods you eat, even by one each week for a few months. Not only will you experience some new flavours, but you may also broaden and increase your nutrient intake in the process.

Consider whether you might need to supplement your nutrient intake with good quality (and preferably food-based) supplements with concentrated levels of the nutrients your body needs.

Stop counting calories and focus instead on supplying your body with the kind of food your body has all of the equipment (digestive enzymes) to break down. I'll give you a hint — it's not processed foods! Research is starting to show that there are substances in some processed foods that we have no ability to digest. Food is the only place you obtain energy from, so why on earth would you want to mess with that? Think about that. Everything in life is more difficult when you are exhausted. Supply your body with whole, real food for the best health and energy, and also to avoid hidden sugars and artificial additives.

Take into consideration how your food has been grown and produced — not just for your own health but also for that of your family, the planet and the other animals who share it with us. Wherever possible choose certified organic produce that has been grown without the use of hormones and antibiotics (in meat) or potentially harmful substances such as pesticides and herbicides (in plants). Opt for local and seasonal produce, if it's available to you, for better nutritional value and to be kind to the

Earth. Think about how, when you eat, you're also consuming what your food has eaten and that this is either supporting your body systems or potentially adding more pressure to them.

Try not to get caught up in food trends and fads — all whole, real foods are superstars! Could you grow your own produce? Or some herbs to flavour and add additional nourishment to your meals? Remember that the nutrient density of plants diminishes from the moment they are picked and continues to decline. If growing your own is not an option, utilise community gardens, or visit farmers' markets and buy spray-free food, paying the farmer directly for their invaluable contributions.

Eat until you are just full, and in a way that fuels robust metabolic activity via increasing (or maintaining if it's already high) muscle mass. Pay attention to any feedback your body gives you when you are eating certain whole, real foods so that you can begin to find out what is best for you, remembering that this can change over time unless it's a true allergy — these are (currently) lifelong. It may help to initially keep a journal so you can keep track of any patterns such as when your abdomen is bloated.

Do what is common sense to you. Based on other information you have read in this book about the relationship between Irish heritage, gut symptoms, iron and B_{12} deficiencies, and autoimmune conditions, you may feel that gluten is no problem for you, or you may feel like you want to do a four to eight-week gluten-free dietary trial.

Consider 'how' you're eating and do your best to eat in a calm state to maximise nutrient uptake. Remember that you can have too much of a good thing and anything in excess can be harmful to our health. When it comes to eating frequency, start to pay attention to what best serves your health and do that. See unresourceful or out-of-control snacking as feedback that something needs to change and try to get to the heart of what's driving this behaviour. If you eat excessive amounts of sweet food or you crave it and feel out of control with your choices, explore what this is really about — a physical or an emotional need — and apply a strategy to help alter this. Bring curiosity rather than judgement. Treat yourself and your body with kindness.

If you eat meat, ensure that it is organic and pasture-fed, not grain-fed. Buy what your budget allows and explore if you can attribute funds from other less important expenses towards your food budget. You might need an iron supplement if you don't obtain 18 milligrams per day (for a menstruating female; post-menopausal women and men require 8 milligrams per day). It is important to check your iron levels with your GP before supplementing, as an excess of iron in the body is also problematic.

If a particular way of eating suits your body or your beliefs — such as vegetarian, vegan, low carbohydrate — be mindful to ensure you are obtaining all of the nutrients your body needs for optimal health and function. If you want to apply a TCM principle, limit damp-inducing foods, avoid cold, raw foods and eat seasonally.

When travelling, make a concerted effort to choose extra vegetables, plus ensure you get enough vitamin C and zinc — even more so if you have travelled on a plane to get to your destination.

Eat amounts that meet your own individual needs, remembering that this can change. Apply the principles related to fist size guides and fat consumption to get you started if you struggle with this (from page 283) and begin to notice how you feel after every meal. Refer to the food matrix (page 288) if you feel that you need more specific guidance at this stage in your nourishment journey.

Remember the ripple effect that your relationship with food has on future generations. Treat yourself with kindness and explore your relationship with your body and yourself to help your ripple to evoke self-care in others, too.

Eat whole, real foods that create robust health and energy for you, not what someone else told you to do that doesn't feel right. To paraphrase a quote often attributed to Buddha, believe nothing, no matter where you read it or who said it, no matter if I have said it, unless it agrees with your own reason and your own common sense. Foster more trust with your own inner wisdom.

And lastly, choose love. It's time to stop living in fear that everything you put into your mouth will affect the size of your body and, with love in your heart, remind yourself that no matter what, you're worth taking care of and you deserve to be nourished.

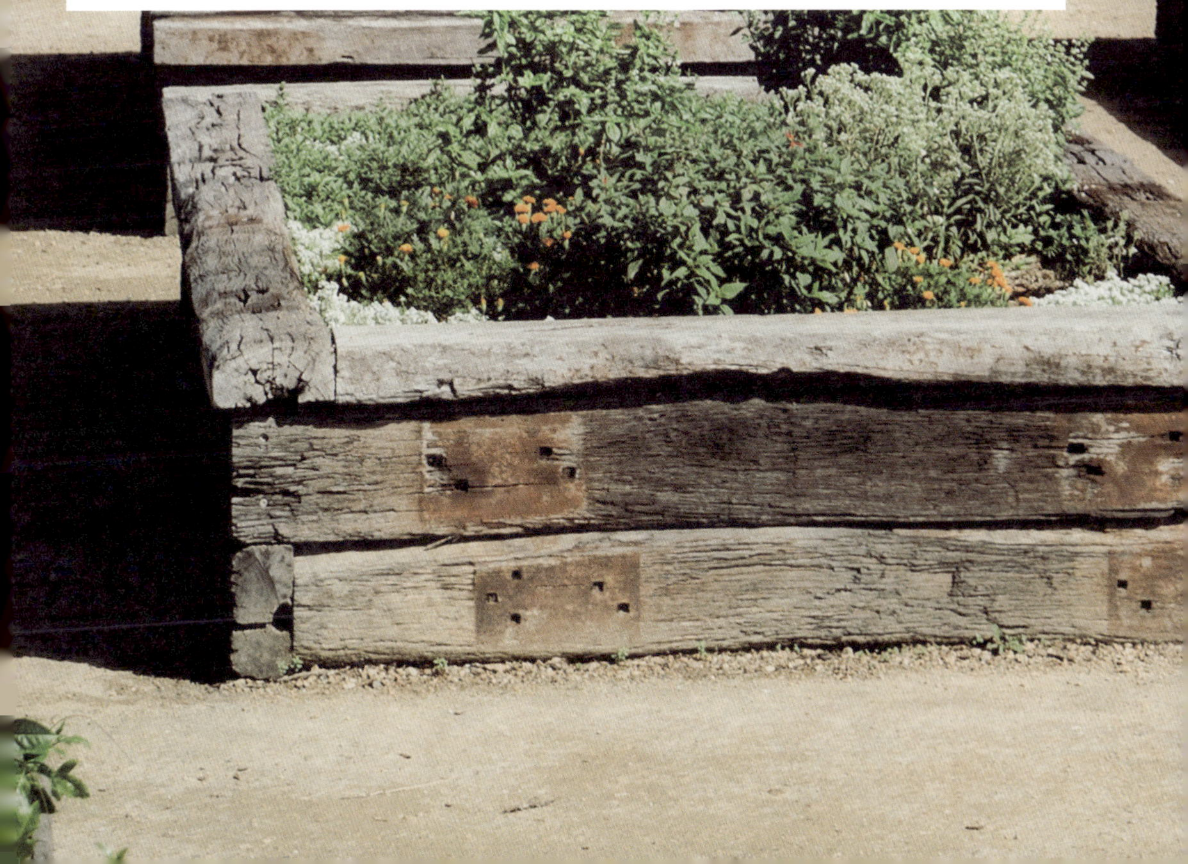

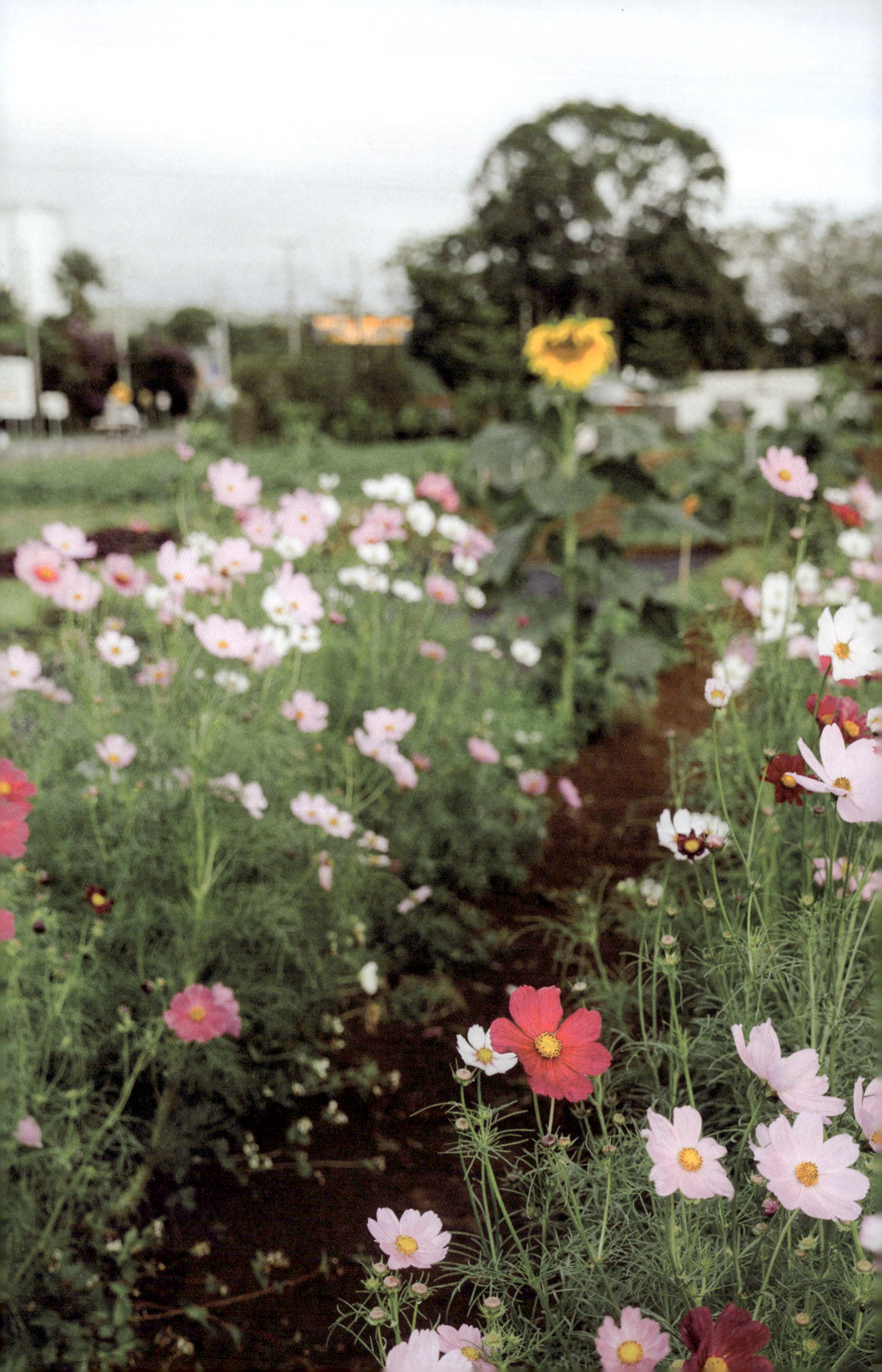

One final note

After opening this book with food information and a big focus on what your body — Earth suit — requires (we cannot fight our biological need for nutrients, for example), we took a journey from your head to your heart. Sure, you might have specific dietary needs, current or long term, that must be met for your health to be optimal. Yet beyond that, you have an inner knowing about what best nourishes you.

Live each day in touch with that wisdom guiding your choices. Apply common sense. Be so kind to yourself. No long-term change I have ever witnessed has stemmed from a place of deprivation. Remember that if you eat or drink emotionally, it is never about the food — you are distancing yourself from the way you perceive things are when they aren't how you want them to be. Bring curiosity, never judgement, to your choices and allow your insights to flow.

Live each day truly, madly, deeply in touch with how precious life is, how precious you are — and treat yourself accordingly.

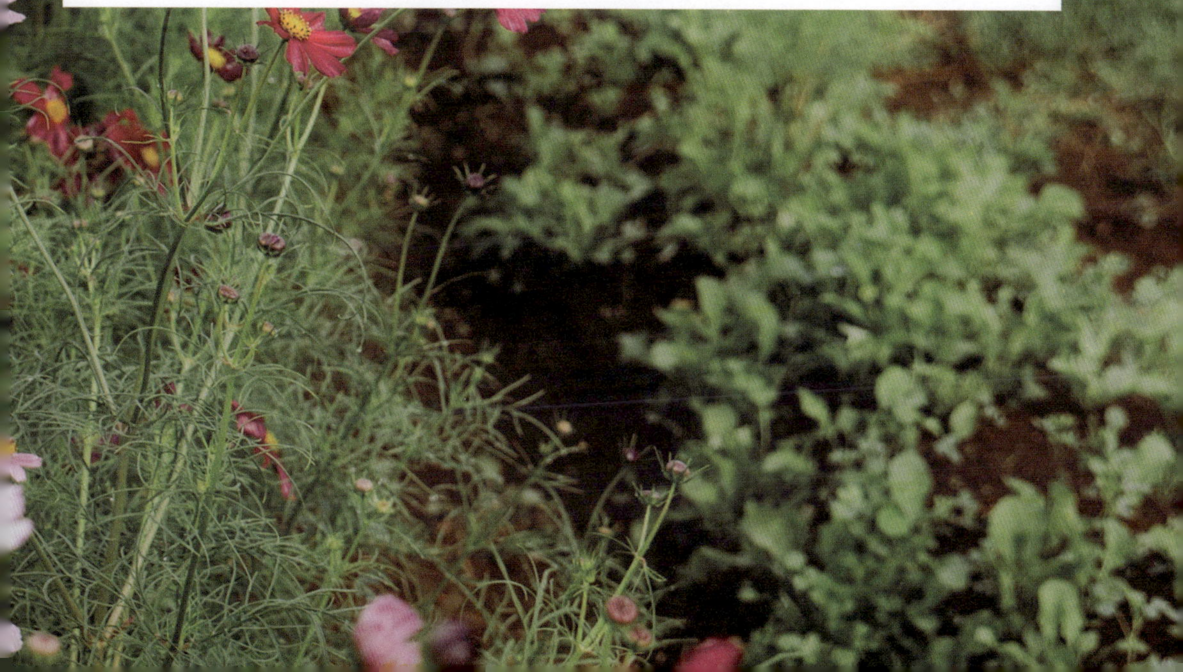

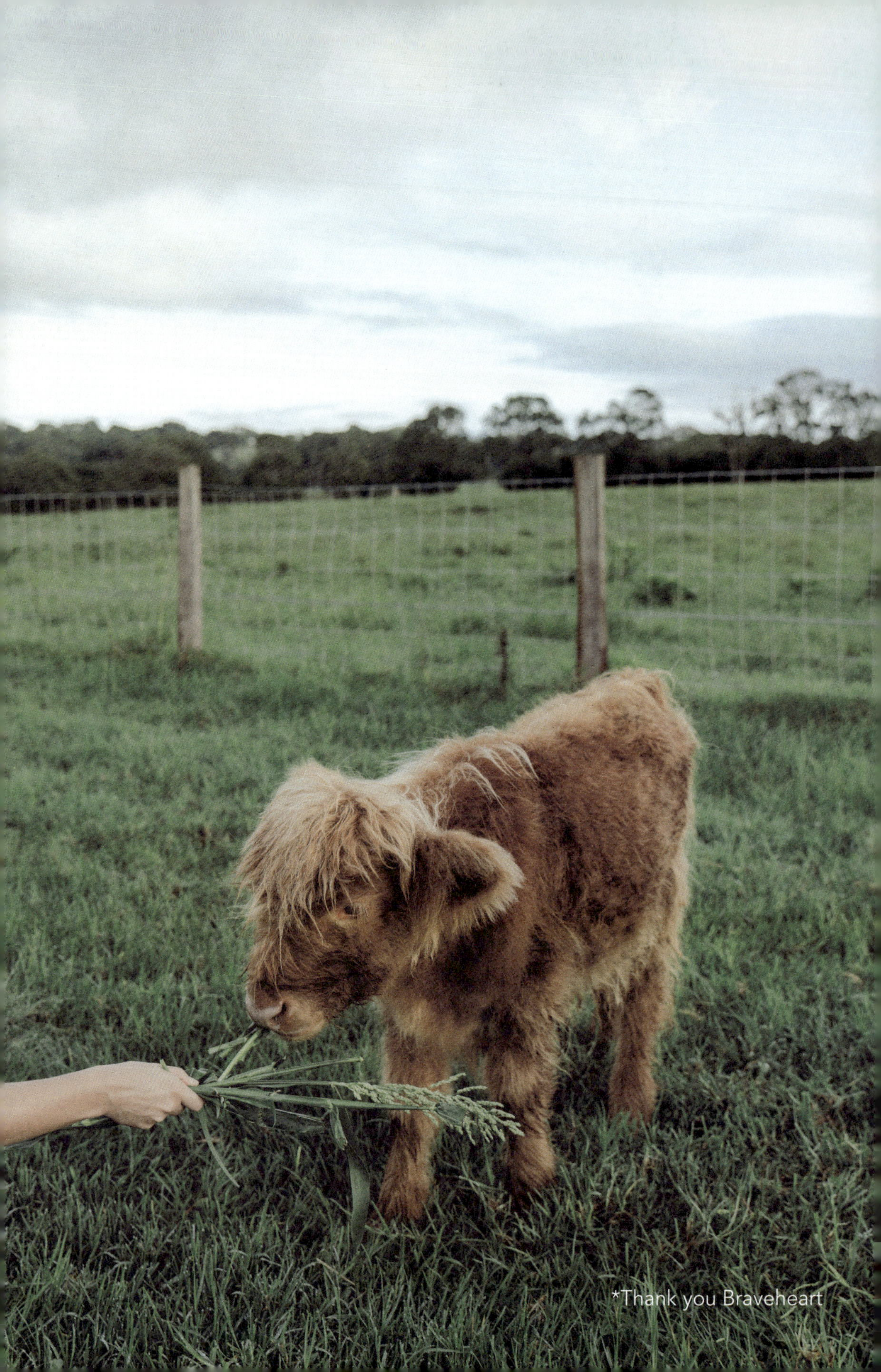
*Thank you Braveheart

Acknowledgments & thank you

I am so fortunate to work (and play) with a team I love and appreciate deeply. Maddy, Sarah, Bree and Chris thank you for making this book all that it is. Thanks to Kate for her edit. Thank you to Steph for her beautiful design, to Sabine for her gifted photography and to The Farm at Byron Bay for generously allowing us to capture such special moments. We all hope that a beautiful book enhances your reading experience, your learning and your care for others, yourself and the planet.

The gift that is life

Don't let it take a health crisis or a threat to your mortality to wake you up to make the changes to your lifestyle that you know in your heart you need to make today.

You know when you are having too much of something or too little of something else.

Take care of your inner body systems, to feel and look your best, and to live a long and robust life of meaning.

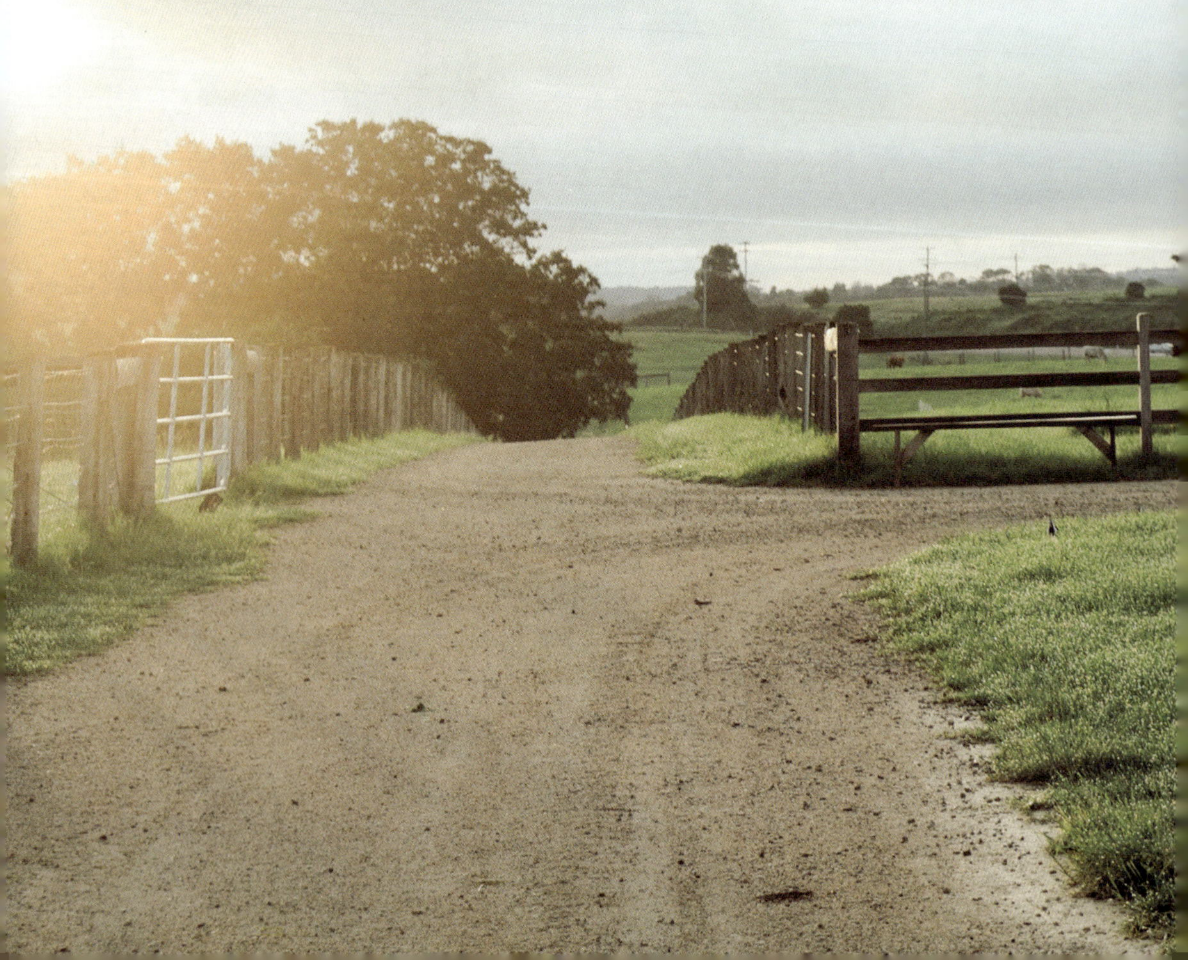

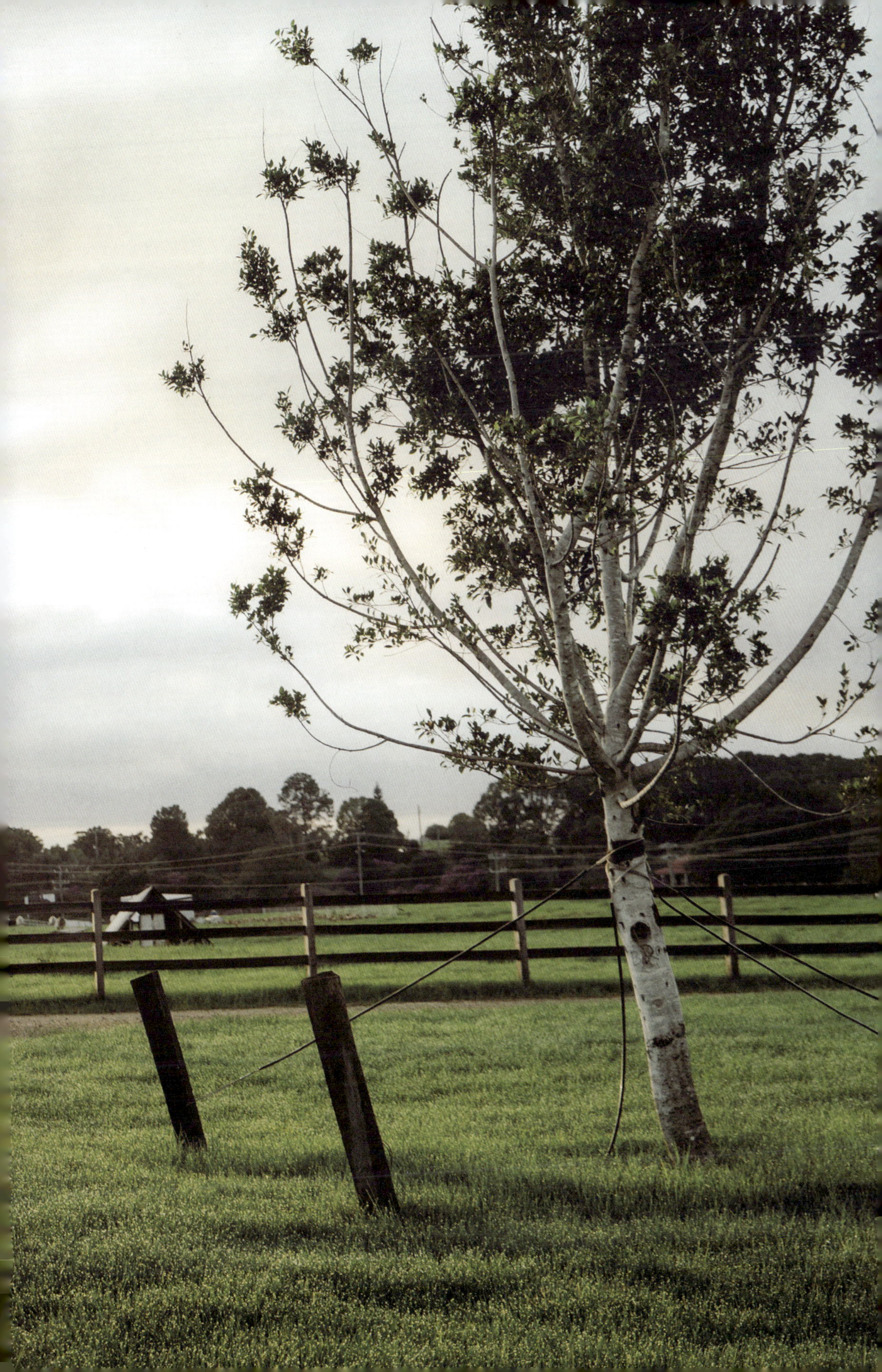

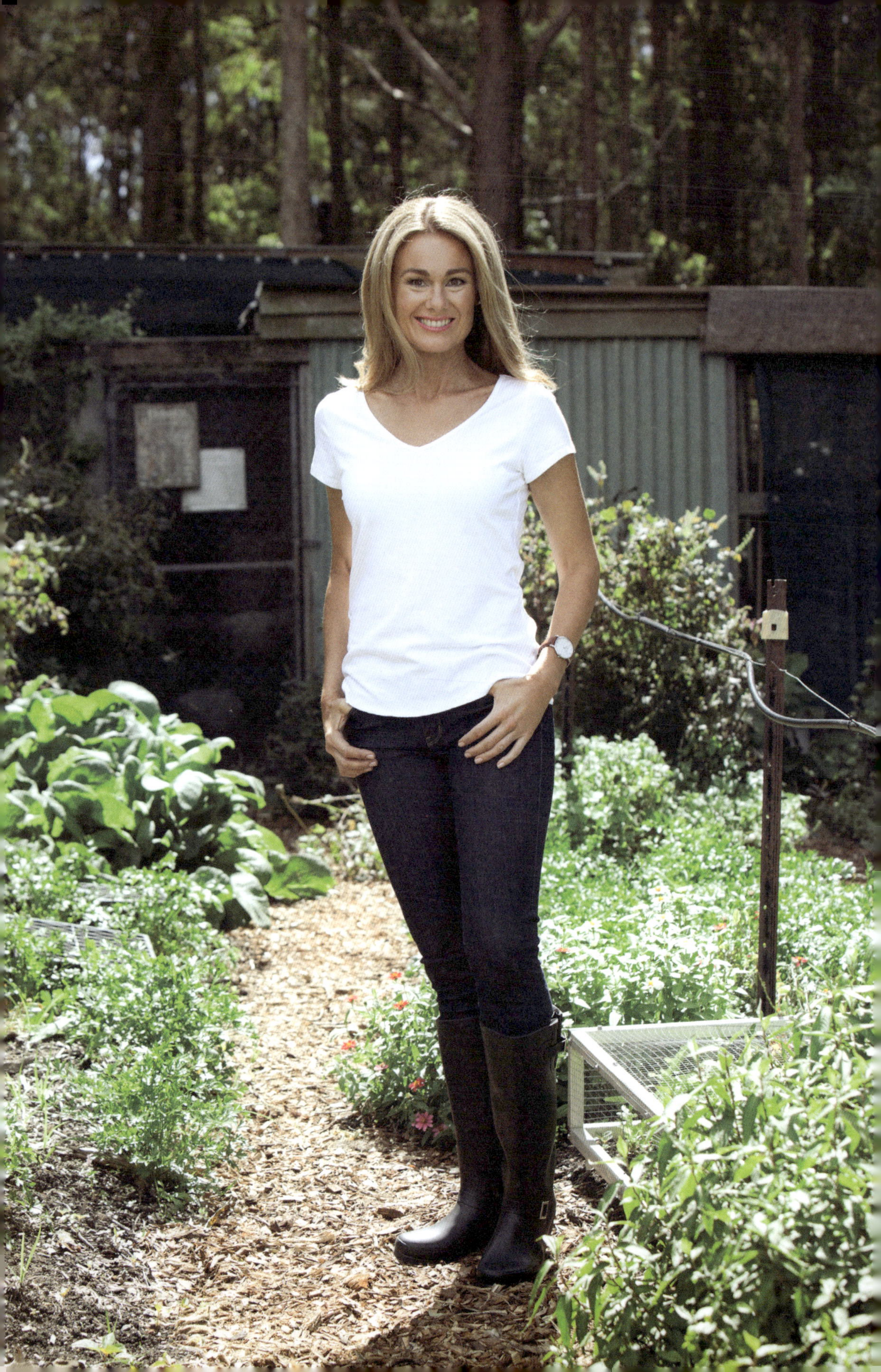

About Dr Libby

NUTRITIONAL BIOCHEMIST, AUTHOR AND SPEAKER

Dr Libby Weaver (PhD) is one of Australasia's leading nutritional biochemists, an author, a speaker and founder of the food-based supplement range, Bio Blends.

Armed with an abundance of knowledge, scientific research and a true desire to help people regain their energy and vitality, Dr Libby empowers and inspires people to take charge of their health and happiness through her books, live events, online courses and nutritional support range.

> "A one-stop shop in achieving and maintaining ultimate health and wellbeing."

Having sold over 300,000 books across New Zealand and Australia, she is a ten-times bestselling author.

A respected international speaker, Dr Libby's expertise in nutritional biochemistry has led her to share the stage with Marianne Williamson, Sir Richard Branson, Tony Robbins and Dr Oz. She is regularly called on as an authoritative figure in the health and wellness industry and has been featured in numerous media publications including *The Times, The Huffington Post, Sydney Morning Herald,* the *Australian Women's Weekly* and she appears regularly on breakfast radio and television.

With a natural ability to break even the most complex of concepts into layman's terms, Dr Libby's health messages embrace her unique three-pillared approach that explore the interplay between nutrition, emotions and the biochemistry of the body.

It's no surprise that when it comes to achieving and maintaining ultimate health and wellbeing, Hollywood stars Deborra-lee Furness and Hugh Jackman describe her as a "one-stop shop in achieving and maintaining ultimate health and wellbeing".

Also by Dr Libby Weaver

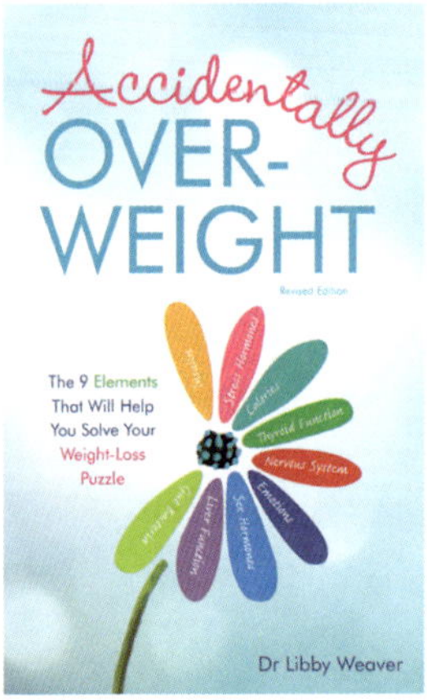

Accidentally Overweight

Accidentally Overweight explores the must-know nine factors essential to successful and sustainable weight loss. They include stress hormones, sex hormones, thyroid function and gut bacteria.

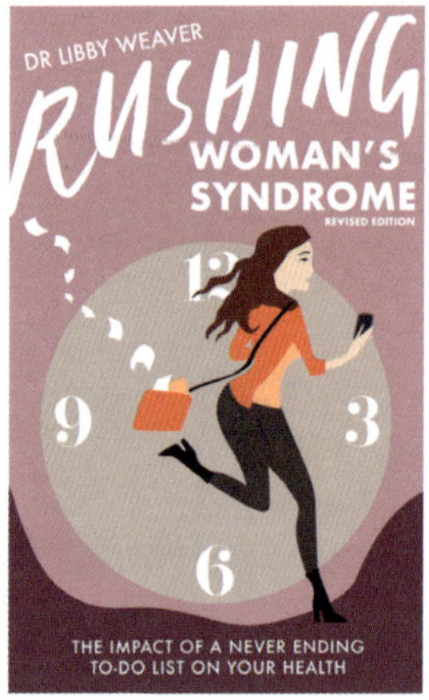

Rushing Woman's Syndrome

Rushing Woman's Syndrome offers you real solutions to both the biochemistry and the emotional patterns of the rush. What you need to do in a day may not change but how you show up can revolutionise how you experience each day and how others experience you.

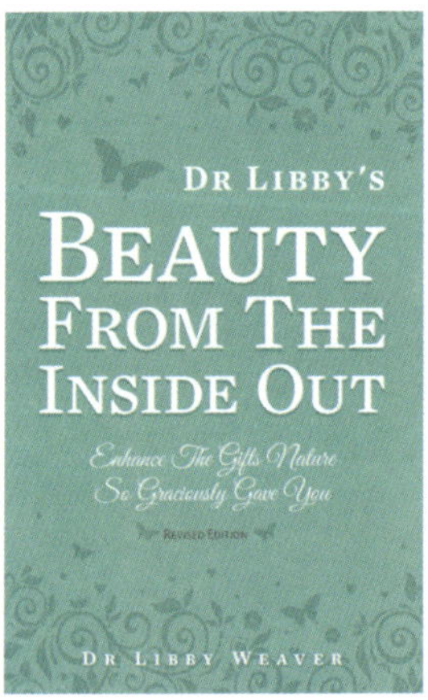

Beauty from the Inside Out

Beauty from the Inside Out is a must-have beauty book for women of all ages. Enjoy radiating your own unique sparkle from the inside out, and learn how everything from nutrients to emotions impacts what is displayed on the outside.

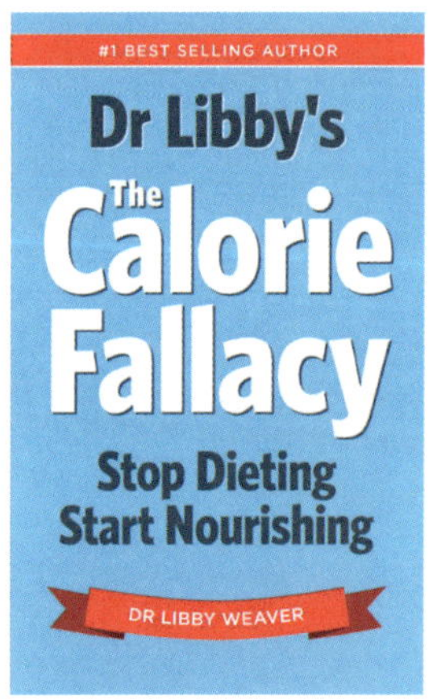

The Calorie Fallacy

This book arms you with the wisdom to stop dieting and depriving yourself and start thriving. Stop dieting and start nourishing and start living with a new freedom with your relationship with food and your body.

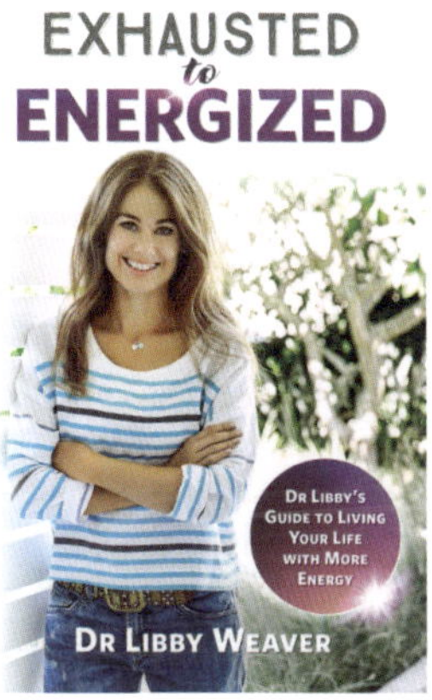

Exhausted to Energized

Everything in life is more difficult when we are exhausted. *Exhausted to Energized* offers you simple but powerful strategies to help liberate you from exhaustion and live a life with more energy.

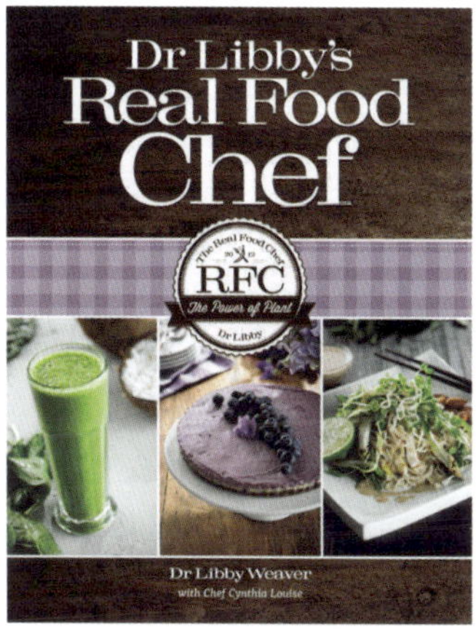

Real Food Chef

The *Real Food Chef* is a beautiful book that will revolutionise the way you are nourished. Filled with delicious and nutrient dense meals, drinks, snacks and sauces, this book educates and supports you to embrace a real food way of eating.

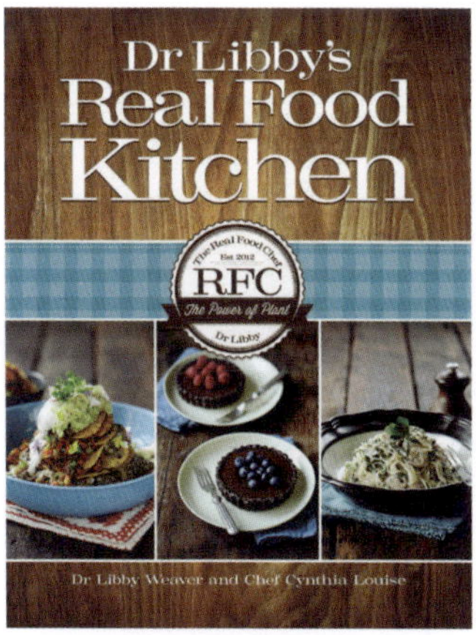

Real Food Kitchen

The *Real Food Kitchen* will inspire you to take better care of yourself with the delicious and nutritious recipes featured. Packed with even more nutritional information as well as recipes that are firm family favourites that have been 'real food chef-ified', you will love using this beautiful cookbook.

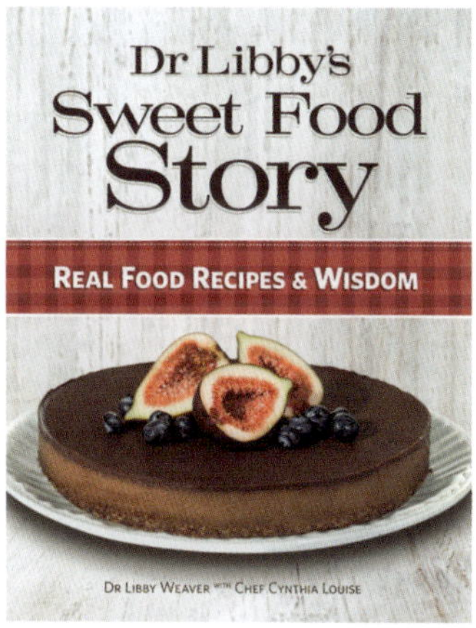

Sweet Food Story

Many people make great food choices for breakfast and lunch, and then at 3 o'clock in the afternoon they feel like someone else has taken over their body, their desire for sweet food can be so intense. The *Sweet Food Story* cookbook was created with this in mind, as a way of educating and supporting you to eat sweet food that serves your health.

Also by Dr Libby Weaver

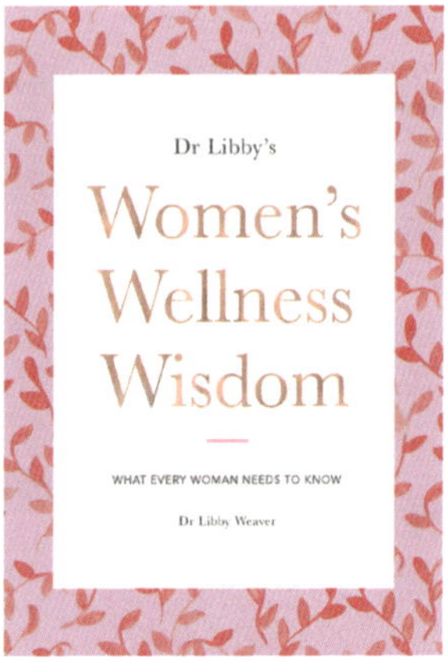

Women's Wellness Wisdom

A definitive guidebook for women, *Women's Wellness Wisdom* includes beautiful imagery, step-by-step guides, worksheets and real-life examples, helping you uncover the sources of your challenges and empowering you with the knowledge to better understand your body. Learn what women of all ages need to know from this inspiring book.

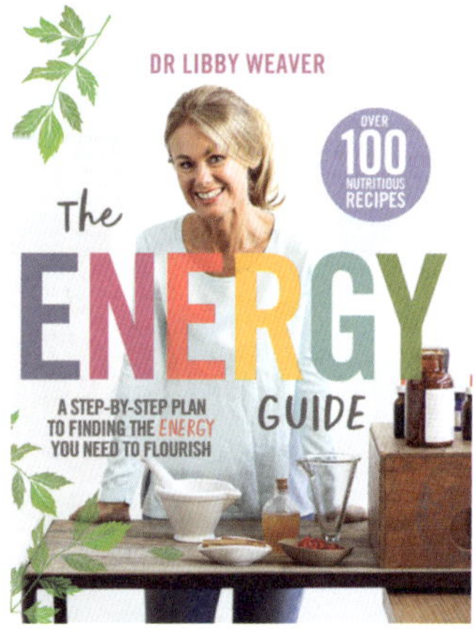

The Energy Guide

Authoritative and compassionate, *The Energy Guide,* which includes over 100 recipes and meal ideas, will help you to reboot your diet, improve your sleep, understand your hormones, reduce your stress and transform the way you think about your energy and your wellbeing.

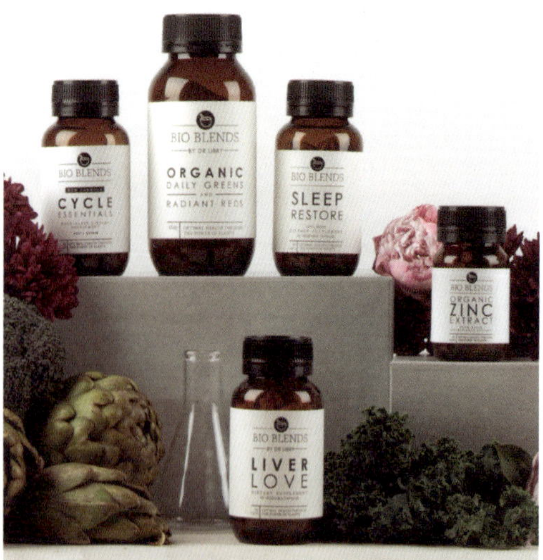

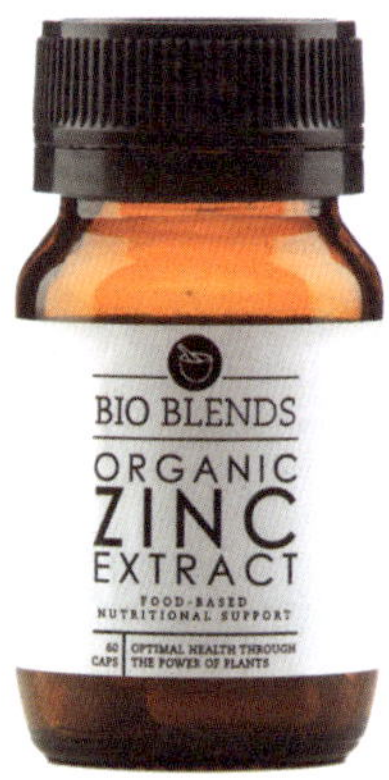

Organic Zinc

Zinc is involved in over 300 processes inside your body and most people today aren't getting enough of it. This superstar nutrient works with your body to help you have a healthy immune system, experience great energy, achieve optimal digestion and have radiant hair, skin and eyes.

Bio Blends

FOOD-BASED SUPPLEMENTS

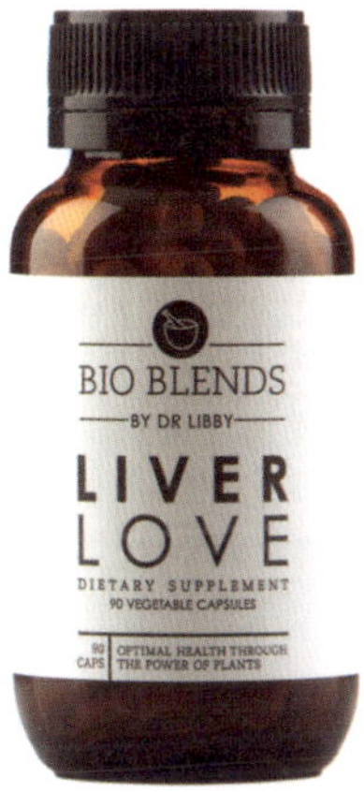

Liver Love

Supports liver regeneration and detoxification and assists your liver to process the harmful liver loaders that could be contributing to your headaches, gut problems, such as bloating and constipation, irritability, fatigue, congested skin, and unexplained weight gain.

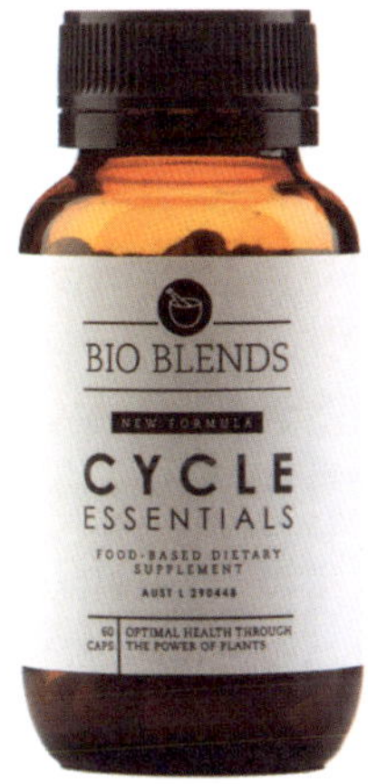

Cycle Essentials

A potent blend of foods, plants and herbs which promote healthy progesterone production and help you address PMS, period pain, bloating, sugar cravings and mood fluctuations, leading to a period that simply shows up.

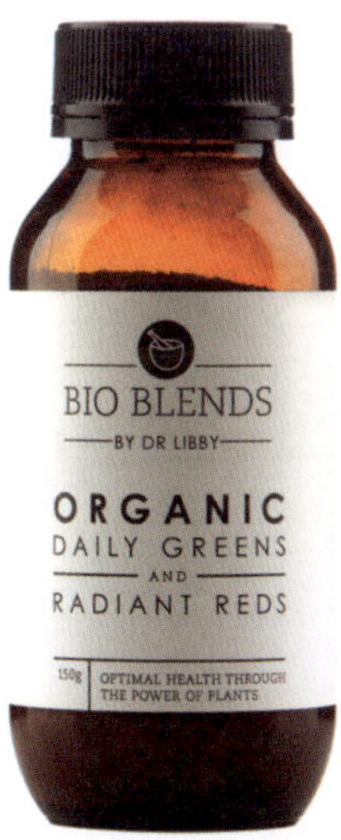

Organic Daily Greens & Radiant Reds

Precisely formulated to contain a powerhouse of nutrients and antioxidants, this delicious powder is designed to optimise digestion and elimination pathways, plus ensure you get a concentrated dose of nutrients that are vital for supporting many body systems.

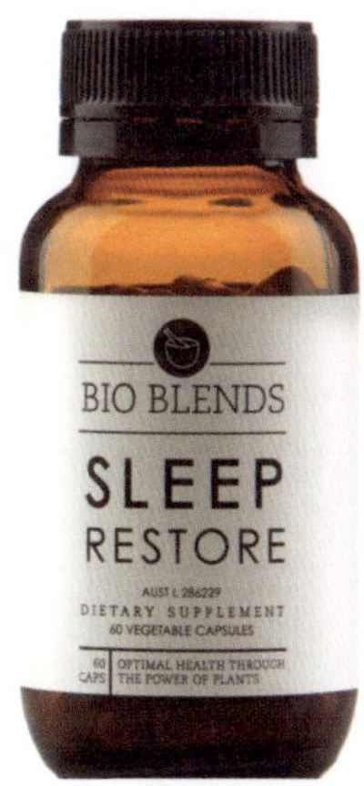

Sleep Restore

The potent combination of herbs has a sedative action on our nervous system, calming, easing anxiety and most importantly helping to uncoil a busy mind to support short-term through to long-term sleep challenges, including insomnia.

Find out more at www.bioblends.com

REFERENCES AND RESOURCES

I am regularly touched by the number of people who, after reading one of my books, write to me saying that it's like I've described their life or peeked at the pages of their journal. If, after reading *What Am I Supposed to Eat?*, you would like to delve further into your physical or emotional health, I encourage you to check out my website where you will find all of my other book titles, weekend events, tours and courses. If body fat or energy challenges are a daily battle for you, you might benefit from Weight Loss for Women, which is a nine-week practical online course overflowing with guidance and tuition to help you solve your weight loss puzzle.

Take a look at the blog too at:

www.drlibby.com

I also post health information each weekday on social media. Connect with me there at:

www.facebook.com/DrLibbyLive
www.twitter.com/DrLibbyLive
And on Instagram, find me as @drlibby

My passion is to educate and inspire, and to help people change the relationship they have with their bodies and their health, and put the power of choice back in their hands. It is an honour to assist you in your optimal health journey.

I have cited some books and papers in this text and they are listed in full here if further reading in a particular area interests you.

Over the last 25 years I have read in excess of 10,000 books and research papers that have inspired and shaped my work. I have done my best to include below those who have been instrumental in contributing to my work, as well as to this book.

There is additional referencing on my website: **www.drlibby.com**

Books

Bennett, Jane and Pope, A. (2008). *The Pill. Are You Sure It's For You?* Sydney: Allen & Unwin.

Bourbeau, Lise. (2011). *Just Listen to your Body and Eat.* Saint-Jerome: Les Editions.

Carson, Rachel. (1962) *Silent Spring.* Boston: Houghton Mifflin.

Gray, Louise. (2016). *The Ethical Carnivore.* London: Bloomsbury.

Hay, Louise. (2004). *You Can Heal Your Life.* Carlsbad: Hay House.

Isaacson, Walter. (2015). *Steve Jobs.* New York: Simon & Schuster.

King, George. (2015) *The Diabetes Reset.* New York: Workman Publishing.

Price, Weston. (2004) *Nutrition and Physical Degeneration: 6th edition.* USA: Price-Pottenger Nutrition Foundation.

Roth, Geneen. (2011). *Women, Food and God.* New York: Scribner.

Journal publications

Abramovitz BA, Birch LL. (2000). "Five-year-old girls' ideas about dieting are predicted by their mothers' dieting". *Journal of the American Dietetic Association* 100:1157-63.

Beydoun MA, & Wang Y. (2009). "Parent-child dietary intake resemblance in the United States: Evidence from a large representative survey". *Social Science & Medicine* 68: 2137-44.

Eastman, C. and Zimmermann, M. (2017) "The iodine deficiency disorders" cited in De Groot, L. et al. (editors) (2000-2017) *Endotext,* accessed online at: https://www.ncbi.nlm.nih.gov/books/NBK285556/

Field AE, Austin SB, Striegel-Moore R et al. (2005). "Weight concerns and weight control behaviors of adolescents and their mothers". *Archives of Pediatric and Adolescent* Medicine 159:1121-6.

Kurenbach, B, Marjoshi, D et al. (2015). "Sublethal exposure to commercial formulations of the herbicides dicamba, 2,4-dichlorophenoxyacetic acid, and glyphosate cause changes in antibiotic susceptibility in Escherichia coli and Salmonella enterica serovar Typhimurium". mBio: *American Society for Microbiology Online Journal* 6; 2: 9-15.

Smolak L, Levine MP & Schermer F. (1999). "Parental input and weight concerns among elementary school children". *International Journal of Eating Disorders* 25: 263-71.

Wertheim EH, Mee V, & Paxton SJ. (1999). "Relationships among adolescent girls' eating behaviors and their parents' weight-related attitudes and behaviors". *Sex Roles* 41: 169-87.

Articles and online articles

Bowden, Jennifer "A Word from the Wiser" *The NZ Listener November 19, 2016.*

http://coconutresearchcenter.org/articles-and-videos/coconut-information/coconut-oil-and-medium-chain-triglycerides/default.htm

http://earthisland.org/journal/index.php/eij/article/in_the_marrow_of_our_bones/

http://innerlight-wellness.net/chinese-medicine-diet/

http://sustainability.hawkesbury.nsw.gov.au/products/avoid-products-with-excessive-packaging

http://sustainablecities.org.nz/wp-content/uploads/earlethesis.pdf

http://www.coeliac.org.nz

http://www.healthyfoodguide.com.au/articles/2011/january/mothers-and-daughters-how-be-healthy-eating-role-model

http://www.nutritionaustralia.org/sites/default/files/Iron-2014.pdf

https://iquitsugar.com/luxury-ubiquity-brief-history-sugar

https://www.betterhealth.vic.gov.au/health/conditionsandtreatments/iron-deficiency-adults

https://www.coeliac.org.au/

https://www.elephantjournal.com/2014/06/tips-for-raising-a-child-to-have-a-healthy-relationship-with-food-and-their-body-dr-stacey-rosenfeld/

https://www.forbes.com/sites/judystone/2015/04/01/antibiotic-resistance-from-unexpected-sources/#4103f6ecdbca

https://www.glnc.org.au/grains/allergies-intolerances/gluten-in-grains/

https://www.shape.com/weight-loss/tips-plans/how-having-daughter-changed-my-relationship-food-forever

Dr Libby live events and online courses

Available at www.drlibby.com
I regularly do speaking tours, so check my website for topics, dates and venues. I also run weekend events that offer participants a wonderful restorative experience coupled with in-depth learning of holistic health: the biochemical, the nutritional and the emotional. The *Beautiful You Weekend* is such a special event.

Online courses and webinars include:

Rushing Woman's Syndrome Quickstart Course

Condition the Calm Course

30 Essential Beauty Gems Course

New Year New You Webinar

Sensational Sleep Webinar

TEDx: *The Pace of Modern Life Versus our Cavewoman Biochemistry* https://www.youtube.com/watch?v=tJ0SME6Z9rw

Understanding the Mysteries and Magic of the Female Body Webinar

Weight Loss for Women

Notes

Notes

Notes